COST-EFFECTIVENESS ANALYSES IN HEALTH

A PRACTICAL APPROACH

Third Edition

Peter Muennig
Mark Bounthavong

T0337993

JB JOSSEY-BASS™
A Wiley Brand

Published by Jossey-Bass
A Wiley Brand
One Montgomery Street, Suite 1000, San Francisco, CA 94104-4594—www.josseybass.com

Jossey-Bass books and products are available through most bookstores. To contact Jossey-Bass directly call our Customer Care Department within the U.S. at 800-956-7739, outside the U.S. at 317-572-3986, or fax 317-572-4002.

Wiley publishes in a variety of print and electronic formats and by print-on-demand. Some material included with standard print versions of this book may not be included in e-books or in print-on-demand. If this book refers to media such as a CD or DVD that is not included in the version you purchased, you may download this material at **http://booksupport.wiley.com**. For more information about Wiley products, visit **www.wiley.com**.

Library of Congress Cataloging-in-Publication Data

Muennig, Peter, author.
  Cost-effectiveness analyses in health : a practical approach / Peter Muennig, Mark Bounthavong.—Third edition.
       p. ; cm.
  Includes bibliographical references and index.
  ISBN 978-1-119-01126-2 (paper), 978-1-119-01127-9 (epdf), 978-1-119-01128-6 (epub)
  I. Bounthavong, Mark, 1976–, author. II. Title.
  [DNLM: 1. Cost-Benefit Analysis—methods. 2. Health Care Costs. 3. Quality of Life. W 74.1]
  RA410.5
  338.4′33621—dc23
                                                    2015036511

Cover design: Wiley
Cover image: © ilolab/Shutterstock

THIRD EDITION
Printed in the United States of America
PB Printing 10 9 8 7 6 5

CONTENTS

LIST OF TABLES, FIGURES, AND EXHIBITS

Tables

Figures

Exhibits

Personalized medicine has evolved to where genomic testing can tailor treatments to individual bodies rather than populations, pharmaceutical treatment can now essentially cure hepatitis C, and a cancer vaccine can increase the life of a terminally ill prostate cancer patient. The downside is that these improvements in health outcomes are expensive. Moreover, they are taking place in the context of poorly functioning healthcare delivery systems that cannot marshal market forces to bring in value and health at the same time. For example, the healthcare delivery system in the United States has ballooned to an unimaginable $2.9 trillion—an amount that will soon surpass the entire gross domestic product (GDP) of France. This comes even as the life expectancy in the United States is declining relative to nations that do a better job of spending their money on treatments that matter.

Cost-Effectiveness Analyses in Health: A Practical Approach was written in order to prepare you, our dear reader, for the inevitable need to evaluate the interventions and programs meant to improve health. This book is meant to teach students how to begin to conduct their own cost-effectiveness analyses.

Rather than go deep into abstract theory or complicated models, this book teaches you how to work with the fundamentals. Consider this book a road map that will guide you through the processes for developing your own cost-effectiveness analysis. With this book, you will be able to develop a research question, find and evaluate data, build a decision model, stress-test the model, interpret the results, and summarize your findings in a report using the most up-to-date techniques and software. We will even walk you step-by-step through an entire analysis. The only skills that you will need are basic math skills and some knowledge about using spreadsheets.

Students and professionals with some knowledge of biostatistics and epidemiology can skip Chapters 11 and 12, which provide a short review of fundamentals. If you're unfamiliar with these subjects, don't worry. Chapters 11 and 12 offer a basic introduction to biostatistics and epidemiology that will be useful when reviewing the literature and performing a cost-effectiveness analysis.

We wrote this book with the public health student in mind, but healthcare professionals and students, policymakers, formulary managers, pharmacoeconomists, healthcare payers, directors of departments and hospitals, and even curious patients will find the information and lessons accessible and easy to understand. We do not expect you to become world-class experts after reading this book. However, you will feel more confident about understanding cost-effectiveness analysis and conducting basic analyses. You will also be prepared to tackle advanced materials if you choose to.

In short, *Cost-Effectiveness Analyses in Health: A Practical Approach* was written to provide a how-to guide to performing cost-effectiveness analysis. The examples used in this book provide simplified scenarios in order to teach the material, but readers should be able to apply these methods to their own research questions of interest.

How to Use This Book

In addition to introducing the cost concepts of cost-effectiveness analysis, this book walks students through basic cost-effectiveness analyses. To fully benefit from the book, students should complete the exercises in each chapter; these exercises guide students through the process of obtaining electronic data, analyzing the medical literature, building a decision analysis tree, and conducting a sensitivity analysis.

Different students have different needs. The following points should help you make the most effective use of this book:

• *Using this book for theoretical study alone.* Health managers and clinicians often wish to understand cost-effectiveness analysis methods but do not wish to conduct research. This book has been designed to allow students to understand the field of cost-effectiveness analysis methods using an applied approach.

• *Using this book as a textbook.* Instructors teaching courses that have biostatistics and epidemiology as prerequisites may skip Chapter 11; however, this chapter provides an excellent review of those concepts applicable to cost-effectiveness research. Introductory courses in cost-effectiveness analysis should skip Chapter 12, which is intended only for students who are actively working on a research project.

• *Using this book for self-study.* Those who are actively working on a cost-effectiveness research question will find Chapter 12 invaluable but might not need as much background information (found in Chapters 1 through 3) as beginning students.

- *Using Internet resources.* This book provides links to data sources, journals, and other useful cost-effectiveness information on the Internet. The Internet is a critical resource for cost-effectiveness research, but as we all know, the addresses for web pages sometimes change. For this reason, links to specific web pages are provided alongside links to the organizations that host these pages and are maintained at www .wiley.com/go/muennig3e.

A Note on Methods

In 1996, the U.S. Public Health Service's Panel on Cost-Effectiveness in Health and Medicine released methodological standards for conducting cost-effectiveness analyses. These standards were developed in response to a wide degree of variation in the ways in which such analyses were conducted. The use of disparate approaches to cost-effectiveness analysis sometimes leads to widely different study results when different research groups examine the cost-effectiveness of a single screening test or medical treatment.

Since the First U.S. Panel on Cost-Effectiveness in Health and Medicine in 1996, the field of cost-effectiveness analysis has evolved considerably. This prompted the formation of the Second U.S. Panel on Cost-Effectiveness and Health. This revised edition incorporates these changes.

ACKNOWLEDGMENTS

The writing of this book required the assistance of a large supporting cast. It's impossible to list everyone. But here's our humble attempt to do so.

We would both like to acknowledge the late Andy Pasternack, of Jossey-Bass/Wiley. Andy first stole Peter away from a contract with Oxford University Press, and Peter has never looked back. Andy was a gentle man with a big heart and great vision who passed away while this book was in the planning stages.

The rest of the staff at Jossey-Bass/Wiley provided an immeasurable amount of assistance, in particular: Seth Schwartz, who took over Andy's role and worked tirelessly to bring this text into being; Melinda Noack for keeping us on track (and catching those pesky mistakes); and the production editor Kumudhavalli Narasimhan and copyeditor Ginny Carroll, who ensured that the text was comprehensible and lucid to all readers other than ourselves.

The TreeAge example wouldn't be possible without the contributions and expertise of Andrew Munzer from TreeAge Software, Inc.

We also want to acknowledge the draft manuscript reviewers Sheryl Foster, David J. Vanness, Roger Edwards, and Victoria Phillip (they are the crucial gatekeepers for ensuring that this edition is accurate and trustworthy).

These lessons and ideas needed an audience before we could record them in this book. Therefore, we thank the students and residents who had to endure these instructions as we refined them. All errors and misinterpretations are the responsibility of the authors and not these excellent people.

Disclosures: The authors did not receive any financial compensation from TreeAge Software, Inc. The opinions and views of the authors do not reflect those of the U.S. Department of Veterans Affairs.

From Peter Muennig

I owe everything to Gezi, who lights my way in the dark, creates beautiful objects with me, and always gives me certainty that tomorrow will be as new and wondrous an adventure as today. I would also like to thank Mark for making this book into something much greater than it was before. And, of course, my family of teachers and unyielding emotional pillars (in random order): Radster, Heidi, Felise, Rufie, Dave, Thom, Misha, Jessica, Josh, Danny, Alex, Hong, and Prairie.

From Mark Bounthavong

The origins of this edition came from an innocent e-mail to Peter regarding clarification on a figure. Since then, Peter has been an invaluable friend and mentor in guiding me through the writing process—thank you! I also owe the beginnings of my interest in this field to my two academic advisors during my pharmacy school days: Mark and Anandi. Like all great mentors, they opened the door to a whole different world. And, of course, to my family, friends, teachers, and students, who always encouraged and supported me despite not understanding what I was really trying to say. (I hope it's clearer in this book.)

Peter Muennig

Peter Muennig is a professor in the Department of Health Policy and Management at Columbia University. He studies the ways in which medical and nonmedical social policies can be optimized to maximize population well-being using cost-effectiveness analysis. He is currently directing GRAPH, a center at Columbia University that seeks to provide local and global policymakers with the most efficient policy mix necessary to reduce the global burden of disease. Policies that focus on education, immigration, welfare, the control of industrial pollution, health insurance, and the built environment have the potential to shape the health, social, and environmental fabric of societies globally. Before such policies can be considered, though, comprehensive cost-effectiveness models, due consideration of the policy's unintended consequences, and randomized controlled trials are needed so that policymakers can determine which investments are best to make.

Peter has been doing this work since 1999, when he began advising the Centers for Disease Control and Prevention, Health Canada, the Chilean government, and the Chinese government regarding which policies might be needed to optimize population health. He has published more than 100 peer-reviewed articles in the scientific literature and has written four books (including this one). His work has appeared on NPR, CNN, and MSNBC, and multiple times in major print media sources such as the *New York Times* (14 articles), the *Wall Street Journal*, and a three-part series in *Slate*.

Mark Bounthavong

Mark Bounthavong is a pharmacoeconomist at the Veterans Affairs San Diego Healthcare System and an adjunct faculty member of the Skaggs School of Pharmacy and Pharmaceutical Sciences at the University of California, San Diego. He performs health technology assessments and writes policies to maximize resource efficiency while maintaining high-quality health care at the U.S. Department of Veterans Affairs. Convinced that there are always new things to learn, Mark is currently completing his PhD in the Pharmaceutical Outcomes Research and Policy Program at the University of Washington.

Mark has received the Pharmacy Benefits Management Innovations Award from the U.S. Under Secretary for Health, the Distinguished Service Award from the University of the Pacific, and the Literature Award for Innovation in Pharmacy Practice from the American Society of Health-System Pharmacists. He has published more than 30 peer-reviewed articles in the scientific literature and several book chapters.

CHAPTER 1

INTRODUCTION TO COST-EFFECTIVENESS

Overview

Imagine that you are the director of a large cancer society. Your day-to-day duties require you to conduct some research and oversee employees whose job is to compile data and make health recommendations. One morning you sit down with a cup of coffee and toast, and when you open the morning paper you find that one of your society's recommendations—that women between the ages of 40 and 60 receive screening mammography for breast cancer—has made the headline news. An elderly-rights group is suing your society. This group argues that your recommendation unfairly discriminates against the elderly because you have implied that women over the age of 60 should not be screened for breast cancer.

You rush to the office and find that the teams who made the recommendation are already in a heated meeting. They have split into two factions, and each group is now accusing the other of making bad decisions. But did they? You manage to calm everyone down and review the process they used to arrive at their recommendation. You learn that both groups were concerned that recommending mammograms for women over a wider age range might become very costly, thereby jeopardizing screening for women who might benefit from screening mammography the most.

One group argued that it made sense to screen older rather than younger women. Mammography works better in older women, who have less dense breast tissue. Older women, they reasoned, were less likely to have a falsely positive mammogram and therefore would be less likely to suffer unnecessary procedures or surgery.

LEARNING OBJECTIVES

- Explain why cost-effectiveness is useful.

- List the elements of a cost-effectiveness analysis.

- Distinguish between an average cost-effectiveness ratio and an incremental cost-effectiveness ratio.

- Explain the difference between efficacy and effectiveness.

- Describe how cost-effectiveness analysis influences policy.

Unnecessary interventions, they noted, place women at risk for surgical complications, are psychologically traumatic, are costly, and may do more harm than good.

The other group argued that it was unwise to actively screen all elderly women with mammography, because women who had breast cancer would die from other natural causes before the cancer had a chance to spread. After all, breast cancer can take more than a decade to kill, and the life expectancy of older people is limited. Therefore, they reasoned, elderly women would be subjected to an uncomfortable and expensive screening test that would have little impact on the length of their lives. Besides, who would want to undergo chemotherapy in the precious remaining years of their lives?

Both factions made arguments based on sound scientific, economic, and social research, but which group's approach would be best for patients? You and your employees decide to conduct a more extensive analysis of the costs and benefits of breast cancer screening and plan to send out a press release to this effect. But where do you start?

You might start by having a team estimate the likelihood that older women will die of breast cancer if they are not screened and have another team estimate the number of women who are likely to have false-positive mammograms at different ages. You might also wish to obtain information on the number of years of life that mammography will save, the quality of life for women who have different stages of breast cancer, and the psychological impact of a positive test result among women who do not in fact have breast cancer (**false-positive test results**). Because both teams were concerned about the costs of mammography, you may also wish to calculate the cost of screening mammography and the cost of all of the medical care that might be averted by detecting breast cancer at an early stage. Finally, because each team is interested in knowing whether women in both age groups might benefit from mammography, you decide that the costs and health benefits of screening each group should be compared to not screening women at all. If all of these factors were put together in a systematic manner, you would have conducted a cost-effectiveness analysis.

Why Cost-Effectiveness Is Useful

Now let's take a step back and consider why all of this is important in the first place. Certainly you want to know whether mammography is going to lead to net improvements or net declines in health relative to some standard of care. If it's only going to hurt people, we certainly don't want to do it. But if we know it helps, we also want to know whether it is affordable.

What does "affordable" mean when you are talking about human life? Take a moment to imagine what we could do with an infinite amount of money. We could build a huge public transportation system that eliminates car accidents, pollution, and noise. We could use only solar power and switch to 100 percent recycling, eliminating the major remaining sources of pollution; this would greatly reduce environmental carcinogens and oxidizing agents that cause cancer, heart disease, and premature aging. We could completely mechanize industry, eliminating occupational accidents. Finally, we could create a highly advanced health system that provides full MRI body scans and comprehensive laboratory screening tests for everyone in the population to ensure that cancers and other disorders are detected at the earliest possible stage.

As it is, there are very few nations that can even provide safe drinking water to all their citizens. The challenge, then, is to figure out how best to spend the money we have so that the quantity and quality of life can be maximized.

Thus, even if mammography screening for breast cancer is on the whole effective, it is conceivable that the money spent on it could save more lives if it went toward something else. **Cost-effectiveness analysis (CEA)** helps determine how to maximize the quality and quantity of life in a particular society that is constrained by a particular budget.

We'll get deeper into this later in the book, but let's examine the specifics of the example to illustrate how resource allocation might work. Assume that the U.S. Congress decided to allocate $1 trillion to the competing health projects we mentioned. It could choose public transportation, greatly reducing pollution (a cause of pneumonia, cancer, and heart disease) and motor vehicle accidents (the fifth leading cause of death). It could invest in clean energy, reducing dependence on oil while reducing air pollution. Or it could choose the universal MRI strategy, detecting more tumor-producing cancers, some of which can be cured if detected early. If Congress knew the cost per year of life saved, it would know how to maximize the number of lives saved with the $1 trillion investment.

One thing that might strike some readers as a bit strange about this hypothetical situation is that we are essentially deciding who lives and who dies. If we save the mothers and fathers with cancerous tumors by opting for universal MRI examinations, many sons and daughters will die in car accidents as a result. Behind these numbers are real people affected by whatever decision is ultimately made. The more tangible these lives are made to the decision makers, the more difficult the decision becomes.

As one physician, Paul Farmer, points out, you cannot let a person die in front of you when you know that an effective treatment exists (Farmer, 2004). Is the solution, therefore, to start a medical clinic, even if it comes at the expense of a more effective vaccination campaign? We might know that one intervention saves more lives than the other. However, when the most cost-effective intervention saves lives we will never see—lives that lie abstracted in numbers—it is more difficult to rationalize the choice.

Nevertheless, policymakers must often make abstracted decisions based on data from cost-effectiveness analysis, and these sometimes involve decisions that improve survival for one group at the cost of survival for another. (We'll see an actual example of this later in the book.) These decisions become more abstract when quality-of-life issues are added to the mix of life-and-death issues.

The sad reality is that making decisions based on "gut feelings" leads to more suffering and more death than making decisions based on science. While the US tends to operate on "gut policy," other rich nations use science to allocate scarce resources. This may partly explain why health and longevity are declining in the US but are increasing in other rich nations.

Elements of Cost-Effectiveness Analysis

Just as a driver really only needs to know about the accelerator, brake, and gearshift before driving a car for the first time, this section provides the basic parts of a cost-effectiveness analysis that you need to have in your head before you can start getting down to business. As we get further into the book, you'll be introduced to more advanced and complex methods that will build on the foundations of earlier chapters.

Health Interventions

A **health intervention** is a treatment, screening test, or primary prevention technique (for example, vaccinating children to prevent measles). Health interventions typically reduce the incidence rate of disease or its complications, improve the quality of life lived with disease, or improve life expectancy. Most produce some combination of these benefits. The benefits of a health intervention are referred to as **outcomes**. Health outcomes can assume any form, but the most common health outcomes are big-picture items, such as hospitalizations prevented, illnesses avoided, or deaths averted (as opposed to little-picture items, such as stomachaches reduced).

The first question that should pop into mind when speaking of the cost-effectiveness of a particular intervention, such as mammography, aimed at improving a health outcome, is "Relative to what?" Mammography will certainly appear cost-effective if we compare it to a total body scan for breast cancer. But it might not be cost-effective relative to educating women to perform breast self-examinations in the shower on a regular basis. The intervention to which you are comparing the intervention of interest is called the **competing alternative**.

The Competing Alternative

Improvements in health states and improvements in length of life do not always go hand in hand. For instance, we perform mammography even though the procedure produces discomfort. Likewise, we provide steroids to patients with asthma even though this medication can be harmful over the long term. Such complications shouldn't be a deterrent. The whole point of cost-effectiveness, after all, is to examine the optimal course of action when there is considerable uncertainty. (Otherwise, why bother with the analysis in the first place?)

Virtually all health interventions cost something up front. But they also affect the amount of money spent on future medical care. For instance, a woman who is found to have breast cancer at an early stage will likely incur the cost of hospitalization and surgery in addition to the mammography, but the cancer may be cured, averting the future cost of more severe disease. Thus, mammography can produce value by averting disease and future costs. In short, the overall cost and overall effectiveness of any given alternative strategy are not often apparent on first glance.

So what is the net (overall) cost of mammography, and how much benefit can we expect? To answer this question, we first want a sense of how much of an improvement in health states we'll get from mammography over the long term.

Health States

While health outcomes such as deaths are concrete overarching measures of health, it is also important to examine more specific improvements in one's state of health, such as reduced pain or improved ability to walk. Specific states of health are quite logically referred to as **health states**. (Whoever said cost-effectiveness was difficult?)

Figure 1.1 shows how a health intervention improves health states. Here, we see that people having an asthma attack arrive at the emergency room with difficulty breathing (Health State 1). The health intervention is to provide intravenous steroids and aerosolized medications to help such

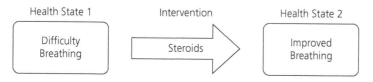

Figure 1.1 Example of the Effect of a Health Intervention on the Health States of Patients Admitted to the Emergency Room for an Acute Asthma Attack

patients breathe. Typically, patients experience dramatic improvements in breathing once treated (Health State 2).

Simple. So why the fuss? We wish to first think about this in very simplistic terms because we will later need to think about the various ways in which health states change when a medical intervention occurs, which can be somewhat complex. Collectively, changes in health states add up to changes in one's **health status**.

Health Status

A person's health status is the sum of his or her health states. Changes in health states are associated with an intervention are not always positive. Steroids can lead to an improved health state, but, over the long-term, can negatively impact health status. Conversely, mammography will often lead to a decline health states over the short-term in the hope of garnering long-term benefits. The vast majority of patients told that they might have breast cancer actually have a false positive test result, leading to psychological distress. If someone can jog and isn't anxious or depressed, we might say that the person has an excellent health status based on those two health states alone.

In a cost-effectiveness analysis, a researcher gathers information on the ways in which a health intervention changes the average health status of a group of people alongside costs (Figure 1.2). Imagine for a moment you are evaluating a treatment for bacterial pneumonia and comparing it to no treatment at all. In Figure 1.2, Health Status 1 represents the collective health states of untreated people, and Health Status 2 represents the collective health states of treated people.

Suppose we're looking at treatment of bacterial pneumonia with antibiotics. Someone with bacterial pneumonia might have pain with breathing and a fever and be confined to bed. Someone who has been treated would have less pain and less fever and might be able to get around. In other words, the treated person would experience an improvement in health status.

Because health status is an amorphous concept, there is no direct way to measure it. Instead, cost-effectiveness analysis examines the quantity of life (mortality) alongside a measure of the quality of life (morbidity)

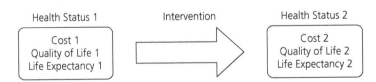

Figure 1.2   Components of a Cost-Effectiveness Analysis

associated with a given health status. The point of a cost-effectiveness analysis is therefore to estimate what an improvement in health status will produce in terms of quality and quantity of life and how much it will cost to achieve these improvements.

We must also look at how health status (the collection of health states) changes over time. For instance, suppose you are again at your job at a major cancer society, and you are trying to decide whether to recommend screening mammography. Cancer evolves over many years. So we'll want to know how it will affect everything from a patient's ability to perform daily activities to her mental health as time goes on.

Take another look at Figure 1.2. The quality of life in Health Status 1 for women screened for breast cancer is higher over the short term than it is in Health Status 2. Women in Health Status 1 have not undergone the pain of having their breast squeezed between two metal plates and do not have to face the pain and suffering associated with the diagnosis (or a misdiagnosis) of breast cancer if it is detected. In fact, since the cancer is producing no symptoms and the women do not know that they have breast cancer, they will be as subjectively healthy as anyone else over the short term. But the women in Health Status 2 (undetected cancer) may not have to face the pain and suffering associated with advanced breast cancer in the future.

Finally, the length of life is shorter for women who have not received a mammogram (Life Expectancy 1) than for those who have (Life Expectancy 2). This is a critical factor that must be considered in any cost-effectiveness analysis. But what do we do with all this information on health status and life expectancy? Enter the **quality-adjusted life-year (QALY)**.

The Quality-Adjusted Life-Year

Consider the nuanced changes in the quality of life that occur when a person with diabetes is given a medication to lower blood sugar. At first, the patient has to take a pill and may think of herself as sicker than she did before being given the prescription. But over time, this pill might prevent a myocardial infarction, which would have a grave impact on the person's perception of her health and her ability to get around or to do other things she enjoys. In other words, it affects many different dimensions of this person's health, or many different health states. Together, real-world improvements in these health states, along with their effect on life expectancy that occurs when a health intervention is applied, constitute the effectiveness of that intervention.

Just to drill the point home, a health outcome (such as a myocardial infarction) leads to changes in one's health states (ability to walk, work, or even to have sex), which in turn affect the person's quantity and quality of life. If we could somehow combine a measure of quantity of life adjusted for the quality of life, we would be just about set in terms of measuring the effectiveness of any given health intervention.

As it turns out, we have just such a thing: the quality-adjusted life-year, which is more affectionately known as a QALY. The QALY is a year of life lived in perfect health. How does the QALY work? Imagine that your last year of life wasn't such a great one. Your spouse left you alone and took your beloved dog. You became depressed. There were times when you were just fine and times when you wanted to die, but on average you felt like it was worth a lot less than other years you have had. There is a magic fraction that is used to account for the total value of the life that was worth living over that year. We will get into how this (questionably) magic number is calculated later, but for now assume that it is 0.5. You are otherwise in outstanding health, but the depression made the year only worth the equivalent of half the prior years in which you were both in good physical and mental health. Even though you lived a full year, it was just one-half a year (0.5 × 1 year) of perfect health.

At any given age, the average number of years we can expect to live is our life expectancy. Therefore, the average number of QALYs we can expect to live is our **quality-adjusted life expectancy (QALE)**. For example, as with a single QALY, if a person is expected to live for 10 years with a quality of life that is reduced by one-half due to a disease, then her total QALE is 5. QALE is the average number of years one can expect to live adjusted for quality of life for those expected lived years. Throughout this book, you'll become increasingly familiar with what a QALY is, how it is calculated, and how it is used. In addition to the QALY, measurements of benefits and efficacy can also include life-years (LYs) and disability-adjusted life-years (DALYs). We will discuss this in more detail in Chapter 8. For now, just accept that a QALY is a year lived in perfect health.

Costs

For a moment, let's consider the changes in costs associated with mammography. The total cost of mammography includes those costs associated with the mammogram as well as future medical costs incurred as a result of this screening test. These future costs will include the value of lost work and the medical costs associated with treating cancer that was detected early.

Failing to provide a screening test also costs something. These costs include those associated with treating breast cancer that is so advanced that it is self-evident to the patient or is easily detectable on physical examination. People with advanced breast cancer will incur higher medical costs and miss more work than will those who were diagnosed early in the course of illness. All of these costs must ultimately be considered.

When comparing mammography to no mammography, the difference in costs, morbidity, and mortality is captured in the *incremental cost-effectiveness ratio*. This tells you how much you will need to spend to realize a unit gain in effectiveness.

The Average and Incremental Cost-Effectiveness Ratio

Ratios put medical information into perspective. For instance, if a physician knows that there are 180,000 new cases of breast cancer a year in the United States, she will not be able to provide much information to a woman worried about developing that disease. If the physician knows that there are 11 new cases per 10,000 women each year, she will have a much better idea of how to communicate the risk. Similarly, the average cost-effectiveness ratio provides the consumers of our research with information that describes the average cost-per-treatment effect for a given strategy. In most cases, this will be the average cost per QALY.

The average cost-effectiveness ratio is the net cost of an intervention divided by its net benefit gain versus the no-intervention option. When the net costs and benefits are compared to *another* competing strategy, we end up calculating the **incremental cost-effectiveness ratio (ICER)**. So, instead of just calculating the average cost and QALYs among women who receive breast mammography relative to no mammography, the ICER provides the relative difference in cost associated with one strategy (say self-screening) versus the difference in effectiveness of the competing alternative. In other words, it tells you how much you will spend to buy additional QALY (benefits) relative to the competing alternative.

Let's take an example other than mammography to give you a break from that topic. Suppose you are working for a pharmaceutical company that just came out with a powerful new antibiotic for treating staphylococcus infection, Staphbegone. It is more effective than other antibiotics at saving life, but it's also much more expensive than what is now being used, Staphbeilln. But it will also get people out of the hospital faster, so it will reduce hospitalization costs and produce improvements in health-related quality of life.

We want to compare Staphbegone to Staphbeilln. We put Staphbeilln on the right-hand side of the equation because it is less effective (this ensures that the ratio will be positive if the intervention costs money but improves health and negative if the intervention saves money and improves health). If we call the old drug "intervention 1" and the new drug "intervention 2," the ICER takes the form:

$$\frac{(Cost\ of\ intervention\ 2 - Cost\ of\ intervention\ 1)}{(QALE\ 2 - QALE\ 1)} \quad (1.1)$$

Recall that QALE refers to quality-adjusted life expectancy, or your remaining life expectancy in perfect health.

Here, quality-adjusted life expectancy is used in the denominator because this is the standard unit of effectiveness (more on standardization in Chapter 2). However, in some cases (also discussed in Chapter 2), other measures of effectiveness might be used. We interpret the ICER as the additional costs invested in one strategy versus a competing strategy for an additional gain in benefit (e.g., QALY). In other words, we would have to invest in some cost for Staphbegone to receive a benefit equivalent to one additional QALE gained relative to Staphbeilln. Depending on our budget constraint, Staphbegone may be considered cost-effective relative to Staphbeilln.

Now you should have a general idea of what cost-effectiveness is. You should also have an idea of what the incremental cost-effectiveness ratio means. In the next section, we move from what cost-effectiveness is to why cost-effectiveness analysis is a critical part of any well-functioning society.

Exercises 1 and 2

1. Suppose that a complete course of Staphbegone costs $12,000 and a complete course of Staphbeilln costs $4,000. The average hospitalization costs $1,000 per day. Patients given Staphbegone have an average length of hospitalization of 5 days and Staphbeilln have an average hospitalization of 10 days. What is the incremental cost of Staphbegone?

2. Persons given Staphbegone have a higher survival rate than those given Staphbeilln. On average, those given Staphbegone can expect to go on to have a quality-adjusted life expectancy of 35 QALYs, while those given Staphbeilln go on to live 34.5 QALYs. Using the answer from Exercise 1, what is the incremental cost-effectiveness of Staphbegone?

TIPS AND TRICKS

Answers to all self-study questions are presented in Appendix A.

Why Conduct Cost-Effectiveness Analysis?

There are a number of ways to prevent or treat most diseases. For instance, breast cancer can be detected by self-examination, examination by a medical practitioner, screening mammography, ultrasound, spiral computed tomography (CT), or magnetic resonance imagery (MRI). It is also possible to compare different levels of intensity of a single health intervention. For example, screening mammography might be performed every six months, every year, or every two years. Each of these competing alternatives is associated with a different effectiveness and a different cost (Mandelblatt et al., 2004). In the real world, many different approaches are used to diagnose or treat disease (Krumholz, 2013; Newhouse & Garber, 2013; Wennberg & Gittelsohn, 1982), some by crackpot medical practitioners.

Many students of cost-effectiveness analysis rightly question the logic of choosing interventions based on both cost and effectiveness criteria rather than effectiveness alone. It seems to many people that we should purchase the most effective screening or treatment procedure irrespective of its cost. In the first section of this chapter, we saw that there is an almost infinite number of lifesaving expenditures, including some combination of screening modalities. The question, then, is "Which ones can we afford?" To answer this question, let's first consider what we mean by *cost* and what we mean by *effectiveness*.

Costs Matter

Even when the most effective modality is known, it may have unforeseen effects on heatlh and longevity if its use takes vital resources from other social programs. First, consider your personal budget. Suppose that you make $2,000 a month. Now suppose that your rent, minimum food purchases, basic utilities, and transportation come to $1,800. You could spend some of the $200 on going out to the movies and save the rest. Alternatively, you could live it up and go out to a fancy dinner and the theater five nights a month and live without electricity, go on an expensive vacation and not pay your rent, or blow the whole wad on that haute couture suit you've always wanted. Some of us can accept that it's not possible to consume everything we want. But when the goods and services we are consuming define who lives and who dies, the choices become much more difficult.

Consider the case of a tiny country with 100 people and a total health budget of $10,000 per year. If the country paid for expensive organ transplants, it could spend its entire budget on one person, leaving nothing for clean water, vaccinations, primary care, or other medical services that greatly prolong the quality and quantity of life for everyone in the country. If it instead spent $1,000 per year to keep vaccinations up to date, $7,000 per year for all needed antibiotics and basic primary care, and $2,000 per year on emergency surgery, many more lives would be saved. The value of goods and services in their best alternative use is the **opportunity cost** of an investment, such as a medical intervention.

Thus, just as your electricity bill has an opportunity cost, so does vaccination.

THE CASE FOR EDUCATION AS A HEALTH EXPENDITURE

Basic schooling is thought to greatly reduce morbidity and mortality in both the industrialized and the developing context. Education provides the cognitive skills and the social credentials needed for survival and adaptation to any ecological niche (Wilkinson, 1999). For instance, middle-class neighborhoods tend to have lower rates of crime victimization, access to healthier foods, and better housing. None of this is likely possible without an adequate education. Similarly, cognitive skills allow people to better assess hazards (such as taking the train instead of a bus in India) and may even reduce errors in medication dosage or compliance with medical prescriptions. As it turns out, education not only saves lives; it saves money (Muennig, 2015; Muennig & Woolf, 2007). Therefore, it can be argued that basic education should be prioritized over the provision of basic medical services when resources are slim (Muennig & Woolf, 2007).

In circumstances where health funds are limited, cost-effectiveness analysis can provide information on how to realize the largest health gains with the money that you have (Gold, Siegel, Russell, & Weinstein, 1996; Neumann, Sanders, Russell, Siegel, & Ganiats, 2016; Ubel, DeKay, Baron, & Asch, 1996). For instance, in a country with a national health system, interventions can be ranked in order of their cost-effectiveness. If we know how much will be spent on each health intervention, it becomes possible to go down the list until the money runs out. This is also known as **appropriate technology utilization**; if a government barely has money to pay for vaccination (an appropriate technology), it does not make sense to pay for heart-lung transplants (a technology that is inappropriate given the budgetary constraints).

The use of appropriate technology isn't always popular. A person who needs a heart and lung transplant and is dying in the hospital evokes more sympathy than the unseen hundreds of people who might benefit from all of the vaccines that could be purchased with the same sum of cash. However, in the absence of sufficient funding to cover all known treatments for all known diseases, prioritizing expensive and less effective interventions will ultimately lead to more illness and death.

In the United States, medical care is almost never denied to anyone who can afford it, and there is no absolute cap on how much is spent on health care. In this setting, cost-effectiveness analysis can provide clinicians, policymakers, and insurers with general guidelines on which interventions might generally be preferable. For instance, an intervention that costs $100,000 for each QALY it produces relative to the next most effective alternative might be seen as expensive by some but might be purchased by others.

While highly anecdotal, this lack of an emphasis on cost-effectiveness likely provides a partial explanation for why the United States spends the most on health care as a proportion of gross domestic product but ranks about fifty-third among nations worldwide in terms of life expectancy in 2015. To get the latest data, you can search for "life expectancy rank of all nations" on the Wolfram|Alpha web site (Wolfram|Alpha, 2015). You will almost certainly note that it the US has fallen even more by the time you read this.

In developing nations, where government health budgets may be as low as $5 per person, the need for cost-effectiveness analysis becomes critical (Attaran & Sachs, 2001). In the African continent, per capita government health-related expenditures ranged from US$2 to US$612, and 56 percent of nations had a per capita government health-related expenditure of US$20 (Sambo, Kirigia, & Orem, 2013). When budgets are small, the use of inappropriate technologies can greatly increase mortality in the population as a whole. Why more so than in industrialized nations? Simply because forgoing the least expensive and most effective interventions such as vaccinations produces more harm than forgoing interventions that produce less spectacular gains and cost more, such as dialysis. The basis for such decisions, therefore, has at least as much to do with its effectiveness at a population level as its cost.

Effectiveness Versus Efficacy

Usually tests, treatments, or interventions are measured in terms of their **efficacy**. Efficacy reveals how a test, treatment, or intervention works under experimental conditions. Experiments tend to work better under the watchful eye of researchers in a controlled laboratory setting than in the real world. Subjects are watched to make sure they take their medications and that laboratory specimens are properly frozen and shipped immediately for testing. In the real world, conditions tend to be less ideal.

Experiments that measure efficacy also tend to look at only short-term outcomes. There is often one best test, treatment, or public health intervention with respect to short-term efficacy. But can we say that the use of the most efficacious interventions will detect the most cases of disease, have the highest rate of treatment success, or prevent the most diseases in the real world?

Sometimes, the answer is no. Not only are tests performed differently or medications taken in different doses in the real world relative to within precise scientific experiments, but a number of other unexpected things happen as well. For instance, screening tests and treatments are sometimes associated with hidden dangers. As we saw in the screening mammography example, a false-positive mammogram can lead to unnecessary surgery and psychological stress. If the woman is unlikely to have breast cancer, we have to ask whether the risks outweigh the benefits. Many societies promote testing for diseases for which there is no cure and early cancer detection does nothing. Screening for pancreatic cancer can be accomplished by CT scans, spiral CT scans, or MRI testing, sure, but these tests buy you no additional life even if the disease is detected. These sad cases usually arise because some well-intentioned family who lost a loved one donated a good deal of money to a cause without really understanding the science behind it.

Moreover, most treatments can produce debilitating or fatal side effects in a fraction of the people taking them. Therefore, when we examine the effectiveness of a treatment at extending human life expectancy, we have to consider that the treatment can prolong life in one way but reduce life expectancy in another way. Thus, the real-world effects may be smaller than the efficacy of the treatment would suggest.

Side effects from an otherwise very good drug can also reduce the chances that a person will take the drug in the real world. In the published experiment (where people in white coats were watching participants take their medications) the efficacy of such a drug will appear to be quite good in print. But in the real world it may produce little benefit because so few people want to take it. **Effectiveness** indicates how well such tests, treatments, or programs perform in the real world.

By providing data on effectiveness, cost-effectiveness analysis provides information on how interventions are likely to work in everyday use. While supplementing cereal grains with the vitamin folate may greatly reduce neural tube defects in newborns, it may also lead to the underdiagnosis of vitamin B_{12} deficiency among poor or elderly populations (Haddix, Teutsch, Shaffer, & Dunet, 1996). When vitamin B_{12} deficiency is not diagnosed and treated early, it too can lead to severe complications. Thus, the efficacy of a given treatment in preventing a disease may not be representative of its overall effectiveness at preventing death due to that disease.

The Reference Case Analysis

Cost-effectiveness analyses can take many subtly different forms. Consider the case of a local health department that wishes to know the cost of screening people for tuberculosis in its clinics. It may examine the cost per case of active tuberculosis prevented when patients are screened in its clinics (relative to not providing these screening exams). This type of analysis would furnish the health department with information useful for making specific internal decisions, such as whether it is worthwhile to spend money on such programs. However, it would not provide a good deal of information on the overall benefits of screening to the population it serves. This is because it does not provide any information whether it is more valuable to treat a case of tuberculosis or better to invest in some other disease.

Or the health department may wish to expand the analysis in order to obtain information on both the cost-effectiveness of its operations and its broader mission of improving the longevity of the population it serves. For instance, it may wish to determine the cost of the program per year of life saved as well as the cost per case prevented. This would also provide information for internal decision making and on how the programs are benefiting the populations that they serve.

Finally, tuberculosis is a severe disease that can require burdensome treatments and long stints in hospitals (sometimes in an isolated room), and it can have an impact on people's quality of life. The health department may therefore also wish to examine the cost of tuberculosis screening relative to improvements in the quality and quantity of life of the population it serves. This type of information would allow them to assess the impact of tuberculosis on mortality. It would also allow them to compare the cost of tuberculosis screening programs to programs that predominantly affect the quality of life, such as mental health programs.

While some health events, such as high-rise construction accidents, predominantly affect the quantity of life, others, such as repetitive stress injuries at work, predominantly affect the quality of life. When a measure of quality of life is added to a cost-effectiveness analysis, it becomes possible to compare health interventions across the spectrum of disease. (Recall that one QALY is a year of life lived in perfect health.)

The ability to make comparisons across different diseases opens up the possibility of standardizing cost-effectiveness analyses, so that the incremental gains associated with virtually any intervention can be compared with those of another. If the health department conducted its analysis based on the cost per active case of tuberculosis prevented, it would provide some information on how the new intervention compares with what it is doing now. But it wouldn't be able to compare its new intervention with other programs in the health department because the denominator is different. If it used life expectancy, the denominator would be the same. Therefore, it could compare the cost per life saved of the tuberculosis program with a program that aimed to prevent window falls.

But you would still miss the boat. A program designed to reduce repetitive stress injuries at work wouldn't save many lives. Therefore, no matter how good the program is, it will always seem less cost-effective than a program designed to prevent window falls. Here again, the QALY saves the day. By comparing interventions across a term that captures both quantity and quality of life, it becomes possible to measure the relative cost-effectiveness of each program in the health department—provided that costs, quality measures, and life-years gained are all calculated in a similar way in each of the analyses. Under these conditions, it is possible to compare the incremental cost per QALY gained for health interventions as different as vaccination and migraine prevention. Of course, you need a standard set of methods to refer to if you are going to do this. This more or less standardized set of methods is called the **reference case analysis** (Gold et al., 1996; Neumann et al., 2016).

The use of disparate approaches to cost-effectiveness analysis some-times leads to widely different study results. For example, in the introduction to their book, the first Panel on Cost-Effectiveness in Health and Medicine notes that the published cost-effectiveness of screening mammography for the detection of breast cancer varies from cost saving to $150,000 per life-year saved (Gold et al., 1996; Neumann et al., 2016). (In that example, we adjusted the cost to 2017 US dollars so that you can get a better idea of what the range would look like today.) This huge variation was due to differences in what was and what was not included in the analysis. The panel set methodological standards for conducting cost-effectiveness analyses in hopes of preventing this kind of variation in cost-effectiveness ratios. Thus, the **reference case** was born.

The reference case standardizes the types of costs that should be included and requires the use of the QALY as the unit of effectiveness to ensure that all studies have comparable outcomes. The reference case also requires that two analyses be performed. In one analysis, the study must include all costs (regardless of who pays). In the second analysis, it requires the use of costs specific to the health sector. In this book we focus on reference case analyses.

FOR EXAMPLE: WHAT'S IN A NAME?

A lot of fuss is made over the distinction between *health* interventions and *medical* interventions (Gold et al., 1996; Neumann et al., 2016). *Health* generally refers to public health programs, such as the provision of clean water or laws requiring grains to be fortified with vitamins. *Medical interventions* specifically refer to things that medical providers do, such as selecting the most appropriate antibiotic. In practice, the distinction is blurry. For instance, checking blood pressure might be considered a health intervention if it is done as part of a screening program, but a medical intervention if it is done to ensure that a patient is receiving the proper dosage of medication. In this book, we usually refer to both types of interventions under the general heading of "health."

Why would you want to conduct any type of cost-effectiveness analysis besides the reference case analysis? Consider the health department used as an example at the beginning of this section. If the department is interested only in internal decision making, a reference case analysis would provide superfluous information, such as private sector costs and patient costs. Therefore, a reference case analysis is not necessarily the best approach in all situations. (For more information, see "A Note on Methods" in the Preface to this book.)

You now should have a sense of what cost-effectiveness is, why it is important, and for whom it is important. In the next section, we move on to how cost-effectiveness analysis is used to make policy decisions in health.

Cost-Effectiveness Analysis and Policy

We have noted that cost-effectiveness analyses are used primarily to compare different strategies for preventing or treating a single disease (such as tuberculosis). In addition, they can be used to maximize the quantity and quality of life within a given budget. In this section, we briefly explore how policy decisions are sometimes made using cost-effectiveness analyses, as well as some of the controversies that have arisen as a result of such policy decisions.

Prioritizing Health Interventions

It is possible to use cost-effectiveness analysis to purchase the most health under a fixed budget. If the incremental cost-effectiveness of everything that is done in medicine were known, we would have a sense of the opportunity cost of any health investment we might make (Jamison, Mosley, Measham, & Bobadilla, 1993). It would therefore be possible to list all interventions in a table and then draw a line between what is and is not affordable. When incremental cost-effectiveness ratios for different interventions are listed in a table, it is sometimes called a **league table** (Mauskopf, Rutten, & Schonfeld, 2003).

FOR EXAMPLE: COST-EFFECTIVENESS IN DEVELOPING COUNTRIES

Nowhere else is cost-effectiveness analysis more important than in developing countries. With annual health budgets as low as $5 per person, efficiency is critical. Recognizing the need for better health purchases, the World Health Organization developed CHOosing Interventions that are Cost-Effective (CHOICE). CHOICE is a program that contains information on costs, mortality, quality-of-life measures, and completed cost-effectiveness analyses for each region of the world (http://www .who.int/choice/en/).

League tables can also be used to place a given intervention in context. For instance, suppose we know that mammography costs $30,000 per QALY gained relative to no mammography. We can't be sure whether this is expensive or cheap relative to other things done in medicine. However, suppose we know that treating an otherwise fatal bacterial pneumonia with a commonly used antibiotic costs $25,000 per QALY gained relative to no treatment. Then we know that $30,000 per QALY gained for mammography is in the ballpark of a treatment that most would agree should not be denied. But if treating bacterial pneumonia were found to cost $300 per QALY gained and heart-lung transplants in active chain smokers were found to cost $15,000 per QALY, then perhaps mammography wouldn't be such a reasonable thing to do. We should, instead, invest in treating pneumonia and heart-lung transplants.

Let's take a look at how else a league table might be used. Table 1.1 represents a hypothetical league table for a village in Malawi with a total health budget of $58,000. In this table, we rank a number of interventions by their incremental cost-effectiveness ratio relative to not providing the treatment at all. This ratio tells us how much it costs to buy one year of perfect health.

If we know the size of the affected population and the total cost of the intervention, we know how much we will spend per year on any given strategy and the total number of QALYs we'll save. In this case, we only have $58,000, so we can't even provide the first four treatments, which

Table 1.1   Hypothetical League Table for a Village in Malawi with a $58,000 Health Budget

Intervention	Incremental Cost-Effectiveness Ratio[a]	Size of Affected Population	Total Cost per Year
Measles vaccine	$375	5,000	$15,000
Sexually transmitted disease treatment	$420	300	$2,100
Pneumonia treatment	$428	150	$1,800
Mosquito nets	$846	22,000	$44,000
HIV treatment	$3,000	100	$30,000
Total			$92,900

[a] The reference intervention is to do nothing.

collectively cost nearly $63,000. We might use this table to advocate for more funding or to figure out how we might reassess our interventions. For instance, prioritizing mosquito bed nets for children, who have not yet developed immunity to malaria, may be more cost-effective than providing them to family members who are older and less likely to succumb to the disease.

Exercises 3 and 4

3. How many QALYs will $1,000 worth of measles vaccine purchase in this village (the ICER for measles vaccine is $375 per QALY gained)?

4. A nongovernmental organization geared toward providing mosquito nets comes to a similar village in Malawi to the one represented in Table 1.1. This village has no health budget but wishes to provide $1,000 worth of mosquito nets (the ICER for mosquito nets is $846 per QALY gained). How many QALYs will be forgone as a result of spending the money on nets rather than on the measles vaccine?

However tempting it might be to create a list of interventions based on their cost-effectiveness, decisions surrounding the allocation of social resources cannot be made based on numbers alone. For example, HIV medications in Table 1.1 purchase a large amount of health for a small group of people, which might not be seen as fair for the village as a whole. Cost-effectiveness analysis does not provide ethical information; it is just one handy tool policymakers might use when deciding on which interventions they will fund (Gold et al., 1996; Neumann et al., 2016). (Other examples of league tables can be found at: https://research.tufts-nemc.org/ cear4/. From there, navigate to League Tables. (For further discussion, including the limitations of league tables, please see Mauskopf et al., 2003.)

FOR EXAMPLE: CHILE'S STORY: HOW TO SUCCEED BY NOT BEING COST-EFFECTIVE

Chile created a national health plan, called the Universal Access with Explicit Guarantees (AUGE) program, that in part used a league table to achieve its policy objectives. The idea was to start covering a small number of conditions and then scale up the program as time went on. Rather than choose the most cost-effective interventions to start with, however, those who designed the plan deliberately chose inefficient but heartwarming treatments, such as chemotherapy for children. The result? An astounding success: The president invited the cured children and other patients for a press conference to tout the success of the program. This single media event defeated the resistance of insurance companies and the national medical association. In 2013, the Ministry of Health increased the number of priority health conditions from 66 (in 2010) to 80. The AUGE program demonstrated that prioritization of treatment is multidimensional and does not rely on a single factor (e.g., cost-effectiveness). Instead, other criteria are used for coverage decisions such as high costs, social consensus, rule of rescue, inequality, effectiveness, capacity of the healthcare system, and burden of disease (Bitrán, Escobar, & Gassibe, 2010; Frenz, Delgado, Kaufman, & Harper, 2013; Vargas & Poblete, 2008). This is how cost-effectiveness analyses are meant to be used—as important pieces of a complex policy decision.

Do Cost-Effectiveness Analyses Actually Change the Way Things Are Done?

Examples of policy decisions that have been influenced by cost-effectiveness analysis include strategies for reducing parasitic infections in immigrant populations (Muennig, Pallin, Sell, & Chan, 1999), conducting cervical cancer screening among low-income elderly women (Fahs, Mandelblatt, Schechter, & Muller, 1992), and adding folate to cereal grains in the United States (Haddix et al., 1996). These studies appear to have sparked changes in the way that patients received medical care in local health departments, changes in Medicare reimbursement policies, and changes in the rules set by the U.S. Department of Agriculture. Still, although Canada, Australia, and a number of European countries use cost-effectiveness to help decide what should be paid for and what should not, Medicare has not yet officially incorporated cost-effectiveness analysis into its payment policies (Neumann, Rosen, & Weinstein, 2005).

Cost-effectiveness analyses can also lead to policy changes with broader implications than the authors intended. For instance, when supplementing cereal grains was found to be a cost-effective strategy for preventing neural tube defects in the United States, not only did cost-effectiveness analysis help convince the food industry that it was worth the cost, but other countries also considered similar interventions (Schaller & Olson, 1996; Wynn & Wynn, 1998).

Cost-effectiveness analysis has also proven to be a controversial tool when used without taking the broader social implications of health interventions into account. For example, in the state of Oregon in the United States, cost-effectiveness analysis was used to prioritize health interventions paid for by the state government using a league table. Those interventions deemed unaffordable were not paid, creating a large statewide and national outcry from groups denied treatment on these grounds. Some of the cost-effectiveness rankings seemed unintuitive when taken on face value. For example, braces for crooked teeth were ranked higher than treatments for Hodgkin's disease. (Hodgkin's disease is one of the few curable cancers.) In addition, the cost-effectiveness computations used to determine the priority list resulted in unintuitive ranks where having crooked teeth was ranked higher than Hodgkin's disease (Oregon Health Services Commission, 1991; Oregon Office for Health Policy and Research, 2001; Penner & McFarland, 2000).

These real-world examples highlight some of the promises and pitfalls of cost-effectiveness analysis for policy. Students embarking on this endeavor may one day find themselves facing tough ethical decisions for which there is no right answer. For instance, you may be working for a government that wishes to base immigration policies on preexisting conditions for applicants. Or you might be working for an insurance company that wishes to deny an effective treatment based on its cost-effectiveness. In such instances, consultation with all stakeholders (physicians, policymakers, payers, and patients) can help you come up with a strategy that better balances everyone's needs. In practice, this is not always easy to do, and oftentimes you are required to make decisions with only the best available evidence on hand.

To end this section on a positive note, though, let's return to Oregon for a moment. Recently, researchers and policymakers collaborated to put Medicaid to the test. Excess funds were used to randomly assign thousands of participants to either receive the opportunity to sign up for Medicaid or to receive whatever medical care they were already managing to scrounge up. The study started a political firestorm because it found that, while Medicaid increased preventive screening, produced financial protections, and reduced depression, it did nothing to actually improve physical health (Baicker et al., 2013). Medicaid opponents therefore argued that Medicaid should be cut. Why is this a happy note? Cost-effectiveness analysis showed that these other benefits actually make Medicaid more than worth the initial investment (Muennig, Quan, Chiuzan, & Glied, 2015).

What Does the Future Hold?

Cost-effectiveness is all fine and well, but most patients in the United States don't want to be told that they can't get an annual physical with their doctor because it isn't "cost-effective." (In fact, not only is it expensive and not helpful, annual physicals may actually be harmful because the doctor can find things that are not a problem and might even eventually require invasive procedures to detect these phantom ailments.) Since insurers already charge patients part of the medical bill to reduce the cost of care (a fee called a "copayment"), one fix to this problem is to just charge less for cost-effective care and more for cost-ineffective care. Of course, we need a good jargon-y name for any such thing, and this idea has a good one: "value-based insurance design" (Fendrick, Smith, Chernew, & Shah, 2001). Several providers have implemented this approach, and preliminary data show that it saves money (Farley, Wansink, Lindquist, Parker, & Maciejewski, 2012; Frank, Fendrick, He, Zbrozek, Holtz, Leung, & Chernew, 2012; Maciejewski, Wansink, Lindquist, Parker, & Farley, 2014).

The Patient Protection and Affordable Care Act (PPACA), more commonly known as "Obamacare," was written into law in 2010. Obamacare is actually a long list of incremental changes to the U.S. healthcare system that are supposed to add up to something big. One such change is to set up a Patient Centered Outcomes Research Institute (PCORI). This institute funds research that will guide patients and providers toward making more informed decisions. PCORI is tasked with performing *comparative*-effectiveness research; that is, it is prohibited from using the dollars per quality-adjusted life-year metric in determining thresholds for selecting the most cost-effective strategy (Neumann & Weinstein, 2010). In other words, the U.S. approach suggests that one should always select the most effective treatment no matter what the cost. Of course, there is no such thing as a bottomless budget. So this approach ends up costing lives by paying for things that we can't afford at the expense of those things that we can.

This is in contrast to other countries, such as the U.K.'s National Institute for Health and Care Excellence (NICE), which use cost-effectiveness analyses to determine coverage decisions for pharmaceutical agents and new technologies. Similarly, Canada and Australia have established agencies that evaluate the submission of pharmaceutical agents for inclusion into the public formularies. In Canada it is the Common Drug Review, and in Australia it is the Pharmaceutical Benefits Advisory Committee. These agencies play critical roles in controlling expenditures, while maintaining or increasing the overall societal values of new pharmaceutical agents. The advantage to these approaches versus the one adopted by the United States is that they can save more lives within a fixed budget. Nice!

Still, public debates over cost-effectiveness have given the field a bit of a black eye. This is unfair in part because those making the argument are ill informed and in part because it is difficult to defend something so complex. After all, you can't win a rhetorical war when you first have to explain the incremental cost-effectiveness ratio. Unlike cost-effectiveness analysis, however, comparative-effectiveness analysis is in theory more individualized. While cost-effectiveness analysis just provides information on what is best for the average person out there, comparative-effectiveness considers "effectiveness, benefits, and harms of treatment options" for the *individual*, not just the average person (Agency for Healthcare Research and Quality, 2015). This does not eliminate the need to evaluate cost; however, it does limit how we use the results from comparative-effectiveness research when making decisions about which treatment options provide the overall greatest benefit to patients, providers, and society.

As future studies on comparative-effectiveness research incorporate cost, the debate will once again return to the question of rationalizing health care and its inherent moral and ethical (and political) problems. Currently, there is great interest in identifying the strategy with the highest value but at the lowest cost. Cost-effectiveness analysis is an important tool for carrying out this task.

Another thing that the future might hold is that cost-effectiveness analyses could increasingly be applied to social policies rather than just comparing medical treatments. This is exciting, because many nonmedical investments that the government makes actually produce health and might do so with more value than investments in the medical system itself (Muennig & Woolf, 2007; Woolf & Aron, 2013). The great upside of this is that governments could make the best use of all of the taxpayer money that is spent. The downside is that modern cost-effectiveness research protocols don't teach students how to actually do these types of studies.

One important difference is that, like new drugs, social policies can produce unintended "side effects." For instance, many policymakers respond to road congestion by building more roads (Sterman, 2006). Road congestion is a terrible problem because people waste a lot of their precious time sitting in their cars while polluting the air and warming the planet. The problem with building more roads is that it increases the demand for cars.

Not only do more people drive, but cities tend to sprawl outward as people have access to cheaper property in the suburbs and exurbs. So people spend more, not less, time in their cars as more roads are built. In addition, accidents, obesity, and pollution tend to get worse than they would have had the money been spent on public transit instead. Unlike a cost-effectiveness analysis of a drug that has been tested using randomized controlled trials, these unintended consequences are not known and must be thought out. However, they can also be modeled using specialized software.

The "science" of thinking these problems out is known as *complex systems dynamics*, among other titles. Throughout this book we will slowly introduce this very cool science to you.

Summary

Due to the increasing costs and limited resources of health care, there had to be some way to objectively determine how much health care we can afford to provide while maintaining (or enhancing) its quality. Cost-effectiveness analysis combines health interventions, competing alternatives, health states, health status, costs, and benefits (e.g., QALYs) in order to calculate the incremental cost-effectiveness ratio, the difference in cost needed to realize an incremental gain in benefit between two strategies. This provides us with a guide to help make coverage decisions for pharmaceutical drugs and costly interventions. However, making these decisions is a multidimensional task and requires us also to consider social preferences, burden of disease, and the capacity of the healthcare system.

Further Readings

Those who are interesting in reading more about Value-Based Insurance Design are encouraged to visit the Center for Value-Based Insurance Design hosted by the University of Michigan (http://www.sph.umich.edu/vbidcenter).

David M. Eddy (Eddy, 1991a, 1991b, 1991c) and Thomas Bodenheimer (Bodenheimer, 1997a, 1997b) wrote several papers about the early phases of the Oregon State Health Plan.

For more information regarding Chile's Health Plan Reform and AUGE, please refer to Vargas and Poblete's review. It provides an excellent explanation of prioritization by Chile's Ministry of Health (Vargas & Poblete, 2008).

References

Agency for Healthcare Research and Quality. (2015). Effective Health Care Program. Retrieved March 22, 2015, from http://effectivehealthcare.ahrq.gov.

Attaran, A., and J. Sachs. (2001). Defining and Refining International Donor Support for Combating the AIDS Pandemic. *Lancet* 357(9249): 57–61. http://doi.org/10.1016/S0140-6736(00)03576-5.

Baicker, K., S. L. Taubman, H. L. Allen, M. Bernstein, J. H. Gruber, J. P. Newhouse, . . . A. N. Finkelstein. (2013). The Oregon Experiment—Effects of Medicaid on Clinical Outcomes. *New England Journal of Medicine* 368(18): 1713–1722. http://doi.org/10.1056/NEJMsa1212321.

Bitrán, R., L. Escobar, and P. Gassibe. (2010). After Chile's Health Reform: Increase in Coverage and Access, Decline in Hospitalization and Death Rates. *Health Affairs* 29(12): 2161–2170. http://doi.org/10.1377/hlthaff.2010.0972.

Bodenheimer, T. (1997a). The Oregon Health Plan—Lessons for the Nation. First of two parts. *New England Journal of Medicine* 337(9): 651–655. http://doi.org/10.1056/NEJM199708283370923.

Bodenheimer, T. (1997b). The Oregon Health Plan—Lessons for the Nation. Second of two parts. *New England Journal of Medicine* 337(10): 720–723. http://doi.org/10.1056/NEJM199709043371021.

Eddy, D. M. (1991a). Clinical Decision Making: From Theory to Practice. What's Going On in Oregon? *Journal of the American Medical Association* 266(3): 417–420.

Eddy, D. M. (1991b). Oregon's Methods. Did Cost-Effectiveness Analysis Fail? *Journal of the American Medical Association* 266(15): 2135–2141.

Eddy, D. M. (1991c). Oregon's Plan. Should It Be Approved? *Journal of the American Medical Association* 266(17): 2439–2445.

Fahs, M. C., J. Mandelblatt, C. Schechter, and C. Muller. (1992). Cost Effectiveness of Cervical Cancer Screening for the Elderly. *Annals of Internal Medicine* 117(6): 520–527.

Farley, J. F., D. Wansink, J. H. Lindquist, J. C. Parker, and M. L. Maciejewski. (2012). Medication Adherence Changes Following Value-Based Insurance Design. *American Journal of Managed Care* 18(5): 265–274.

Farmer, P. (2004). *Pathologies of Power*. Berkeley: University of California Press.

Fendrick, A. M., D. G. Smith, M. E. Chernew, and S. N. Shah. (2001). A Benefit-Based Copay for Prescription Drugs: Patient Contribution Based on Total Benefits, Not Drug Acquisition Cost. *American Journal of Managed Care* 7(9): 861–867.

Frank, M. B., A. M. Fendrick, Y. He, A. Zbrozek, N. Holtz, S. Leung, and M. E. Chernew. (2012). The Effect of a Large Regional Health Plan's Value-Based Insurance Design Program on Statin Use. *Medical Care* 50(11): 934–939. http://doi.org/10.1097/MLR.0b013e31826c8630.

Frenz, P., I. Delgado, J. S. Kaufman, and S. Harper. (2013). Achieving Effective Universal Health Coverage with Equity: Evidence from Chile. *Health Policy and Planning*, 29(6): 717–731. http://doi.org/10.1093/heapol/czt054.

Gold, M. R., J. E. Siegel, L. B. Russell, and M. C. Weinstein. (1996). *Cost-Effectiveness in Health and Medicine*. New York: Oxford University Press.

Haddix, A., S. Teutsch, P. Shaffer, and D. Dunet. (1996). *Prevention Effectiveness: A Guide to Decision Analysis and Economic Evaluation*. New York: Oxford University Press.

Jamison, D. T., W. H. Mosley, A. R. Measham, and J. L. Bobadilla. (1993). *Disease Control Priorities in Developing Countries*. New York: Oxford University Press.

Krumholz, H. M. (2013). Variations in Health Care, Patient Preferences, and High-Quality Decision Making. *Journal of the American Medical Association* 310(2): 151–152. http://doi.org/10.1001/jama.2013.7835.

Maciejewski, M. L., D. Wansink, J. H. Lindquist, J. C. Parker, and J. F. Farley. (2014). Value-Based Insurance Design Program in North Carolina Increased Medication Adherence but Was Not Cost Neutral. *Health Affairs* (Project Hope) 33(2): 300–308. http://doi.org/10.1377/hlthaff.2013.0260.

Mandelblatt, J. S., C. B. Schechter, K. R. Yabroff, W. Lawrence, J. Dignam, P. Muennig, . . . M. Fahs. (2004). Benefits and Costs of Interventions to Improve Breast Cancer Outcomes in African American Women. *Journal of Clinical Oncology* 22(13): 2554–2566. http://doi.org/10.1200/JCO.2004.05.009.

Mauskopf, J., F. Rutten, and W. Schonfeld. (2003). Cost-Effectiveness League Tables: Valuable Guidance for Decision Makers? *PharmacoEconomics* 21(14): 991–1000.

Muennig, P. (2015). Can Universal Pre-Kindergarten Programs Improve Population Health and Longevity? Mechanisms, Evidence, and Policy Implications. *Social Science & Medicine* (1982), 127: 116–123. http://doi.org/10.1016/j.socscimed.2014.08.033.

Muennig, P., D. Pallin, R. L. Sell, and M. S. Chan. (1999). The Cost Effectiveness of Strategies for the Treatment of Intestinal Parasites in Immigrants. *New England Journal of Medicine* 340(10): 773–779. http://doi.org/10.1056/NEJM199903113401006.

Muennig, P., R. Quan, C. Chiuzan, and S. Glied. (2015). Considering Whether Medicaid Is Worth the Cost: Revisiting the Oregon Health Study. *American Journal of Public Health* 105(5): 866–871. http://doi.org/10.2105/AJPH.2014.302485.

Muennig, P., and S. H. Woolf. (2007). Health and Economic Benefits of Reducing the Number of Students per Classroom in US Primary Schools. *American Journal of Public Health* 97(11): 2020–2027. http://doi.org/10.2105/AJPH.2006.105478.

Neumann, P. J., A. B. Rosen, and M. C. Weinstein. (2005). Medicare and Cost-Effectiveness Analysis. *New England Journal of Medicine* 353(14): 1516–1522. http://doi.org/10.1056/NEJMsb050564.

Neumann, P. J., and M. C. Weinstein. (2010). Legislating against Use of Cost-Effectiveness Information. *New England Journal of Medicine* 363(16): 1495–1497. http://doi.org/10.1056/NEJMp1007168.

Neumann, P. J., G. D. Sanders, L. B. Russell, J. E. Siegel, and T. G. Ganiats. (2016). *Cost-Effectiveness in Health and Medicine*. New York: Oxford University Press.

Newhouse, J. P., and A. M. Garber. (2013). Geographic Variation in Medicare Services. *New England Journal of Medicine* 368(16): 1465–1468. http://doi.org/10.1056/NEJMp1302981.

Oregon Health Services Commission. (1991). Oregon Medicaid Priority Setting Project. Oregon State Government.

Oregon Office for Health Policy and Research. (2001). Oregon Health Plan. Retrieved from http://www.ohppr.state.or.us/.

Penner, N. R., and B. H. McFarland. (2000). Background on the Oregon Health Plan. *New Directions for Mental Health Services* (85): 23–32.

Sambo, L. G., J. M. Kirigia, and J. N. Orem. (2013). Health Financing in the African Region: 2000–2009 Data Analysis. *International Archives of Medicine* 6(1): 10. http://doi.org/10.1186/1755-7682-6-10.

Schaller, D. R., and B. H. Olson. (1996). A Food Industry Perspective on Folic Acid Fortification. *Journal of Nutrition* 126(3): 761S–764S.

Sterman, J. D. (2006). Learning from Evidence in a Complex World. *American Journal of Public Health* 96(3): 505–514. http://doi.org/10.2105/AJPH.2005.066043.

Ubel, P. A., M. L. DeKay, J. Baron, and D. A. Asch. (1996). Cost-Effectiveness Analysis in a Setting of Budget Constraints—Is It Equitable? *New England Journal of Medicine* 334(18): 1174–1177. http://doi.org/10.1056/NEJM199605023341807.

Vargas, V., and S. Poblete. (2008). Health Prioritization: The Case of Chile. *Health Affairs* 27(3): 782–792. http://doi.org/10.1377/hlthaff.27.3.782.

Wennberg, J., and A. Gittelsohn. (1982). Variations in Medical Care Among Small Areas. *Scientific American* 246(4): 120–134.

Wilkinson, R. G. (1999). Health, Hierarchy, and Social Anxiety. *Annals of the New York Academy of Sciences* 896: 48–63.

Wolfram|Alpha. (2015). Computational Knowledge Engine. Retrieved March 22, 2015, from http://www.wolframalpha.com/.

Woolf, S. H., and L. Aron. (2013). *US Health in International Perspective: Shorter Lives, Poorer Health*. Washington, DC: National Academic Press.

Wynn, M., and A. Wynn. (1998). The Danger of B_{12} Deficiency in the Elderly. *Nutrition and Health* 12(4): 215–226.

CHAPTER 2

PRINCIPLES OF COST-EFFECTIVENESS ANALYSIS

Overview

So far, you have learned what cost-effectiveness is and how it is used to affect policy. This chapter introduces the basic concepts behind cost-effectiveness analysis. We explore the different types of analyses, how costs are tabulated, how health-related quality of life is measured, and how QALYs are generated. You will also learn how to interpret cost-effectiveness ratios in more detail.

The Perspective of a Cost-Effectiveness Analysis

Terry Jones, the chief executive officer of a large insurance company, has received hundreds of requests for contraceptive reimbursement from the company's enrollees. He is interested in improving the company's services for the enrollees but is concerned that the costs might be prohibitive. Nevertheless, because the company must pay for pregnancies when they occur, reimbursing patients for contraceptives might reduce the company's expenditures on hospitalization costs.

Jones realizes that if the company does not reimburse for the birth control pill, most of the company's clients who wish to protect themselves from pregnancy will purchase the contraceptives on their own. However, some people will have unwanted pregnancies because it was either too inconvenient or too expensive for them to purchase contraceptives. Because pregnancy occasionally results in medical complications or even death, the company's failure to pay for contraceptives could theoretically

LEARNING OBJECTIVES

- Identify different perspectives for cost-effectiveness analysis.

- List the costs that are associated with the different perspectives.

- Define and distinguish QALY and QALE.

- Differentiate between direct, indirect, and intangible costs.

- Explain the incremental cost-effectiveness ratio (ICER).

- Differentiate between cost-effectiveness analysis, cost-utility analysis, cost-benefit analysis, and cost-minimization analysis.

result in litigation as well. Therefore, Jones commissions an analysis examining the cost of providing contraceptives per pregnancy prevented when the insurance company pays for contraception versus a no-pay policy.

Jo Jo Thompson is the commissioner of a local health department in Saratoga, Illinois. Thompson receives a report indicating that the maternal mortality rate among low-income women in Saratoga has increased over the past year. Many low-income women simply cannot afford contraceptives. Thompson wishes to know whether his health department can afford the program and whether it will be effective at reducing maternal mortality.

Finally, Tina Johanas is a U.S. senator interested in enacting legislation mandating that all insurance companies pay for contraceptives. Johanas's primary interest is to improve the quality of life of her constituents, but she is also concerned about the overall impact of the proposed legislation on the healthcare system. Therefore, she commissions a cost-effectiveness analysis examining the incremental cost per QALY gained when insurance companies are mandated to pay for contraception relative to the cost per QALY gained of the current policy of letting insurance companies decide whether to pay for contraceptives.

In the analysis conducted from the perspective of the insurance company headed by Jones, the relevant question is whether the company pays for all of the contraceptives or none of the contraceptives. Jones decides not to include any costs incurred by patients in the analysis because such costs do not appear on his company's budget. He would be interested in knowing whether paying for contraceptives might reduce pregnancy-associated costs, because such costs do account for a portion of his company's expenditures.

Commissioner Thompson is interested in costs specific to the health department. He wishes to include only medical services and goods for which the health department will pay. These might include the cost of medical services that occur in health department clinics and the cost of the contraceptive itself. Unlike Jones, Commissioner Thompson does not wish to include the costs associated with pregnancies that occur among privately insured women since they do not appear on his balance sheet.

Finally, Senator Johanas is worried about the overall costs of her legislation to everyone in society. She wishes to ensure that the interests of health departments, insurance companies, and regular citizens are met. Therefore, she wishes to include all costs relevant to enacting the legislation or failing to enact the legislation. Moreover, Johanas is worried about the overall health and well-being of her constituents rather than just the number of pregnancies prevented. Because unwanted pregnancy can cause emotional as well as physical harm, she wishes to ensure that the overall quality of life of women with unwanted pregnancies is accounted for in the analysis. Commissioner Thompson and Senator Johanas realize that the state also pays for half of all Medicaid costs. So, they also want to conduct an analysis that includes costs relevant to the health system.

The party interested in the study can have an influence on which costs and which effectiveness outcomes are included in an analysis. When a particular organization includes only costs and outcomes relevant to its needs, the analysis is said to have been conducted from that party's perspective. For example, when the study applies only to a government agency, the study is said to assume a **governmental perspective**. When the study applies to society as a whole, it is said to assume a **societal perspective**. When costs are considered from the health care sector, it is called a health care sector perspective. Table 2.1 illustrates the different types of costs that might be included in a study from the perspective of an insurance company, a government agency, or society as a whole.

In Table 2.1, each of these three entities is paying for the cost of the contraceptive, medical visits, and hospitalization. Because insurance companies do not have to compensate patients for their time or pay transportation costs or environmental costs, these costs would not be included in a study that assumes the perspective of the insurance company. However, the government would be interested in some of these costs. For example,

Table 2.1   Costs Included in a Cost-Effectiveness Analysis of Free Contraception, Conducted from Three Perspectives

Cost	Insurance	Government	Society	Health Sector
Contraceptive pill	All costs	All costs	All costs	All costs
Medical visit	All costs	All costs	All costs	All costs
Hospitalization	All costs	All costs	All costs	All costs
Patient time	No costs	Some costs	All costs	No costs
Transportation	No costs	Some costs	All costs	Ambulance costs
Environment	No costs	All costs	All costs	No costs
Education system	No costs	Most costs	All costs	No costs

because the local government disproportionately hires low-income women, some of the women seeking contraception might be government employees and will take time off from work to receive medical care.

From the societal perspective, all costs must be included regardless of who pays for them. "Society" refers to everyone who might be affected by the intervention. Thus, costs relevant to the government, employers, patients, insurance companies, and anyone or anything else should be included as long as they are likely to be large enough to make a difference in the analysis. Usually the term *society* refers to everything within the borders of a country (Drummond, Sculpher, Torrance, O'Brien, & Stoddart, 2005).

Since different perspectives require including or excluding different costs, the only way to standardize cost-effectiveness analyses is to require that all of these analyses assume the same perspective. For this reason, among others, the reference case scenario of the Panel on Cost-Effectiveness in Health and Medicine requires that the societal perspective be adopted (Neumann, Sanders, Russell, Siegel, & Ganiats, 2016). The societal perspective is important because it tell us what we all have to pay when a particular policy, treatment, or screening procedure is changed. But in reality, the tradeoffs are not balanced between all social expenditures. For instance, money is not taken from housing or from the military and allocated to vaccinations. For this very practical reason, the new Panel now recommends that a health sector perspective is included alongside a societal perspective.

To publish cost-effectiveness analyses, it is best to include a reference case analysis so that your results can be placed in the context of other studies. Recall from Chapter 1 that the reference case includes all relevant costs (regardless of who pays) and QALY as the unit of effectiveness. When all costs are included, it is a simple task to exclude some of the costs not of interest to one party or another. This way, you can easily add another perspective (e.g., governmental as well as societal) to your study.

In the insurance company's case, it might conduct a reference case analysis and then calculate cost-effectiveness ratios from the company's perspective by leaving out the costs mentioned in Table 2.1 that aren't relevant. If the company were to publish the study in the medical literature (perhaps to attract attention to its good deeds), it could simply present the reference case results along with the results of interest to the company.

THE THEORY BEHIND COST-EFFECTIVENESS ANALYSIS

One theoretical framework for cost-effectiveness is based upon something called the von Neumann–Morgenstern utility maximization theory (Garber & Phelps, 1997; von Neumann & Morgenstern, 1953). (Those are their names. Really.) The idea is that a "rational" person will purchase as much happiness (sometimes referred to as utility) as possible with the money that they have. The incremental benefit that they get from their purchase would have to be balanced by the incremental cost. Sound familiar? This is the structure of the incremental cost-effectiveness ratio (ICER) you learned about in Chapter 1. It is also the main idea behind welfare.

There are two schools of thought on welfare, and they are of course divided. One school is "welfarism." The other is "extra-welfarism." Under the welfarist school of thought, benefits are converted into dollars (or "monetized" in technical terms). In this case, a cost-benefit analysis makes more sense because the consumer only needs a final decision: do it or not, based upon whether it is cost-saving. This assumes that we know how much health is "worth." However, extra-welfarists measure health benefits in terms of health (or QALYs). So, while welfarists are worried about utility, extra-welfarists are worried only about health. In a cost-effectiveness analysis, separating out QALYs from easier to measure economic benefits allows the consumer to figure out how many QALYs can be saved under any given budget if perfect investments are made. Cost-effectiveness has the advantage of allowing one to rank a bunch of interventions and then draw a budgetary line below which we cannot afford to make an investment.

Later in this chapter we will expand on both cost-benefit analysis and cost-effectiveness analysis.

Capturing Costs

Before we go on, take another look at Equation 1.1 from Chapter 1:

$$\frac{(Cost\ of\ Intervention\ 2 - Cost\ of\ Intervention\ 1)}{(QALE\ 2 - QALE\ 1)} \tag{2.1}$$

Let's call doing nothing "Intervention 1" and mammography for women over the age of 50 "Intervention 2." (Remember that the intervention strategy goes on the left of the equation and the reference case goes on the right.) In this instance, our research question is "What happens when women who would not otherwise have received a mammogram are given one?"

We saw in Figure 1.2 that the new intervention (in this case, mammography) moves women with breast cancer from Health Status 1 (undetected cancer) to Health Status 2 (cancer detected early). Since this is the "capturing costs" section of the book, our job here is to think only about costs. We need to consider three factors: (1) the costs associated with Health Status 1, (2) the costs associated with the intervention, and (3) the costs associated with Health Status 2.

The total cost of doing nothing is equal to the total cost of Health Status 1. In Health Status 1, women who do not have breast cancer will go on with their lives without incurring any costs whatsoever. Those who do have cancer but don't know it will incur the future costs associated with more advanced disease.

The total cost of the mammography intervention is the cost of mammography itself plus the total cost of Health Status 2. The total cost of Health Status 2 may be something less than the total cost of Health Status 1 because it is generally less expensive to treat less advanced disease than it is to treat more advanced disease. Or it may cost more because screening leads to false positives.

The cost of medical visits, hospitalizations, X-rays, and other goods and services are referred to as **direct costs.** Consider the cost of time lost in going to the doctor's office or time spent away from the beach due to breast cancer. The Americans have the saying "Time is money," and in cost-effectiveness analysis we attempt to place a monetary value on this time. Lost time is an **indirect cost.** Such costs are called "indirect" because they don't involve the consumption of goods or services. Another way to think about indirect costs is in terms of worker productivity. Society relies on you to be a healthy contributor to the workforce. If you are sick or ill for a given period of time, then your productivity decreases during that period. Conversely, if you are healthy, then you are contributing some measure of productivity during that time. Indirect costs capture your productivity during a specific period to society.

While indirect costs still involve the consumption of something that is measurable (for example, the time spent doing something), there are costs that can't be easily accounted for. Such costs, referred to as **intangible costs,** are those that cannot be measured by any conventional metric. Examples of intangible costs are pain, suffering, or the monetary value of a year of healthy life. In cost-effectiveness analysis, intangible costs related to pain and suffering (quality of life) are also often referred to as **morbidity costs,** and costs related to death are sometimes called **mortality costs.**

In cost-effectiveness analysis, intangible costs are not monetized. Rather, such costs can be captured in the quality-of-life measure used to calculate QALYs.

Capturing Quality

Recall that a QALY is one year of life spent in perfect health. The trick is to come up with some subjective measure of how to convert a year of life lived with disease into a year of life lived in perfect health. This is done through the use of a **health-related quality-of-life (HRQL) score.**

The HRQL (sometimes abbreviated as HRQoL) score measures the effect of a disease on the way a person enjoys life. This includes the way illness affects a person's ability to live free of pain, work productively, and interact with loved ones. In other words, the HRQL score translates a person's perception of his or her quality of life with a particular illness into a number.

For example, on a scale from 0 to 1, individuals who consider themselves to be in perfect health would rate their life as a 1, and someone who would just as soon be dead might rate his or her life as a 0. Another person with a chronic debilitating disease might rate life as a 0.7, indicating that she values her life as worth only seven-tenths of a year of life lived in perfect health (see Figure 2.1).

In this example, one year of perfect health is therefore simply 0.7 × 1 year = 0.7 QALY. Two years in this state is 0.7 × 2 years = 1.4 QALYs. In other words, while the QALY represents a year of perfect health, the HRQL score represents the proportion of time lived in perfect health.

You will learn how one comes by this proportion in Chapter 7. For now, let's leave it at this: It's probably more accurate to place a 0 to 1 value on the trade-off between life and death than it is to place a monetary value on the trade-off. Therefore, we use this number rather than a dollar value.

Aha! Now you know why the HRQL score is discussed within a section of the book about costs. Let's take a second to look at an example of how this is used. Before you do, close your eyes, clear your head, and recall just three things: (1) The HRQL score tells you what proportion of your time is spent in the equivalent of perfect health; (2) the QALY is a year of life spent in perfect health; and (3) one year at an HRQL of 0.7 is equal to 0.7 QALYs.

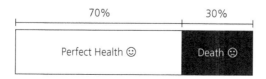

Figure 2.1   Graphical Representation of an HRQL Score

Suppose that we are evaluating a new drug that greatly reduces the morbidity associated with adult-onset diabetes. Suppose further that, although this new drug has a dramatic effect on morbidity, it has no effect on mortality. We wish to compare this new drug with current medications. If we want to know how this new drug might change the total QALYs lived from the average age of onset for diabetes (67 years) to the average age of death (77 years) in a hypothetical group of women, we would add up the differences in QALYs lived each year (see Table 2.2).

The total number of years each group of women would have lived is the same (10 years). However, when quality of life is considered, the women without treatment would have gained just 6.2 QALYs. The treated women gained 8.6 QALYs over those 10 years. Therefore, although their life was just as long, the treated women experience a gain in years of perfect health equal to 8.6 QALYs – 6.2 QALYs = 2.4 QALYs. Figure 2.2 illustrates the difference in total QALYs between the two strategies.

Now let's think about this on a larger scale. Appendix B contains life tables for the U.S. population, which include life expectancy at a given age. If the average HRQL at birth is 0.82 and the average life expectancy is 77.5,

Table 2.2   Hypothetical Differences in Health-Related Quality of Life over 10 Years for Diabetic Women and Women in Perfect Health

Year	Diabetic Women	Treated Women
1	0.8	0.9
2	0.8	0.9
3	0.7	0.9
4	0.8	0.9
5	0.6	0.9
6	0.6	0.9
7	0.5	0.8
8	0.6	0.8
9	0.4	0.8
10	0.4	0.8
Total QALYs	6.2	8.6

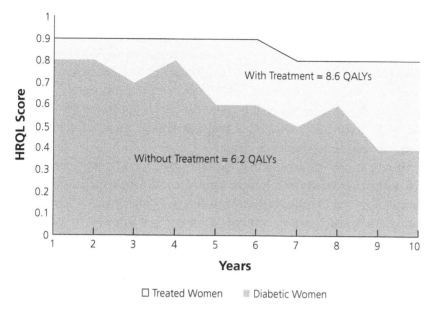

Figure 2.2   Difference in Total QALYs Between Women Treated and Not Treated for Diabetes over 10 Years

how many QALYs does the average American live? This is a matter of simple multiplication: $77.5 \times 0.82 = 63.6$ QALYs.

In Chapter 7, we will see that the way an HRQL score is measured can bias the calculation of QALYs. Because there is no perfect way to measure a person's HRQL score and because the HRQL can affect the way in which denominator "costs" are counted, it is important that HRQL scores are obtained and used in a consistent way. In fact, the use of something as subjective as an HRQL score affects the overall usefulness of reference case cost-effectiveness analyses (Gold & Muennig, 2002; Neumann et al., 2016). Still, the only way to compare different interventions across different diseases is to include HRQL in the cost-effectiveness analysis.

Ask yourself, "how much would you pay to get rid of a really bad headache?" The answer might be relatively straightforward, at least for you personally. But the much bigger question is "how much should society pay to help alleviate headaches in general?" That is much less straightforward. It becomes even less straightforward when we think about how much we might pay to save a year of life. The HRQL score is meant to capture such morbidity and mortality (intangible) "costs."

The HRQL score makes the accounting of tangible, direct costs (e.g., the cost of a doctor's visit) and intangible costs (e.g., getting rid of a headache) much more easy to manage. Rather than trade money for sickness, HRQL allows people to make tradeoffs using longevity as a "currency." When people are asked to generate an HRQL score, they must deeply imagine what it is like to have the health state that they want to get rid of. They then make trade-offs between that health state (e.g., a headache, lost limb, or depression) and a chance of death.

It was previously argued that indirect costs, namely, those associated with **lost productivity** and **leisure time,** are at least partially captured in the HRQL score. The idea is that if you deeply enough imagine your health state, you will also take into account its impact on your ability to work or to enjoy your time away from work. But, starting with new recommendations by the second Panel on Cost-Effectiveness in Health and Medicine, it is now recommended that these costs be measured separately (Neumann et al., 2016).

Lost productivity and leisure time refer to the time that one loses when he or she is sick. Illness can affect how well you do your work. Sick people cannot work to their full ability, and they work fewer hours. These costs are included in the numerator of a cost-effectiveness analysis when an analysis assumes the societal perspective.

They are usually *not* included when you assume the health sector perspective. Why? They are included in the societal perspective because one's illness impacts everyone in society. (If you can't work as productively, it has an impact on the economy.) However, from the health sector perspective, we don't care about the economy as a whole. We only care about those costs that are specific health care delivery. We might include lost productivity costs in rare instances (like in SARS or Ebola outbreaks when health workers are impacted), but these types of analyses are rare.

> **TIPS AND TRICKS**
>
> Cost of caring
>
> The Panel on Cost-Effectiveness in Health and Medicine recommends that it is important to value the time of people who are caregivers but who are not paid for their work when assuming the societal perspective. After all, they are making a real contribution, even if there is no actual exchange of money. The time of caregivers is equal to the pre-tax wages of caregivers plus overhead.

The use of QALYs allows researchers to combine the effects of quantity of life (for example, years of life gained by an intervention) with quality of life in a single measure. But how is something as subjective as quality measured, and how are measures of quantity and quality of life combined? In Chapter 7, we will learn how quality is measured in cost-effectiveness analysis, and we will then learn how QALYs are calculated in Chapter 8.

As mentioned earlier, in 2017, the recommendations for costs and the analytic perspective changed. Exhibit 2.1 shows how the recommendations for previous and current analyses have changed.

EXHIBIT 2.1. HOW THE RECOMMENDATIONS FOR NUMERATOR AND DENOMINATOR VALUES IN THE INCREMENTAL COST-EFFECTIVENESS RATIO HAVE CHANGED WITH THE NEW RECOMMENDATIONS IN 2017.

Pre-2017 Recommendations

	Societal Perspective	Health Sector Costs
Numerator	Direct Costs	Optional
	Indirect Costs	Optional
Denominator	Health-Related Quality of Life	
	Years of Life Remaining	
	Lost Productivity/Leisure Time	

Post-2017 Recommendations

	Societal Perspective	Health Sector Costs
Numerator	Direct Costs	Direct Costs
	Indirect Costs	Not Included
	Lost Productivity	Not Included
Denominator	Health-Related Quality of Life	
	Years of Life Remaining	

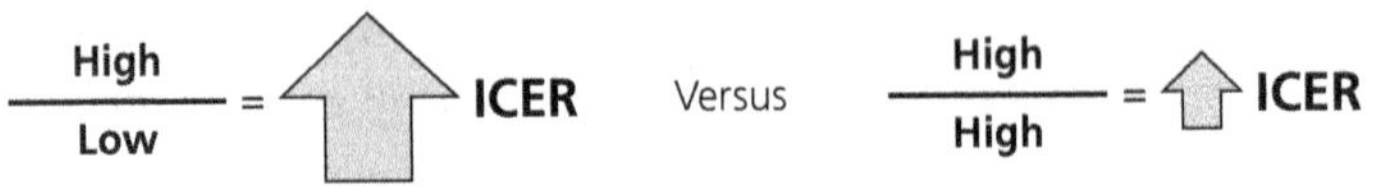

Figure 2.3   Graphical Representation of the Impact of High and Low Numerators and Denominators in Calculating Incremental Cost-Effectiveness Ratios

Interpreting the Cost-Effectiveness Ratio

Let's revisit Equation 1.1 from Chapter 1 yet again:

$$\frac{(Cost\ of\ Intervention\ 2 - Cost\ of\ Intervention\ 1)}{(QALE\ 2 - QALE\ 1)} \tag{2.2}$$

Notice that if the incremental cost in the numerator is high but the number of QALYs gained by the intervention is low, the ratio becomes very large (Figure 2.3). If the cost is high but the number of QALYs is also high, the ratio will be smaller. So you can see that very expensive interventions that are also very effective may still be cost-effective relative to less expensive but less effective interventions.

Researchers do not generally state whether an intervention is cost-effective in medical publications because their area of expertise is research, not policymaking. Instead, it is generally preferred to simply document how the interventions studied compare with other interventions. The most practical strategy for putting the results of an analysis into context is to compare the results of the study at hand to the results of other studies in the same country to provide some basis for comparison (Gold et al., 1996; Neumann et al., 2016). In the United States, the CEA Registry (https://research.tufts-nemc.org/cear4/) has simplified this task by presenting cost-effectiveness ratios for many different interventions that comply with the reference case.

FOR EXAMPLE: HOW MUCH DOES A DRUG REALLY COST?

Newer anticancer drugs such as Provenge (Sipuleucel-T) cost upward of $93,000 for a one-month course of therapy (Simoens, 2012). The money spent on coming up with the name alone might be worth it, but costs like that raise serious questions about affordability. The Centers for Medicare and Medicaid Services has decided to pay for Provenge for some indications (Chambers & Neumann, 2011). But should such drugs be avoided because of their cost? Cost-effectiveness analysis can be used to indicate how chemotherapy with these drugs compares to chemotherapy without them. If they produce a large number of QALYs, such drugs may well be worth the investment. If they do not, cost-effectiveness analysis can also provide information regarding what one might reasonably pay for the drug. Armed with this information, governments and private insurers can negotiate fair prices with the companies that manufacture the drugs.

Exercises 1 and 2

1. Oseltamivir is a medication that can be used to treat symptomatic infection with the influenza virus (Treanor et al., 2000). (You may have heard about this drug when supplies dried up during the avian influenza scare of 2005–2006.) Doctors know that this drug is effective at shortening both the duration and the severity of influenza symptoms, but the medication is expensive and probably not lifesaving when given to youngsters, so the standard of care for treating influenza among healthy adults is to recommend that the person stay home, get some rest, drink plenty of fluids, and have some soup. The cost of not providing the medication can thus be called providing "supportive care" and consists mostly of lost productivity and leisure time.

    Suppose that the average cost of providing oseltamivir to an individual is $100 and the average cost of providing supportive care to an individual is $10. Suppose further that oseltamivir will result in a gain of 0.5 QALYs per person treated and that providing supportive care alone results in a gain of 0.1 QALYs (relative to nothing at all). What is the incremental cost-effectiveness of providing oseltamivir to persons with influenza relative to providing supportive care alone?

2. Suppose that the average cost of vaccinating an individual is $150 and that vaccination results in the gain of 0.75 QALYs per person relative to supportive care. Using information from Exercise 1, calculate the incremental cost-effectiveness of the influenza vaccination relative to treatment with oseltamivir.

Defining the Comparator

Currently a fraction of the population receives the influenza vaccine at the beginning of the influenza season. If we recommend that everyone receive vaccination at the start of the season, this baseline rate of vaccination might increase only a little. Why? Because only some people would heed the recommendation. Our incremental cost-effectiveness ratio will therefore be very different if we compare a recommendation for vaccination to current practice than if we compare receiving the vaccination to not receiving it at all.

In the first case, we are talking about a slight increase in the rate of vaccination relative to what is now done. In the second, we are making a much more absolute comparison between doing nothing and giving everyone a vaccination. The comparison intervention is sometimes referred to in economics as a **counterfactual**. The counterfactual represents a group that is very similar to the intervention group in every way (including exposure to a disease), but that did not receive the intervention.

When comparing interventions, it is important to know how much more or less costly and effective one intervention is relative to what is considered the current standard of care. **Standard of care** refers to that which is generally agreed on to be the best practice. It is also good to know how an intervention stacks up against the **status quo,** or what is actually done in the real world. (Sadly, the standard of care and the status quo are often quite different in medical practice.)

A cost-effectiveness analysis provides the most useful information when it indicates how much more an intervention costs when compared to current medical practice (Neumann et al., 2016). By including current practice in our analysis, we are calculating a meaningful baseline cost and baseline effectiveness against which we can evaluate the real-world effects of our intervention (e.g., the effect of a recommendation for vaccination relative to the current vaccination rates in the population). In Chapter 1, we call this the incremental cost-effectiveness ratio (ICER).

It is also helpful to include a "no-intervention" or "do-nothing" comparator. A no-intervention comparator will provide to the consumer the cost-effectiveness analysis with a concrete point of reference (Gold et al., 1996; Neumann et al., 2016). If we are to build a league table of incremental cost-effectiveness ratios for setting funding priorities, each ratio must represent the incremental cost-effectiveness of an intervention relative to a common denominator.

Exercise 3

3. What is the policy implication of a research question focusing on vaccinating everyone in the general population?

Finally, we may wish to know how the incremental cost-effectiveness of vaccination or treatment compares to other interventions that might realistically be used to treat or prevent influenza. Although cost-effectiveness analyses should ideally compare all realistic alternatives to the current standard of care, this is not always possible. At a minimum, the reference case suggests that the most realistic alternatives to the current standard of care should be examined (Gold et al., 1996; Neumann et al., 2016).

Interpreting Incremental Changes in Cost and Effectiveness

If one intervention is more effective and less expensive than another and the intervention is ethically and socially acceptable, there should be no question that the more cost-effective intervention is preferable. Usually, though, interventions that are more effective are also more costly than the standard of care. When this occurs, the consumer of the cost-effectiveness analysis must decide whether the added effectiveness is worth the added cost.

If a particular intervention is going to cost us money but will improve health relative to the counterfactual, we have to decide whether we are willing to pay the increased price. Basically, it depends on whether or not we are willing to pay for this added benefit. If the intervention is going to save money and improve health, it is clear that it's worth doing so long as it doesn't produce any ethical dilemmas and is generally acceptable. In this case an intervention is said to be **dominant** (Drummond et al., 2005; Neumann et al., 2016). (See Table 2.3.) If the intervention is more expensive and less effective than the comparator, it is said to be **dominated.** (Whoever said cost-effectiveness researchers were a boring lot?)

An important concept of cost-effectiveness is the **willingness-to-pay**. This is the maximum amount that a patient, payer, or society is willing to invest for a gain in benefit. Let's suppose that we are comparing the cost-effectiveness of oseltamivir to standard care. The incremental cost-effectiveness ratio is $50,000 per QALY gained. If the willingness-to-pay were $100,000 per QALY gained, then oseltamivir would be considered a cost-effective strategy versus standard care. As long as the incremental cost-effectiveness ratio comparing oseltamivir to standard care is less than the willingness-to-pay, then oseltamivir is cost-effective. When the incremental cost-effectiveness ratio is greater than the willingness-to-pay, oseltamivir is not cost-effective.

Table 2.3   Decision Matrix for Various Cost-Effectiveness Scenarios

Cost	Effectiveness	Label	Decision
Lower	Higher	Dominant	Implement
Lower	Lower	Trade-off	Depends on willingness to pay
Higher	Higher	Trade-off	Depends on willingness to pay
Higher	Lower	Dominated	Do not implement

Types of Economic Analysis

Most people are familiar with the term *cost-benefit analysis*, but few can concretely describe the differences between a cost-effectiveness analysis and a cost-benefit analysis. In this section, you will learn how cost-effectiveness analysis differs from the other types of economic analyses and about the related field of burden-of-disease analysis. Other types of economic analyses complement cost-effectiveness analysis because they provide policymakers and clinicians with different types of information.

Cost-Effectiveness and Cost-Utility Analysis

Although the terms are often used interchangeably (as is the case in this book), health economists distinguish **cost-utility analysis** from cost-effectiveness analysis. From a practical standpoint, a cost-utility analysis can be considered a specific type of cost-effectiveness analysis in which some quality-of-life measure is included in the analysis. A **cost-effectiveness analysis** is a more general term for an analysis that compares the relationship between costs and any outcomes. For example, a cost-effectiveness analysis might compare the cost per number of hospitalizations avoided, cost per number of life-years gained, or cost per number of vaccine-preventable illnesses averted. Cost-effectiveness analyses may or may not include a quality measure.

There are also a number of ways in which quality measures, such as HRQL scores, are combined with quantity measures, such as the number of years of life gained by an intervention. Together these measures of quantity and quality fall under the generic category of health-adjusted life-years (HALYs), which include QALYs, disability-adjusted life-years (DALYs), and healthy-years equivalent (HYE).

So what's the difference among these types of HALYs? It mostly comes down to how health-related quality of life is measured. You'll learn about this in Chapter 7.

When to Use Nonreference Case Cost-Effectiveness Analyses

We have already looked at examples of how a health department might conduct a cost-effectiveness analysis on deciding whether to provide contraceptives. Let's revisit that idea using a different example. Suppose a health department was interested in knowing how many vaccine-preventable diseases could be averted if a vaccine campaign were initiated. By definition, the relevant outcome in this analysis would be the cost per illness averted. A full reference case cost-effectiveness analysis would provide information regarding the effect the vaccine would have on the quality of life of everyone vaccinated and would include costs to employers and other segments of society. However, these outcomes are not relevant to the research question posed by the health department in this example. An alternative would be to use a nonreference case analysis, which is generally easier to complete because they require less information, and they may be more useful in circumstances where there is only one relevant outcome.

If a student wishes to conduct a cost-effectiveness analysis that does not incorporate quality-of-life measures using the societal perspective, special considerations must be made. If the outcome of interest is the number of years of life lost to disease instead of QALYs, morbidity costs (pain and suffering) are counted in the numerator. The reason is that the HRQL score that theoretically incorporates a subjective measure of these costs is excluded. Students who wish to conduct this type of analysis can otherwise follow the procedures outlined in this book.

If the study is conducted from a specific perspective or includes other measures in the denominator, such as "hospitalizations averted," the costs included and the end points of the study must be carefully thought through. The following exercises should help guide you.

Exercises 4 and 5

4. You are working for a pharmaceutical company that wishes to examine the cost per illness averted for its new human papilloma virus vaccine from the perspective of an insurance company. What morbidity costs do you include?

5. Your boss at La Mega pharmaceutical corporation wishes to add some pizzazz to marketing for a powerful new antibiotic the company developed. She feels that the public won't understand QALYs, so she asks you to present the results of the study in life-years gained. Will this change how you will calculate the cost-effectiveness of the new antibiotic? How?

Other Measures

The DALY is frequently used for studies in developing countries and might serve as an international standard for cost-effectiveness analyses (Murray & Lopez, 1997). It may also be used to study immigrants to industrialized nations (Muennig, Pallin, Sell, & Chan, 1999). Unfortunately, there are technical problems with this measure that limit its usefulness and render it incompatible with the reference case scenario (Gold et al., 1996; Neumann et al., 2016; Muennig & Gold, 2001). Students wishing to use the DALY may follow all of the procedures outlined in this book and simply use the HRQL scores tabulated for DALYs by Murray and Lopez (the latest values can easily be found online). For technical reasons, DALY scores must be subtracted from 1.0 before they can be used. (See Chapter 8). The HYE falls to the other extreme. Although it is highly regarded from a technical standpoint, it is difficult to use and might not be an appropriate measure for most studies, such as those conducted in developing countries. For these reasons, the use of quality-of-life measures other than the QALY will be discussed only briefly in this book in the context of cost-effectiveness analysis.

Cost-Benefit Analysis

An alternative to cost-effectiveness analysis that economists sometimes favor is cost-benefit analysis. In this type of analysis, a dollar value is placed on both the costs and the effectiveness of an intervention. In a cost-benefit analysis, all costs are included in dollar terms, even the intangible costs associated with the disease. The final outcome is reported as a monetary value. Any intervention associated with cost savings (a net benefit) should be undertaken, and any intervention associated with (excess) costs should not. Why? Because everything is properly accounted for, including the amount people are willing to pay to get rid of the disease. Therefore, any treatment with a cost greater than $0 means that the treatment costs more than it's worth.

Some economists argue that cost-benefit analysis is preferable to cost-effectiveness analysis because it produces a more definitive end point. Moreover, it is universal. Since cost-effectiveness is mostly used in health and education, we often can't compare investments in medical care to other health investments, such as freeway safety improvements, without conducting entirely new analyses. However, a cost-benefit analysis requires that disease and suffering be valued. Some argue that it is so difficult to place a dollar value on human life and human suffering that most cost-benefit analyses will produce inconclusive results (Gyrd-Hansen, 2005).

There is a lot of debate associated with putting a dollar sign on human life. Even though cost-effectiveness analyses separate out costs and QALYs, some believe that we should not estimate costs at all and instead just report QALYs. Currently, this is the position that the Patient-Centered Outcomes Research Institute (PCORI) holds (Neumann & Weinstein, 2010).

The idea that we should just focus on comparative effectiveness rather than costs arose from political rhetoric rather than real scientific or ethical dilemmas. Kevin McCarthy, a Republican, stated that cost-effectiveness "may start us down a treacherous path toward government-encouraged euthanasia." Normally, we cite quoted text, but this statement has since been removed from the Senator's website. This statement, along with notions that a government effort to formally evaluate the cost-effectiveness of medical treatments was tantamount to forming "death panels" that would kill grandmothers did get policy traction. It was part of the rhetoric that was probably intended only as a political weapon, but turned into a policy for PCORI. Most people recognize that cost-effectiveness is a tool for saving lives by allocating resources where they are needed, rather than taking lives by denying treatments.

However, there is a genuine scientific problem with cost-benefit analyses as well. That is that they have never been standardized in the same way that cost-effectiveness analyses have. Recall that health is one of the most difficult things to measure in a cost-effectiveness analysis. If we are going to move collectively toward cost-benefit analysis for simplicity of policy-making, that is great. But the QALY is our best available standard measure of health and longevity. So, a change from complicated cost-effectiveness analyses to simple cost-benefit analysis would require that we place a dollar value on QALYs and that we estimate costs using a set of standards similar to those of the Panel.

Still, most non-health policies are evaluated in terms of cost-benefit analysis. As mentioned earlier, all policies are health policies. Because all policies have the potential to impact human health and longevity, we really need to have a standardized way of accounting across all potential social investments that a government might make. At present, this does not exist.

FOR EXAMPLE: YOUR MONEY OR YOUR LIFE

To convert a cost-effectiveness analysis into a cost-benefit analysis, some researchers have proposed merely placing a monetary value on QALYs and adding this value to the numerator costs of a cost-effectiveness ratio. While many feel that QALYs cannot be valued, there is no shortage of researchers willing to try. In a meta-analysis of the literature to the year 2000, Hirth and colleagues (2000) found that the 1997 valuation of QALYs fell between $25,000 and $428,000 depending on the economic method used to valuate them (Hirth, Chernew, Miller, Fendrick, & Weissert, 2000). (This amounts to $37,000 and $626,000 in constant 2015 U.S. dollars.) Alternatively, Lee and colleagues (Lee, Chertow, & Zenios, 2009) estimated that the value of a statistical year of life using dialysis as a benchmark was $129,000 per QALY in 2003 U.S. dollars, which translates to $189,000 per QALY in 2015 U.S. dollars (adjusted for inflation). Another approach is to monetize statistical lives in terms of value of statistical life year (VSLY), which captures the expected number of life-years remaining for the average person (Copeland, 2010). The Food and Drug Administration (FDA) has used VSLY values ranging from $100,000 to $500,000 per life-year (Robinson, 2007). There are many ways to monetize life; however, it is important that any research in cost-benefit analysis provide justification for the approach used. Comparison with other published literature is a good way to provide credibility for your approach.

Cost-Minimization Analysis

Cost-minimization analysis is useful in cases when the outcome of two interventions is similar but the costs are different (Drummond et al., 2005). For example, patients with bacterial endocarditis (an infection of the heart) often require long-term treatment with intravenous antibiotics. Traditionally, patients with endocarditis were hospitalized while they received therapy. Today antibiotics are sometimes administered at home, potentially reducing the costs associated with this treatment. Because both therapies are equally effective, the only relevant medical issue in evaluating each treatment is the overall cost of administering the treatment at home versus at the hospital. In this situation, a cost-minimization analysis can be used to determine the least costly treatment. Because cost-minimization analysis is easier to conduct than full cost-effectiveness analysis, it should be used whenever two or more interventions of equal effectiveness are being compared.

Burden-of-Disease Analysis

Burden-of-disease analyses do not incorporate information on the cost of a disease. Rather, they are used to determine which diseases are responsible for the most morbidity and mortality within a country and are sometimes used by governments or nongovernmental organizations to allocate health resources.

Traditionally, the burden of a disease was measured by the number of years of life lost to that particular disease. Using that definition, diseases with high mortality rates, such as malaria and tuberculosis, were thought to be the most significant health problems in the world. More recently, the World Health Organization, the World Bank, and Harvard University redefined burden-of-disease analyses by incorporating a measure of quality of life, the disability-adjusted life-year (DALY), into their definition (Murray & Lopez, 1997). Once quality of life was included, depression, which previously ranked near the bottom of the list, moved up to become one of the world's most significant health problems.

The DALY is a controversial but methodologically solid measure. It's solid because it uses a standard life expectancy value and straightforward calculations that can be fairly and easily applied across countries. It is controversial because of the way HRQL is measured.

Because people of different nationalities and cultures have different perceptions of human suffering and quality of life, the limitations in generating the health-related quality of life scores are exaggerated when conducting cross-national comparisons. To get around this limitation and simplify the collection of HRQL scores, quality of life is measured using the input of experts rather than people residing in a specific culture (Murray & Lopez, 1997). For reasons that will be discussed in Chapter 7, this renders the DALY incompatible with the reference case scenario of a cost-effectiveness analysis (Gold et al., 1996; Neumann et al., 2016).

One promising alternative to the DALY's HRQL component is the EuroQol, a QALY-compatible measure that has been applied to a growing number of nations (EuroQol Group, 1990; Rabin & de Charro, 2001). For instance, the EuroQol has been included in the Medical Expenditure Panel Survey in the United States, so the burden of disease can be calculated for just about any demographic group, any illness, and many risk factors (Muennig, Franks, Jia, Lubetkin, & Gold, 2005).

Other alternatives include the Health Utility Index (HUI) (Furlong, Feeny, Torrance, & Barr, 2001) and the Assessment of Quality of Life (AQoL) (Hawthorne, Richardson, & Osborne, 1999). Both have been used to generate utility scores for calculations of QALYs.

Summary

This chapter focused on the heart of the cost-effectiveness analysis—the incremental cost-effectiveness ratio (ICER). The ICER is simply the change in costs between two courses of action divided by the health outcomes associated with those actions. In most cost-effectiveness analyses, these outcomes will be measured in quality-adjusted life-years (QALYs). You also learned the basics of how health-related quality of life (HRQL) is captured and how costs are captured. Critically, those costs associated with pain and suffering are included in the HRQL score. Because the HRQL score is used to calculate QALYs, it is included in the denominator of the ICER. Most everything else costwise is included in the numerator.

You learned that there are several perspectives that you can use when calculating the ICER. Perspectives influence the types of costs used in a cost-effectiveness analysis. For example, direct medical costs are used to capture the medical-related costs from the perspective of someone paying for medical care, such as an insurance company. If you are concerned with the costs that everyone in society pays, then costs due to loss in worker productivity should also be included. Intangible costs such as pain are difficult to measure, but some can be captured within the QALY. Always start off by defining your perspective, and you will be able to easily determine what kinds of cost are needed.

In this chapter, you were also introduced to several types of economic analysis, such as cost-benefit analysis, cost-effectiveness analysis, cost-utility analysis, cost-minimization analysis, and burden-of-disease analysis. You can use these tools to answer your economic question of interest. However, in order for you to conclude that a new intervention is cost-effective compared to standard care, you will need to calculate the incremental cost-effectiveness ratio and see if it is below the willingness to pay.

Further Readings

We encourage students interested in the theoretical framework of cost-effectiveness analysis to read Garber and Phelps's paper (Garber & Phelps, 1997) and Chapter 7 by Meltzer and Smith from the *Handbook of Health Economics*, Volume 2 (Meltzer & Smith, 2012). Discussions about the limitations of the theoretical framework have been provided by Johannesson and Meltzer (Johannesson & Meltzer, 1998), Weinstein and Manning (Weinstein & Manning Jr., 1997), Johannesson (Johannesson, 1995), and Johannesson and Weinstein (Johannesson & Weinstein, 1993). Students who are interested in learning more about welfarism and extra-welfarism should read Brouwer, Culyer, van Exel, and Rutten (Brouwer, Culyer, van Exel, & Rutten, 2008), Birch and Donaldson (Birch & Donaldson, 2003), and Gyrd-Hansen (Gyrd-Hansen, 2005).

Students interested in the development and validation of HRQL instruments should read *Reliability and Validity of Data Sources for Outcomes Research and Disease and Health Management Programs,* edited by Dominick Esposito (Esposito, 2013).

For an updated discussion on the future of QALY in the United States, interested students should read Peter Neumann and Dan Greenberg's article in *Health Affairs,* "Is the United States Ready for QALYs?" (Neumann & Greenberg, 2009).

Students interested in federal guidance on monetizing life should read Copeland's report to the Congressional Research Service entitled "How Agencies Monetize 'Statistical Lives' Expected to Be Saved by Regulations" (Copeland, 2010).

References

Birch, S., and C. Donaldson. (2003). Valuing the Benefits and Costs of Health Care Programmes: Where's the "Extra" in Extra-Welfarism? *Social Science & Medicine,* 56(5): 1121–1133.

Brouwer, W. B. F., A. J. Culyer, N. J. A. van Exel, and F. F. H. Rutten. (2008). Welfarism vs. Extra-Welfarism. *Journal of Health Economics* 27(2): 325–338. http://doi.org/10.1016/j.jhealeco.2007.07.003.

Chambers, J. D., and P. J. Neumann. (2011). Listening to Provenge—What a Costly Cancer Treatment Says About Future Medicare Policy. *New England Journal of Medicine* 364(18): 1687–1689. http://doi.org/10.1056/NEJMp1103057.

Copeland, C. W. (2010). How Agencies Monetize "Statistical Lives" Expected to Be Saved by Regulations, No. 7-5700, p. 44. Washington, DC: Congressional Research Services. Retrieved from www.crs.gov.

Drummond, M. F., M. J. Sculpher, G. W. Torrance, B. J. O'Brien, and G. L. Stoddart. (2005). *Methods for the Economic Evaluation of Health Care Programmes,* 3rd ed. New York: Oxford University Press.

Esposito, D, ed. (2013). *Reliability and Validity of Data Sources for Outcomes Research & Disease and Health Management Programs.* Lawrenceville, NJ: ISPOR.

EuroQol Group. (1990). EuroQol—A New Facility for the Measurement of Health-Related Quality of Life. *Health Policy* (Amsterdam, Netherlands) 16(3): 199–208.

Furlong, W. J., D. H. Feeny, G. W. Torrance, and R. D. Barr. (2001). The Health Utilities Index (HUI) System for Assessing Health-Related Quality of Life in Clinical Studies. *Annals of Medicine* 33(5): 375–384.

Garber, A. M., and C. E. Phelps. (1997). Economic Foundations of Cost-Effectiveness Analysis. *Journal of Health Economics* 16(1): 1–31.

Gold, M. R., and P. Muennig. (2002). Measure-Dependent Variation in Burden of Disease Estimates: Implications for Policy. *Medical Care* 40(3): 260–266.

Gold, M. R., J. E. Siegel, L. B. Russell, and M. C. Weinstein. (1996). *Cost-Effectiveness in Health and Medicine.* New York: Oxford University Press.

Gyrd-Hansen, D. (2005). Willingness to Pay for a QALY: Theoretical and Method-ological Issues. *PharmacoEconomics* 23(5): 423–432.

Hawthorne, G., J. Richardson, and R. Osborne. (1999). The Assessment of Quality of Life (AQoL) Instrument: A Psychometric Measure of Health-Related Quality of Life. *Quality of Life Research* 8(3): 209–224.

Hirth, R. A., M. E. Chernew, E. Miller, A. M. Fendrick, W. G. Weissert. (2000). Willingness to Pay for a Quality-Adjusted Life Year: In Search of a Standard. *Medical Decision Making* 20(3): 332–342.

Johannesson, M. (1995). On the Estimation of Cost-Effectiveness Ratios. *Health Policy* 31(3): 225–229. http://doi.org/10.1016/0168-8510(95)98130-T.

Johannesson, M., and D. Meltzer. (1998). Editorial: Some Reflections on Cost-Effectiveness Analysis. *Health Economics* 7(1): 1–7. http://doi.org/10.1002/(SICI)1099-1050(199802)7:1<1::AID-HEC327>3.0.CO;2-U.

Johannesson, M., and M. C. Weinstein. (1993). On the Decision Rules of Cost-Effectiveness Analysis. *Journal of Health Economics* 12(4): 459–467. http://doi.org/10.1016/0167-6296(93)90005-Y.

Lee, C. P., G. M. Chertow, and S. A. Zenios. (2009). An Empiric Estimate of the Value of Life: Updating the Renal Dialysis Cost-Effectiveness Standard. *Value in Health* 12(1): 80–87. http://doi.org/10.1111/j.1524-4733.2008.00401.x.

Meltzer, D. O., and P. C. Smith. (2012). Theoretical Issues Relevant to the Economic Evaluation of Health Technologies. In *Handbook of Health Economics,* vol. 2, pp. 434–469. Waltham, MA: Elsevier B.V.

Muennig, P., P. Franks, H. Jia, E. Lubetkin, and M. R. Gold. (2005). The Income-Associated Burden of Disease in the United States. *Social Science & Medicine,* 61(9): 2018–2026. http://doi.org/10.1016/j.socscimed.2005.04.005.

Muennig, P., and M. R. Gold. (2001). Using the Years-of-Healthy-Life Measure to Calculate QALYs. *American Journal of Preventive Medicine* 20(1): 35–39.

Muennig, P., D. Pallin, R. L. Sell, and M. S. Chans. (1999). The Cost Effectiveness of Strategies for the Treatment of Intestinal Parasites in Immigrants. *New England Journal of Medicine* 340(10): 773–779. http://doi.org/10.1056/NEJM199903113401006.

Murray, C. J. L., and A. D. Lopez. (1997). Global Mortality, Disability, and the Contribution of Risk Factors: Global Burden of Disease Study. *Lancet* 349(9063): 1436–1442. http://doi.org/10.1016/S0140-6736(96)07495-8.

Neumann, P. J., and D. Greenberg. (2009). Is the United States Ready for QALYs? *Health Affairs* (Project Hope) 28(5): 1366–1371. http://doi.org/10.1377/hlthaff.28.5.1366.

Neumann, P. J., G. D. Sanders, L. B. Russell, J. E. Siegel, and T. G. Ganiats. (2016). *Cost-Effectiveness in Health and Medicine.* New York: Oxford University Press.

Neumann, P. J., and M. C. Weinstein. (2010). Legislating Against Use of Cost-Effectiveness Information. *New England Journal of Medicine* 363(16): 1495–1497. http://doi.org/10.1056/NEJMp1007168.

Rabin, R., and F. de Charro. (2001). EQ-5D: A Measure of Health Status from the EuroQol Group. *Annals of Medicine* 33(5): 337–343.

Robinson, L. A. (2007). How US Government Agencies Value Mortality Risk Reductions. *Review of Environmental Economics and Policy* 1(2): 283–299. http://doi.org/10.1093/reep/rem018.

Simoens, S. (2012). Pharmaco-Economic Aspects of Sipuleucel-T. *Human Vaccines & Immunotherapeutics* 8(4): 506–508. http://doi.org/10.4161/hv.18334.

Tengs, T. O., M. E. Adams, J. S. Pliskin, D. G. Safran, J. E. Siegel, M. C. Weinstein, and J. D. Graham. (1995). Five-Hundred Life-Saving Interventions and Their Cost-Effectiveness. *Risk Analysis* 15(3): 369–390.

Treanor, J. J., F. G. Hayden, P. S. Vrooman, R. Barbarash, R. Bettis, D. Riff, . . . R. G. Mills. (2000). Efficacy and Safety of the Oral Neuraminidase Inhibitor Oseltamivir in Treating Acute Influenza: A Randomized Controlled Trial. US Oral Neuraminidase Study Group. *Journal of the American Medical Association* 283(8): 1016–1024.

Von Neumann, J., and O. Morgenstern. (1953). *Theory of Games and Economic Behavior.* Princeton, NJ: Princeton University Press.

Weinstein, M. C., and W. G. Manning Jr. (1997). Theoretical Issues in Cost-Effectiveness Analysis. *Journal of Health Economics* 16(1): 121–128. http://doi.org/10.1016/S0167-6296(96)00511-5.

DEVELOPING A RESEARCH PROJECT

Overview

This chapter explains how to develop a cost-effectiveness research project. We explore some of the key things to think about as you develop your question, and then go into how to sketch out your model so that you have some idea of what data you'll need to collect.

Eight Steps to a Perfect Research Project

Cost-effectiveness analyses are conducted using a series of intuitive methodological steps, many of which may be generalized to any scientific research project:

1. Think through your research question.
2. Sketch out the analysis.
3. Collect data for your model.
4. Adjust your data.
5. Build your model.
6. Run and test the model.
7. Conduct a sensitivity analysis.
8. Write it up.
9. Have a cup of tea.

In this book, you'll walk through these steps while looking at applied sample cost-effectiveness analyses. We'll periodically remind you where you are with a project map outlining these eight steps.

LEARNING OBJECTIVES

- Identify the steps to a perfect research project.
- Develop a research question by examining its anatomy.
- Develop a process for systematically going through a checklist for a cost-effectiveness analysis.
- Construct a sketch of a simple event pathway model.
- Identify what data will be needed for a cost-effectiveness model.

Let us briefly review each step:

1. *Think through your research question.* A research question is a well-defined statement about your hypothesis on a particular subject or topic. To test your hypothesis, you must clearly indicate which interventions you will be comparing, which subjects you plan to include, which perspective you will use, and how your analysis will be conducted.

2. *Sketch out the analysis.* In designing a cost-effectiveness analysis, a researcher must thoroughly review the background information on the disease and health interventions under study (often using clinical practice guidelines) and then chart the different twists and turns a disease might take when different health interventions are applied. This usually requires sketching out a model on paper.

3. *Collect data for your model.* Data relevant to your analysis may come from published studies, electronic databases, or other sources, such as medical experts. In any cost-effectiveness analysis, you will need to be transparent with your data source. Using the most recently available data will build credibility for your work. However, if antiquated data were collected in a way that is more sound, the researcher has to strike a balance between being up to date and being valid.

4. *Adjust your data.* Few data will be in a form ready for use in your analysis. For instance, some students will be surprised to learn that the amount providers charge for their services is much higher than the amount the providers are actually paid. Therefore, cost data often need to be adjusted to better reflect real-world costs. Similarly, both cost and probability data often need to be adjusted in such a way that they better reflect the demographic profile of your study cohort. Combining data can be tricky and will require you to use weights to properly distribute the influence from independent study results (e.g., estimating the weighted-average effect).

5. *Build your decision analysis model.* This model sometimes takes the form of a graphical representation of how your analysis will unfold. It indicates the chances that subjects will see a doctor, receive a laboratory test, and so forth. It also includes the costs associated with each of these events. When run, it melds this information and produces an incremental cost-effectiveness ratio. Fortunately, it is now possible to easily build decision analysis models using basic and intuitive software packages.

6. *Run and test your decision analysis model.* Before you can be confident that the information your model provides you is accurate, you will need to run some tests. Fortunately, these are usually quite easy to run.

7. *Conduct a sensitivity analysis.* No data are entirely free from error. A **sensitivity analysis** will evaluate how the error in your data might affect the cost or effectiveness of each of the medical interventions you are studying.

8. *Prepare the study results for publication or presentation.* Once you have finished your study, you will need to present it in a way that anyone can understand. Adopting standard publication formats helps you achieve this goal (and get published).

Developing a Research Question

This section looks at the ins and outs of developing a research question for cost-effectiveness analyses. One of the biggest mistakes beginning researchers make is to think of the comparison they wish to make as a complete research question. This can lead to a lot of unnecessary work. By thinking hard about the characteristics of the groups she or he is comparing, for instance, a beginning researcher will avoid collecting the wrong types of data. The section ends with a research checklist to ensure you have proper footing before embarking on a project.

Anatomy of a Research Question

Every research question in cost-effectiveness analysis should have four key components: (1) information about the population you are studying, (2) a clear description of the interventions being compared, (3) the perspective of the study, and (4) a definition of the disease you are studying. When broken down into these basic components, the research question naturally presents itself to both the reader and the researcher.

Defining the Population

Cost-effectiveness analyses usually analyze study outcomes for a hypothetical cohort, or a cohort of defined characteristics using multiple sources of data. Suppose we want to know whether it is a good idea to vaccinate all healthy adults against influenza or forgo vaccination in this population altogether. We must first think through what we mean by "healthy." The influenza vaccine is currently recommended for people with chronic lung disease, diabetes, and heart disease, among other conditions (Centers for Disease Control and Prevention, 2013). Although it may sound crazy, we would still call someone with two broken legs "healthy" as long as he or she didn't have any of the conditions for which vaccination is recommended.

We should also think of the usual demographic characteristics of the population to which we will recommend the vaccine. The most important consideration is age. In this case, we are shooting for people who are over the age of fifteen but under the age of sixty-five. We should also consider whether to include children. Other considerations are income (poor populations are more likely to have most diseases) and gender (some diseases are more common in one gender than the other). All of the studies that you find in the literature should come close to matching the demographic profile of the cohort you are defining in your analysis. If this is not possible, then certain assumptions will need to be made about the generalizability to the target population.

Defining the Interventions Under Study

Some students might be thinking, "If healthy adults are already getting vaccinated, what do we mean when we say that we recommend vaccination?" If you are one of these students, you are on your way to becoming a great research scientist. Two critical questions naturally arise from this: (1) Can we reasonably vaccinate everyone in the real world? (2) If not, how many more people are we going to vaccinate above and beyond the number who are now getting vaccinated?

We could "recommend" vaccination for healthy adults, but in most countries this might lead to only a slight increase in current rates of vaccination. Another alternative is to require influenza vaccinations in schools, the workplace, and doctors' offices. This might push the vaccination rates higher still. Alternatively, we could simply evaluate the effect of vaccinating everyone. Although it isn't reasonable to expect that this would really happen in a democracy, it is conceivable that if enough people were vaccinated, transmission of the virus would grind to a halt. This phenomenon, known as "herd immunity," occurs once a critical tipping point of vaccination is reached—say, 70 percent of the healthy adult population in the United States (Department of Health and Human Services, 2015).

The next question that naturally arises is: Relative to what? We might compare vaccinating everyone to the current baseline rates of vaccination in the population, or we might compare vaccinating everyone to no vaccination.

For the comparators in which some or all subjects go without a vaccine, we must consider what treatment they do get. Unvaccinated people usually get chicken soup when they get the flu. (Some students might choose tofu soup and echinacea.) They also send their loved ones out to the drugstore to buy some medicine that might make them feel better but won't make them recover any faster.

Let's consider one more example. Suppose that you have been asked to evaluate a new antibiotic against community-acquired pneumonia (as opposed to more dangerous forms of pneumonia one might contract in the hospital). You might compare it against not giving an antibiotic at all, against the most commonly used antibiotic, against the preferred antibiotic (which, sadly, is not the most commonly used), or against "usual care."

Recall that "usual care" or "current practice" implies that interventions are being compared to a mixture of medical interventions that reflect the current practice standards (Gold, Siegel, Russell, & Weinstein, 1996; Neumann, Sanders, Russell, Siegel, & Ganiats, 2016). Therefore, usual care might include some combination of treatments (including inappropriate treatments) that we see in everyday medical practice. If we compare the new antibiotic to usual care, we may be deceiving the consumer of your study. Why? Because "usual care" for pneumonia includes misdiagnoses, the use of inappropriate or expensive medications, or other modalities that are either unnecessarily expensive or ineffective. Such a comparator will make the new antibiotic seem unduly effective since you are comparing it to something suboptimal.

Nevertheless, usual care can be a useful comparator in many cases. For instance, with usual care as the comparator, we can provide policymakers with concrete information about the cost-effectiveness of a campaign that is expected to increase influenza vaccination by 10 percent over the current (usual care) baseline.

Finally, remember that any reference case cost-effectiveness analysis should include a do-nothing comparator that compares the intervention to the natural history of disease (Gold et al., 1996; Neumann et al., 2016). This allows interventions to be stacked up against one another in a league table.

Exercise 1

1. You are a policymaker in the Netherlands and wish to know whether it would be a good idea to add a new antibiotic to the drug formulary for community-acquired pneumonia. Currently clinicians use a variety of antibiotics to treat community-acquired pneumonia, but you have the power to change practice. Do you want to know how the new drug compares against the variety of drugs currently prescribed or against what is currently thought to be the best antibiotic?

Defining the Disease You Are Studying

Usually, but not always, this part is straightforward. For instance, influenza-like illness is a cluster of diseases that produce symptoms similar to those people have when they are infected with the influenza virus. These symptoms may be induced by the virus itself or by a number of other respiratory tract viruses or bacteria. The World Health Organization defines influenza-like illness as the presence of fever (over 100°F) plus a sore throat or cough (Hirve et al., 2012). Basically, when we have a cold, feel especially lousy, and have a fever, we say we have the "flu." Alternatively, you might use a stricter definition and call the disease "influenza" only when the presence of the virus has been confirmed by a laboratory test.

Our research question might take the form: "Among healthy adults, should we prevent the infection with vaccination, treat flu infections when they arise, or provide supportive care alone?" It sounds pretty good, but there are still a number of things to consider before we continue.

Research Checklist

When you cook lasagna, you know roughly what you'll need to buy at the grocery store, but if you go without a shopping list, you are bound to forget something important. The same is true with scientific research. Therefore, I provide a sample shopping list for any cost-effectiveness research project.

Most books on cost-effectiveness analysis have a checklist against which you can evaluate your research question or, conversely, the research project of others (Drummond, Sculpher, Torrance, O'Brien, & Stoddart, 2005; Gold et al., 1996; Neumann et al., 2016; Haddix, Teutsch, Shaffer, & Dunet, 1996). More recently, the International Society for Pharmacoeconomics and Outcomes Research (ISPOR) and the Society for Medical Decision Making (SMDM) developed a good research practice task force for using models in decision sciences (Caro, Briggs, Siebert, Kuntz, & ISPOR-SMDM Modeling Good Research Practices Task Force, 2012). We've compiled some of the more important points and added a few of our own.

Have I Included All of the Important Alternatives?

When considering treatment options, we could include the anti-influenza medications in our analysis, such as oseltamivir. We could compare different doses of oseltamivir (Dixit et al., 2014) or include the inhaled cousin of oseltamivir, called zanamivir (Monto, Robinson, Herlocher, Hinson, Elliott, & Crisp, 1999).

In an ideal situation, all comparisons for which uncertainty exists would be included in a cost-effectiveness analysis. The reference case scenario recommends that the standard of care be included as a comparator (Gold et al., 1996; Neumann et al., 2016). It also suggests that the next best alternative to the intervention under study and a no-intervention strategy be included.

Sometimes, you may not know what alternatives are available (or which ones are appropriate). But you can consult with experts to find out what's considered the status quo—the alternative that is most often used.

THE NATIONAL INSTITUTE OF HEALTH AND CLINICAL EXCELLENCE (NICE)

The United Kingdom's National Institute of Health and Clinical Excellence (NICE) has a formal scoping process that identifies which technologies they will evaluate. (Yes, the British do have a good sense of humor.) This scoping process helps them define the intervention and alternative comparators that are currently in use for the given treatment. It also helps identify what alternatives to include based on feedback from stakeholders such as practitioners and experts in the field. You may not need to be this formal when conducting your own research, but it would be good to have some method for getting feedback from experts on your choice of an alternative comparator.

Where Will the Intervention Take Place?

It is sometimes important to consider the place where a patient will receive the interventions you are studying. For example, if patients are to go to their doctor specifically for a vaccination, the cost of vaccination will be higher than if patients are vaccinated at their workplace. Not only are doctors' offices expensive places to get vaccinated, but you have to drive to get there. Moreover, the total time the recipient spends receiving the vaccine is much higher if he or she has to go to a doctor's office. Not only does one have to drive to get there, but there is also usually a wait. As we say, "Time is money." Therefore, the strategy of vaccinating in the workplace is likely going to cost less than making a special trip to the doctor for the vaccination.

You should also consider the country where the intervention takes place. In the United States, access to information may be easier compared to other developing countries. In addition, some countries may not have the resources or infrastructure to acquire and administer any given treatment you are studying. For instance, the cost of administering a vaccine can be much greater in sub-Saharan Africa, where infrastructure such as roads and refrigeration are scarce. In other cases, the health system's purchasing power may determine "costs." For instance, the average cost for etanercept (brand name Enbrel) in 2013, which is used for rheumatoid arthritis, ranged between $1,017 in Switzerland and $2,225 in the United States; the average cost for an MRI ranged between $138 in Switzerland and $1,145 in the United States (International Federation of Health Plans, 2013). Therefore, it is important to include in your research question the country (and, possibly, the state) in which the intervention takes place.

Are Different Levels of Treatment or Different Screening Intervals Relevant?

Preventive interventions, such as screening mammography, must often be repeated throughout the patient's lifetime. But how frequently should this occur? If screening tests are performed frequently, the cost of screening will increase, but the chances of catching the disease early will also increase. Therefore, analyses of screening interventions should usually contain a subanalysis examining the cost of screening at different frequencies (Gold et al., 1996; Neumann et al., 2016). For instance, different institutions or agencies produce very different screening recommendations depending on how conservative or generous they are with their model inputs. These decisions are sometimes more political than scientific. The American Cancer Society recommends annual screening mammography for females who are 40 years and older (Smith et al., 2014). To make matters more complex, the U.S. Prevention Services Task Force recommends that females who are 50 to 74 years old receive biennial screening mammography, but females between 40 and 49 years old should receive screening depending on their circumstances and values (U.S. Preventive Services Task Force, 2009).

If we dig through the USPSTF data (which probably come closest to "state-of-the-art"), we see that more frequent screening will detect more cancer (a major goal of the American Cancer Society). But, as pointed out in Chapter 1, it can also harm women in other ways. More frequent screening could therefore conceivably lead to *higher* overall morbidity and mortality even as more cancer is detected.

What Type of Study Is Appropriate?

This book focuses only on cost-effectiveness analyses with a strong emphasis on cost-utility analysis (because this is the subtype of cost-effectiveness analysis recommended by the Panel on Cost-Effectiveness in Health and Medicine). Nevertheless, keep in mind other ways of evaluating health interventions, such as a cost-benefit analysis (Drummond et al., 2005; Gold et al., 1996; Neumann et al., 2016; Haddix et al., 1996). We discussed some other economic analyses (e.g., cost-minimization analysis and burden-of-disease analysis) in Chapter 2.

If the study is intended for an internal review within a company or government agency but not for publication, then there is less need for a reference case analysis. This relates to the next point: for whom you conduct the study determines how you conduct the study.

For Whom Will I Conduct the Study?

The audience for the study determines which costs and outcomes are to be included. For example, when conducting a cost-effectiveness analysis, an insurance company may be concerned only with how much money it will have to spend and how much it might save on a treatment or preventive intervention. It is unlikely that the insurance company will be very interested in whether a patient has to spend money on gas or take a taxi to get to the hospital for a preventive intervention. The audience of the study therefore also determines the perspective of the analysis (Drummond et al., 2005; Gold et al., 1996; Neumann et al., 2016; Haddix et al., 1996). (Remember that the reference case always uses the societal perspective.)

Recall that in Chapter 2 we discussed some of the potential perspectives you can have: patient, payer, provider, and societal. Societal, by far, is the most comprehensive and is one of recommended by the U.S. Panel on Cost-Effectiveness (Gold et al., 1996; Neumann et al., 2016). However, there are times when this is not appropriate, such as when evaluating a program for a government or an agency that bears costs in different ways from society as a whole. Therefore, it is up to the researcher to identify the perspective up front so that the readers have a clear understanding of the goals of the study.

Recall that the types of costs and outcomes you will want to collect will strongly depend on the perspective you choose. For instance, if a societal perspective is chosen, then direct and indirect costs will need to be determined, and QALYs will need to be estimated from the healthy adult population who receive and do not receive influenza vaccination; whereas, a cost-effectiveness analysis that uses the payer perspective may only be interested in direct medical costs such as the number of hospitalizations prevented because these are costly resources used up that the insurance company pays for. (They don't really pay for lost productivity or transportation costs, for instance.) Last, a study performed using the patient perspective may collect data on out-of-pocket costs and changes in health-related quality of life (HRQL) the patient may experience as a result of being ill or incapacitated. This is reemphasized here because students have a difficult time wrapping their heads around which costs are relevant to include.

Exercise 2

2. Suppose you were going to design a cost-effectiveness analysis on implementing an influenza vaccination program from the payer's perspective. List some of the direct and indirect costs relevant for this type of audience. How different would your answer be if this was from the societal perspective?

How Far into the Future Do I Need to Capture Outcomes?

The **analytical horizon** (or **time horizon**) is the period over which all costs and outcomes are considered (Haddix et al., 1996). In the case of influenza, a person is ill for a short period of time and then recovers. In the case of adult-onset diabetes, the disease usually arises in middle age and sticks around until death. Therefore, the analytical horizon of the analysis might be the mean age of onset of death. The time horizon should be long enough to capture relevant costs and outcomes, but it should also be short enough not to run indefinitely. For example, a cost-effectiveness analysis for an acute infection should have a time horizon that covers approximately 7 to 14 days (depending on the infection). If the time horizon is a year, you run the risk of capturing other costs and outcomes unrelated to the actual disease.

What Do I Include, and What Do I Ignore?

Let's assume for a moment that vaccination occasionally saves the life of a healthy adult. Thirty-year-old people who die today from influenza might have otherwise lived to be seventy-five, so we might count each year of future life lost in the denominator of our cost-effectiveness ratio. However, these deaths are so rare that they will hardly put a dent in the life expectancy of all healthy adults in our hypothetical cohort.

If you don't count these deaths, the analytical horizon is about 5 to 10 days (the duration of the flu). Excluding deaths therefore greatly simplifies the analysis. If you do count these deaths, you have to account for future years of life lost, and the analytical horizon is human life expectancy.

When a cost makes a dent in the incremental cost-effectiveness ratio, it is said to be "relevant." There is no point in including model inputs that are not likely to make a difference in the incremental cost-effectiveness of a given strategy, but determining what is relevant or not can be challenging.

Ultimately deciding what to include and what to exclude should be part of the agenda of your research team. Model inputs should never be excluded simply because they are difficult or impossible to capture, however (Gold et al., 1996; Neumann et al., 2016). Instead, some attempt at deriving a rough estimate is necessary.

It's best to start off with a conceptual model by drawing it out and getting expert opinions to help. This will guide you in determining the data you'll need to effectively perform a cost-effectiveness analysis. In addition, you'll have face validity because you consulted with experts in the field that will support your model.

Are There Enough Data to Answer My Question?

Some cost-effectiveness analysis questions are not possible to answer because the data are unavailable. Cost-effectiveness analyses may use data from electronic databases, the medical literature, ongoing studies, or even expert opinion. When one key data element is missing, it is possible to conduct a **threshold analysis**. A threshold analysis tells how the results would differ under various guesses surrounding the value of a given parameter. If we did not know how many people become infected with influenza each fall, a threshold analysis would reveal the incidence rate at which vaccination would be the more cost-effective option (Gold et al., 1996; Neumann et al., 2016).

Review

Let's imagine that we have settled on a cost-effectiveness analysis comparing vaccination supportive care. When the time comes for your analysis, you'll scratch similar pertinent information down on a handy piece of paper. It will become crumpled and coffee stained as the months go by but will serve as your invaluable research partner over the duration of your analysis. Let's briefly examine what this might look like:

Interventions

- Vaccination required by schools and employers and administered at the worksite or school.

- Assume that vaccine will reduce the incidence of influenza in the general population by 30 percent.

Comparator

- Supportive care is over-the-counter medications plus or minus chicken (or tofu) soup and rest.

Population

- Healthy persons (no chronic lung disease, heart disease, or diabetes) ages 15 to 65 residing in the United States. Also consider secondary transmission to elderly people at risk of complications from influenza (who might benefit from the lower incidence of infection among healthy adults).

Checklist

- All important interventions included? We will not consider oral antiviral medications or laboratory testing for influenza infection.

- Clinical setting? Office, schools, routine medical visits.

- Levels of intervention?

- Vaccination: Mandatory vaccination rather than a recommendation for all employees and schoolchildren.

- Type of study? Reference case cost-effectiveness analysis.

- For whom? Policymakers.

- Analytical horizon? Life expectancy of cohort.

- What to ignore? Include all possible inputs.

- Are there enough data to answer our question? Yes; however, changes in person-to-person transmission will be difficult to estimate.

Designing Your Analysis

Now you have your research question down. The research question is probably the hardest part of an analysis. But once you know what you are about to tackle, it becomes easy to plan your course of attack.

Before you can do that, though, you will need to learn just about all there is to know about the disease. For instance, in the influenza research question, we would need to know the specifics of how influenza is transmitted, how vaccination interrupts transmission of the virus, what the normal course of an infection is, and all of the potential complications of influenza. We will also need information on each of the interventions we are evaluating to prevent or treat it.

Understanding the disease requires reading medical textbooks and review articles. **Clinical practice guidelines** are an important source of information. These guidelines provide perspective on the optimal way to manage a disease in the clinical setting. They are especially helpful because they often contain flowcharts that can be used for inspiration in designing a decision analysis model. One good place to obtain clinical practice guidelines is through the Agency for Health Research and Quality (available at http://www.ahrq.gov). Clinical practice guidelines can also sometimes be downloaded from medical societies such as the American Cancer Society or using a search engine.

Once you have the clinical practice guidelines and other information about the disease in hand, you can chart out the course of the disease when different interventions are applied.

PROJECT MAP

1. Think through your research question.

2. *Sketch out the analysis.*

3. Collect data for your model.

4. Adjust your data.

5. Build your model.

6. Run and test the model.

7. Conduct a sensitivity analysis.

8. Write it up.

The information you'll need to conduct your analysis will probably include incidence rates, mortality data, and costs. These data are obtained from the medical literature, electronic datasets, and other sources. But how do you know exactly what you'll need and where to start? Most people think visually. Therefore, sketching out a chart of events that occur before and after an intervention will provide a framework for your analysis.

Let's again turn to the influenza vaccination example for ideas about how we might approach this question. Figure 3.1 shows one approach to sketching out the course of possible events related to influenza virus infection over the typical flu season.

Why is it possible to develop influenza even if you are vaccinated? In reality, the influenza vaccine isn't 100 percent effective in 100 percent of the people who receive it. The scientists who make the vaccine must try to make an educated guess at which strains of the virus will be circulating during the influenza season. They are sometimes only partly right at guessing. Some years they miss altogether, and the vaccine does no good at all. Figure 3.2 charts the course of the flu among those who receive a vaccination.

In addition to the fact that the influenza vaccination is not always perfectly matched to the virus, some people's immune systems do not make antibodies to the vaccine. In other cases, the vaccine helps the body recognize the live virus, but the person develops a mild illness nonetheless. Most vaccinated people are never aware that they were exposed to the virus at all and develop few symptoms. But the point is that the vaccine will never prevent infection in all the people all the time.

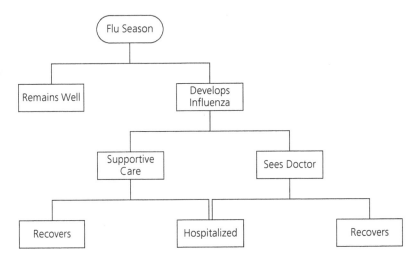

Figure 3.1   Flowchart Indicating the Clinical Course of Influenza Illness

In Figure 3.2, the supportive care tree has been removed for simplicity. Here, we see that the vaccine prevents infection in some people (Works) but does not in others (Fails). Those who develop an influenza-like illness despite vaccination are less likely to need to see a doctor, less likely to be hospitalized, and less likely to die than those who receive supportive care alone.

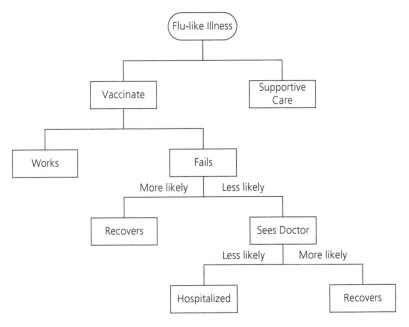

Figure 3.2   Flowchart Indicating the Course of Influenza Infection Among Subjects Who Receive a Vaccination

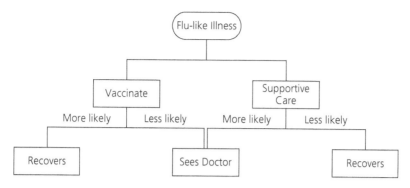

Figure 3.3 Probability of Seeing a Doctor Among Subjects Who Receive Vaccination Versus Those Who Receive Supportive Care

Figure 3.2 is an example of an **event pathway**. An event pathway depicts the course of different events that can occur in a cost-effectiveness analysis. Once each of these events is charted, you will have a much better idea of which data elements you will need to collect for your analysis. For instance, Figure 3.2 helps us see that those who receive the vaccine are more likely to recover once infected with the influenza virus.

Given that vaccinated people are more likely to recover even if they are infected and become symptomatic, we will need a separate set of probabilities in our event pathway for vaccinated and unvaccinated people (see Figure 3.3). For instance, we need to know the probability that those who developed the flu but received only supportive care will need to see a doctor. We also need to know the probability of a doctor's visit among those who were vaccinated but nonetheless developed the flu. Because this second group has partial immunity to the flu, the probability that they will see a doctor is likely to be lower.

Now let's consider another important probability: the chance that the vaccine will work sufficiently well that those who are exposed to the flu will develop few or no symptoms. This probability, referred to as *vaccine efficacy*, will be a key determinant of how much the vaccination strategy will cost. Let's say that we've gone through the medical literature and found the vaccine efficacy, the probability of seeing a doctor, and the probability of hospitalization among people who have been vaccinated but who developed the flu anyway (see Figure 3.4).

One key feature of each of these probabilities (seeing a doctor or not, getting hospitalized or not, and so forth) is that they are mutually exclusive events. For instance, you cannot kind of get hospitalized. Moreover, you cannot partially receive a shot for the influenza vaccine (at least not in our

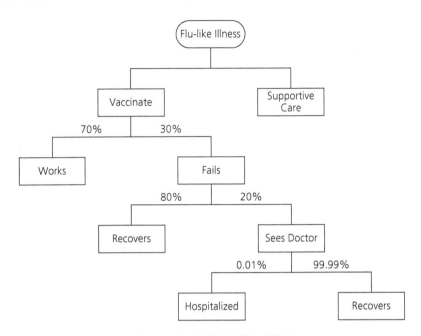

Figure 3.4   Vaccination Strategy Represented with All Probabilities Filled In

model). Therefore, all of the probabilities at any given branch must add up to 1.0. Thus, if we know that the efficacy of the influenza vaccine is 70 percent, the probability of developing the flu despite vaccination must be 100 minus 70 percent, or 30 percent. (This is the complement rule. We'll discuss this more in Chapter 9.)

Almost all of the "events" (represented as boxes in these figures) in an event pathway are associated with a cost. In Figure 3.4, for example, ill people might see a doctor or might recover on their own. If they see a doctor, they will incur the cost of driving to the doctor, the cost of the doctor's visit, and so on. Sometimes these costs are available in the medical literature, but usually they have to be calculated using a dataset, such as the Medical Expenditure Panel Survey (MEPS). We'll learn how to obtain and adjust these costs in Chapter 4.

For now, let's assume that we already have all the costs and probabilities on hand and take a moment to consider how costs and probabilities work together.

Figure 3.5 is a truncated version of the event pathway. Let's call this the "vaccination decision node." (That sounds nice and technical, so it will make all of the academics happy.) Imagine for a moment that we know the cost of vaccine failure ($100 in Figure 3.5). This $100 cost includes the cost of any doctor visits or hospitalizations that occur later, but we'll ignore that

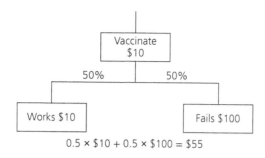

Figure 3.5   Vaccination Decision Node

for now. The cost of vaccination success is simply the cost of the vaccine ($10, which includes the time to administer it and so forth).

Now, let's estimate the overall cost of the vaccination strategy. Pretend that the vaccine was 50 percent effective in the 2006–07 flu season. We see in Figure 3.5 that our overall cost of vaccination is:

$$(0.5 \times \$10) + (0.5 \times \$100) = \$55. \tag{3.1}$$

It quickly becomes apparent that if we change the vaccine efficacy, our costs will be profoundly affected. For instance, if the vaccine is 70 percent effective during the average season, then the average cost is:

$$(0.7 \times \$10) + (0.3 \times \$100) = \$37. \tag{3.2}$$

Likewise, if the vaccine is 100 percent effective, then the total cost is just the cost of the vaccination, or:

$$1.0 \times \$10 = \$10. \tag{3.3}$$

So far, you've learned the basics of how to formulate a research question in cost-effectiveness analysis. You've also learned the basics of how costs and probabilities work together. As you will soon see, the effectiveness portion of a cost-effectiveness analysis works in essentially the same way as costs. Before getting into that, let's take a moment in Chapter 4 to fill in the details of what we've already created and take a deeper look at how costs are actually calculated.

Exercise 3

3.   In Figure 3.4, the event pathways for vaccination include "Works" and "Fails." Suppose you were going to resketch the event pathways. What are some possible pathways that can occur besides "Works" and "Fails"?

Summary

In this chapter, we introduced you to the initial steps for planning your cost-effectiveness analysis. Most important, we provided some guidance on designing your own research question. Unless this is carefully thought out, you will waste hours doing and redoing your analysis until you get the research question right. The research question is an important step and should consider the population, interventions, and the disease of interest. In addition, you will also need to consider the time horizon or the length of the study, the location where the intervention will take place, and the perspective of the cost-effectiveness analysis. This will help you select the appropriate study design (e.g., cost-effectiveness analysis and cost-benefit analysis) from which to answer your question. Finally, having a flow diagram will not only provide a nice visual guide for your audience, but it will help you plan and identify elements that you'll need in your cost-effectiveness analysis.

Further Readings

The International Society for Pharmacoeconomics and Outcomes Research (ISPOR) and the Society for Medical Decision Making have developed a Modeling Good Research Practices Task Force to assist researchers in constructing decision models. These recommendations are available in the ISPOR's Good Practice for Outcomes Research Index site (International Society for Pharmacoeconomics and Outcomes Research, 2015). Students should begin by reading the Modeling Good Research Practices—Overview: A Report of the ISPOR-SMDM Modeling Good Research Practices Task Force—Part 1, which gives a good overview of developing decision models.

References

Caro, J. J., A. H. Briggs, U. Siebert, K. M. Kuntz, and ISPOR-SMDM Modeling Good Research Practices Task Force. (2012). Modeling Good Research Practices—Overview: A Report of the ISPOR-SMDM Modeling Good Research Practices Task Force—1. *Value in Health* 15(6): 796–803. http://doi.org/10.1016/j.jval.2012.06.012.

Centers for Disease Control and Prevention. (2013). Prevention and Control of Seasonal Influenza with Vaccines: Recommendations of the Advisory Committee on Immunization Practices—United States, 2013–2014. *Morbidity and Mortality Weekly Report* 62(7): 1–43.

Department of Health and Human Services. (2015). Healthy People 2020: Vaccination Coverage Objectives. Retrieved August 12, 2015, from https://

www.healthypeople.gov/2020/topics-objectives/topic/immunization-and-infectious-diseases/objectives.

Dixit, R., G. Khandaker, P. Hay, K. McPhie, J. Taylor, H. Rashid, . . . R. Booy. (2014). A Randomized Study of Standard Versus Double Dose Oseltamivir for Treating Influenza in the Community. *Antiviral Therapy.* http://doi.org/10.3851/IMP2807.

Drummond, M. F., M. J. Sculpher, G. W. Torrance, B. J. O'Brien, and G. L. Stoddart. (2005). *Methods for the Economic Evaluation of Health Care Programmes,* 3rd ed. New York: Oxford University Press.

Gold, M. R., J. E. Siegel, L. B. Russell, and M. C. Weinstein. (1996). *Cost-Effectiveness in Health and Medicine,* 1st ed. New York: Oxford University Press.

Haddix, A., S. Teutsch, P. Shaffer, and D. Dunet. (1996). *Prevention Effectiveness: A Guide to Decision Analysis and Economic Evaluation.* New York: Oxford University Press.

Hirve, S., M. Chadha, P. Lele, K. E. Lafond, A. Deoshatwar, S. Sambhudas, . . . A. Mishra. (2012). Performance of Case Definitions Used for Influenza Surveillance Among Hospitalized Patients in a Rural Area of India. *Bulletin of the World Health Organization* 90(11): 804–812. http://doi.org/10.2471/BLT.12.108837.

International Federation of Health Plans. (2013). 2013 Comparative Price Report: Variation in Medical and Hospital Prices by Country. London: International Federation of Health Plans.

International Society for Pharmacoeconomics and Outcomes Research. (2015). ISPOR Good Practices for Outcomes Research Index. Retrieved March 23, 2015, from http://www.ispor.org/workpaper/practices_index.asp.

Monto, A. S., D. P. Robinson, M. L. Herlocher, J. M. Hinson, M. J. Elliott, and A. Crisp. (1999). Zanamivir in the Prevention of Influenza Among Healthy Adults: A Randomized Controlled Trial. *Journal of the American Medical Association* 282(1): 31–35.

Neumann, P. J., G. D. Sanders, L. B. Russell, J. E. Siegel, and T. G. Ganiats. (2016). *Cost-Effectiveness in Health and Medicine.* New York: Oxford University Press.

Smith, R. A., D. Manassaram-Baptiste, D. Brooks, V. Cokkinides, M. Doroshenk, D. Saslow, . . . O. W. Brawley. (2014). Cancer Screening in the United States, 2014: A Review of Current American Cancer Society Guidelines and Current Issues in Cancer Screening. *CA: A Cancer Journal for Clinicians* 64(1): 30–51. http://doi.org/10.3322/caac.21212.

U.S. Preventive Services Task Force. (2009). Screening for Breast Cancer: U.S. Preventive Services Task Force Recommendation Statement. *Annals of Internal Medicine* 151(10): 716–726, W–236. http://doi.org/10.7326/0003-4819-151-10-200911170-00008.

WORKING WITH COSTS

Overview

Sandra Montero returned to her office after dropping off Sandra Jr. at day care. Sandra always tried to incorporate exercise into her work routine, so after giving the security guard a friendly smile, she turned in to the stairwell to make her usual four-flight climb up the stairs, as her doctor recommended. After the first few steps, she felt her thigh muscles ache and suddenly felt tired all over. She lumbered into her office, started to cough, and decided to visit the company physician.

After sitting for almost half an hour in the clinic, the doctor told her that she had the flu. Sandra went home for the rest of the day, with instructions to drink plenty of fluids and take some over-the-counter medications. On her way home, she wearily picked up the medicines at a pharmacy near her house, then drove home and climbed in between her fresh linen sheets. Before dozing off, she remembered that Sandra Jr. would soon need a ride home, so she called her babysitter and asked him to pick her up from day care.

When Sandra decided to see her physician, she set off a chain of events, each associated with a cost. First, the receptionist, the medical assistant, and the doctor each spent time seeing Sandra for her illness. Second, while sitting in the office waiting to see the physician, she unknowingly exposed the receptionist and an elderly file clerk to the influenza virus. The receptionist developed a mild illness that kept her at home for a few days, and the file clerk was eventually hospitalized for bacterial pneumonia that arose as a result of the initial influenza infection. Third, Sandra decided to purchase some over-the-counter

LEARNING OBJECTIVES

- Identify specific costs that will go into a cost-effectiveness analysis.

- Distinguish between micro-costing and gross costing and how they are applied in cost-effectiveness analysis.

- Describe how to apply the cost-to-charge ratio adjustment to certain charges.

- Explain how to use DRG codes to identify costs for certain diseases.

- Distinguish between adjusting for inflation and discounting and how they are applied in cost-effectiveness analysis.

medications as recommended by her physician. Fourth, because of her illness, Sandra would stay home from work for the next three days. Finally, the babysitter had to leave his other job early to pick up Sandra Jr. from day care.

So you can see how a relatively common illness can translate into a diverse range of medical and nonmedical costs. In our analysis, when thinking about the costs associated with an influenza-like illness, we must take all of these possible events into consideration. Of course, this is just one scenario, and a cost-effectiveness analysis deals with population averages.

In this chapter, we'll take a bit of a break from plotting out and executing our analysis to look at how we might place a monetary value on each of the events Sandra put into motion. You will also learn some of the ways in which costs are collected. More detailed descriptions of how costs are collected can be found in Chapter 12.

TIPS AND TRICKS

Internet links change from time to time. Up-to-date links and exercises can always be found at this book's web site: http://www.wiley.com/WileyCDA/WileyTitle/productCd-1119011264.html.

Opportunity Costs

Recall from Chapter 1 that an opportunity cost is the value of goods and services in their best alternative use. If we invest in a mammogram, we are diverting resources from other potentially important investments. When the societal perspective is assumed, goods and services are generally thought of in terms of the social resources that are used rather than prices. By thinking in terms of the resources used when a medical intervention is applied, we will be providing policymakers with better information on whether those resources should be diverted to more efficient projects or interventions.

In sum, the key driver of costs is not the price of the resource, but the amount of resource used. Imagine that you have an amazing cask of wine that will last forever. Now imagine that your intervention is to drink one glass per day for one year. In that case, the resource you are using is one glass of wine per day. The alternative is not to drink the wine. You will be less happy and will have higher blood pressure, but you will also have all of your wine. The opportunity cost of your wine intervention is the value of the wine drained from your cask.

Although there are many esoteric theoretical reasons for thinking in terms of opportunity costs, there is really one practical reason: In health care, market prices rarely reflect what people actually end up paying. For instance, one gynecologist in New York admitted that he charges uninsured patients $175 for a routine visit but accepts payments of $25 from insurance companies for the same services (Kolata, 2001). The patient walking in off the street is not likely to start bargaining with her gynecologist for a better price. If we were to use the $175 figure in our cost-effectiveness analysis, our estimate would be seven times higher than the standard fee that insurance companies pay.

To estimate the cost of this gynecological visit, we might be better off considering the value of the resources that go into a gynecological visit. For instance, we might place a price on the amount of time the doctor spends with the patient, the number and types of laboratory tests the doctor orders, the overall time the patient spends in the clinic, and the amount the patient spends on transportation to and from the clinic.

WHEN TO USE PRICES

What costs do we include in our analysis when valuing drugs? In theory, the opportunity cost of a drug should include just the manufacturing and distribution costs. Manufacturing costs are difficult to obtain, so cost-effectiveness researchers usually use just the wholesale cost of products (such as drugs). This more practical approach makes sense especially when comparing the cost-effectiveness of pharmaceuticals. Consider two drugs of equal effectiveness with similar manufacturing costs. If one is a brand-name drug and costs twice as much as the other on the market, we would naturally want to purchase the cheaper version. However, an analysis based on manufacturing and distribution costs alone might rate the drugs as equally desirable. A meaningful comparison for policy therefore would require the use of the reimbursed price of one drug versus the other.

We generally use the reimbursed cost of drugs, laboratory tests, and so forth to estimate costs in cost-effectiveness analysis. Why? Because the reimbursed cost is more or less representative of the amount we are paying in the real world. Using the amount that a hospital or doctor bills a patient will distort what is actually paid for such services in the real world. But the use of some opportunity costs can also distort the usefulness of a cost-effectiveness analysis.

Fine. So how do we actually get such information? In the United States, the actual amount paid for a service can be obtained from the Medical Expenditure Panel survey, and the average wholesale price (AWP) and wholesale acquisition cost (WAC) of a drug can be obtained from the

RED BOOK™. However, the *RED BOOK* requires a subscription, which may be beyond the ability of a student to pay unless your library happens to carry it. The average sales price (ASP) is provided free of charge by the Centers for Medicare and Medicaid Services (CMS), but it includes only pharmaceuticals associated with Medicare Part B (Centers for Medicare & Medicaid Services, 2014b). (Data outside the United States can be found on this book's web site, http://www.wiley.com/WileyCDA/WileyTitle/ productCd-1119011264.html, as well as in Chapter 12. Sorry for being U.S.-centric.) When medical expenditures are not available in a given country, it is possible to value the cost of services using wages and the estimated costs of the products consumed. In a moment, we'll go into more detail about how wages and wholesale prices can be used to generate an overall cost. But we should first consider which costs we are actually incurring for a given health intervention.

PHARMACEUTICAL BENCHMARK PRICES

Pharmaceutical price benchmarking underwent some major changes on March 30, 2009, when the U.S. District Court Judge Patti B. Sarris, for the District of Massachusetts, issued a final order and settlement to McKesson Corporation, a drug wholesaler, and First DataBank, a drug pricing publisher, for illegally raising the AWP of prescription drugs, which was the common pharmaceutical benchmark at the time.

Reimbursement amounts by the government (e.g., CMS) and third-party payers were done without knowledge of the actual costs of pharmaceuticals. Rather, a benchmark was commonly used to determine the reimbursement amount for drugs administered by providers and sold by pharmacies to patients. For the past 40 years, the AWP was the benchmark used by most third-party payers in their reimbursement calculations. Manufacturers typically sell drugs to wholesalers or distributors at some negotiated price. The wholesalers then sell the drugs to pharmacies and hospitals by setting the price based on the WAC. The pharmacists and hospitals then sell the drugs to patients, who are usually covered by some prescription drug plan through their healthcare insurance company or a government program (e.g., Medicaid), also known as third-party payers. These third-party payers do not know the actual cost of the drugs. However, they could estimate the costs by using the AWP, which was published by certain companies (e.g., First DataBank, *RED BOOK* [Truven Health Analytics], and Gold Standard [Elsevier]).

Since the settlement, there has been a major gap for a standard pharmaceutical drug price benchmark left by distrust associated with the AWP. First DataBank discontinued publication of the AWP on September 28, 2011; however, *RED BOOK* and Gold Standard continue to provide it. Some organizations have started to develop their own benchmarks. For example, CMS has developed the National Average Drug Acquisition Cost (NADAC), which is based on a monthly survey to retail pharmacies across the United States (Centers for Medicare & Medicaid Services, 2015); however, it is not all-inclusive.

So what are we supposed to do? We recommend using the pharmaceutical price that is relevant to your research or work environment. Because of the competitive nature of the marketplace, most institutions are reluctant to make their acquisition costs available. The AWP is still around, but we can consider using the WAC and acquisition costs (if available). We have provided a short list of potential candidates for pharmaceutical drug pricing benchmarks (Table 4.1).

Table 4.1   Comparison of Pharmaceutical Benchmark Prices

Type	Description
Actual Acquisition Cost (AAC)	This is the final price paid by pharmacies and includes the net price after discounts and rebates. This varies across different pharmacies and distributors. In addition, it is not publicly available, thereby making it difficult to acquire. Most institutions are unlikely to share this information.
Average Sales Price (ASP)	The Centers for Medicare & Medicaid Services (CMS) receive a unique price from pharmaceutical manufacturers called the ASP. Manufacturers are required to submit the ASP to CMS on a quarterly basis, which includes discounts and rebates. Each price must be verified by the CEO/CFO of the pharmaceutical manufacturer. This is limited to Medicare Part B drugs, which are approximately 2 percent of outpatient prescriptions and not specific to National Drug Code (NDC) numbers.
Average Wholesale Price (AWP)	This is the list price by the drug price publishers. AWP is calculated using a markup applied to the WAC or direct price from the actual manufacturer. The markup is capped at 1.20 times the WAC. Each AWP is specific to the NDC.
Federal Supply Schedule (FSS)	The federal price negotiated by the Department of Veterans Affairs National Acquisition Center for large-volume purchases of pharmaceutical drugs and other medical items. This is usually based on the most favored commercial customer pricing, which is in the best interests of the federal government.
National Average Drug Acquisition Cost (NADAC)	CMS conducts monthly surveys (Survey of Retail Prices) of retail pharmacies in order to calculate the average drug acquisition costs. This provides a national benchmark, which state Medicaid agencies can use to determine reimbursement amount. NADAC is updated monthly, but there is a two-month delay.
Wholesale Acquisition Cost (WAC)	This is the manufacturer's list price as sold to the pharmaceutical distributor or wholesaler. Unlike AWP, the manufacturer determines the WAC. It is also known as the list price and direct price. Drug publishing companies continue to provide the WAC.

Identifying Costs

In Chapter 3, we saw that vaccination will reduce but not eliminate the likelihood of costly health events. Moreover, people who might never get sick incur the cost of vaccination, so if the incidence of influenza is low, the average cost is high. Recall, too, that we assumed that the cost of each event in the influenza pathway was essentially the same: Whether you've been vaccinated or not, a doctor's visit is still going to set you back $70. However, the probability of incurring a given cost differed depending on the strategy; a vaccinated person is much less likely to get the flu and is therefore less likely to see a doctor.

Since the costs in each pathway are essentially the same, we can merge the vaccination and supportive care strategies when speaking of costs. Figure 4.1 provides a basic framework for identifying the costs that you will use in the analysis. But this is only a basic framework. Within each box, the overall cost comprises a number of smaller costs.

For example, even if she does not see a doctor, Sandra (the subject in the earlier example) will remain at home in bed and will not drive to work while sick. But someone who remains well throughout influenza season will drive to work every day (or take a bus or train). Because the presence or absence of influenza-like illness causes a change in transportation use, the higher rate of transportation among well people could be counted as a cost. Therefore, we might want to change the $0 value in the No Infection box in Figure 4.1.

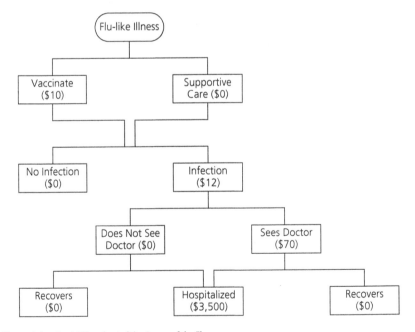

Figure 4.1   Partial Flowchart of the Course of the Flu

Note: Each box represents a cost associated with influenza infection.

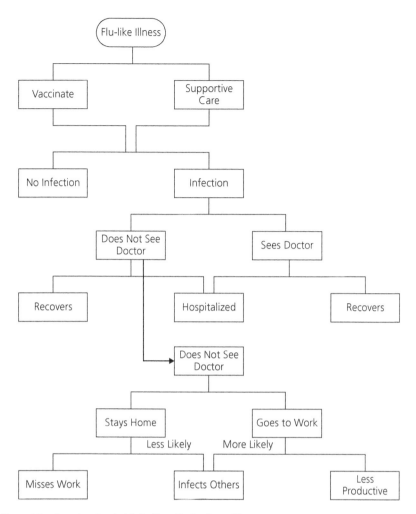

Figure 4.2   Costs Associated with the "Does Not See Doctor" Box

Figure 4.2 provides some examples of the costs associated with the flu even when the subject does not seek medical care. If Sandra stays at home, she is less likely to infect others, which will greatly reduce the overall cost of the supportive care strategy. But she will also miss work, which will partly offset these costs. Don't worry quite yet about how all of these costs are actually captured. Our job for now is to think about what types of costs we might consider so that we can make a list of the data elements we will be collecting later on.

Ideally, we will want to make a list of costs associated with all of the other boxes as well. Using the overall flowchart as a framework, it is a good idea to break down (identify) all of the costs that lead to the overall cost of each event. This allows us to think more clearly about the subtleties of how costs change when we do something in health or medicine. In practice, though, many of the costs will be obtained in aggregate. For instance, we would probably just look up the average cost of a doctor's visit for influenza virus infection using an electronic dataset.

So why bother with all this business about identifying the resources used? If we do not at least identify all of the costs, we will miss some of the costs that were not included in the value we obtained from an electronic dataset. For instance, the dataset will contain information on the cost of a medical visit but no information about the cost of getting to the doctor in the first place. By identifying all of the minuscule costs involved, we won't miss any important costs.

Exercise 1

1. What are some of the costs associated with "Hospitalized" box in Figure 4.1.

Micro-Costing and Gross Costing

TIPS AND TRICKS

It is important to understand what is included in the cost that you use. This book will provide a lot of information about the most common sources of cost data and how to use them. But some students will get costs from a particular institution or other source. These sources might provide the billed cost (what the clinic or hospital charged) or the reimbursed cost (what they actually received from insurance companies), or they might just include the cost of the item in question (e.g., just the cost of a vial of influenza vaccine). Make sure you know what you have before you decide how you are going to use it!

Costs such as the value of an intravenous (IV) bag or a gallon of gasoline are components of larger costs, such as hospitalization or transportation costs. As such, they are called **micro-costs**. Aggregated costs obtained from electronic datasets or from the medical literature are called **gross costs**. The gross cost may not capture all costs in which we are interested. Therefore, it is usually necessary to add some micro-costs to gross cost estimates obtained from electronic datasets or the medical literature. Other events in the event pathway may have to be "micro-costed" (in the grammar of health economics) because no gross cost estimates are available.

One example is the cost of the vaccination itself. We are unlikely to find the actual cost of influenza vaccination anywhere in the medical literature or in an electronic dataset. Therefore, we will need to look up the cost of the vaccine, estimate the time a nurse will take to administer the vaccine, estimate the time it will take to receive the vaccine, and consider other costs, such as the cost of a syringe.

So you just learned that the first step in obtaining costs for your cost-effectiveness analysis is to *identify all of the relevant resources that will be consumed* (Gold, Siegel, Russell, & Weinstein, 1996; Neumann, Sanders, Russell, Siegel, & Ganiats, 2016). You also learned that each cost can be obtained by micro-costing or simply using a gross cost. When micro-costing, we need to add two more steps to the process of identification.

Step 2 is to *quantify the resources used.* For example, to estimate Sandra's transportation costs, we might need to know how many miles she lives from her job, how much fuel her car consumes per mile traveled, and so on. This information can often be obtained from census datasets, estimated by expert opinion, or assumed. (Whenever we make an assumption, we must state what the assumption is and why we chose the value we did so that others can judge whether it was reasonable. More on this later.)

Step 3 is to *place a monetary value on the resources used.* The final step in determining a micro-cost is to place a monetary value on each resource used. For instance, we might determine the market price of a gallon of gasoline and multiply this cost by the number of gallons used in driving to work or to the clinic. For patient time costs, wages are applied to the number of hours spent receiving an intervention or treating a patient. Sandra spent 30 minutes at the clinic before the doctor sent her home. If she made $30 per hour, the value of the time spent at the clinic would be 0.5 hours × $30 = $15.

Now let's take a broader view of the process of identification, quantification, and valuation. Suppose that we were estimating the cost of Sandra's office visit in the example. First, we would identify all of the resources used: the cost of any medical supplies used, any tests performed, Sandra's time, the medical assistant's time, the secretary's time, and the physician's time. To measure the quantity of the resources used, we would estimate the type and number of medical supplies used and the amount of time each person spent treating, or receiving treatment for, the illness. If we were to measure these resources separately, we would assign a wage to each person's time, assign a cost to any tests that might have been performed or supplies used, and then add these costs together. The process of identifying each resource used, measuring these resources, valuing the resources, and adding them together is called **micro-costing**.

Gross costing, using gross costs obtained from a single data source, is generally much easier and less time-consuming than micro-costing,

Table 4.2   Partial List of Costs for Treatment of Influenza Infection

Identify	Quantify	Monetize	Total
Nonmedical costs			
Lost work	5 days	$70/day	$350.00
Patient time	1 hour	$8.75/hour	$8.75
Transportation	10 trips	$1.50/trip	$15.00
Patient time	0.1 hour	$8.75/hour	$0.88
Medical costs			
Receptionist's time	5 minutes	$0.25/minute	$1.25
Physician's time	10 minutes	$2.50/minute	$25.00
Nurse's time	5 minutes	$0.25/minute	$1.00
Vaccine	8	$2.50/minute	$25.00
Syringe	1	$0.5/syringe	$0.50

especially when complex hospital costs are involved. It is often possible to obtain a hospital charge for a particular disease in a matter of minutes over the Internet. Nevertheless, it is easy to overlook important costs when using gross costs.

Another concern is double-counting costs when using gross costs with micro-costs. For instance, the gross cost may not provide you with an itemized list of individual costs. Not knowing what went into a gross cost may predispose you to adding a micro-cost that has already been incorporated. Therefore, we want to make lists of every cost, and we need to know whether or not we use micro-costs or gross costs. Table 4.2 presents a sample of some of the three-step process discussed here.

Getting Cost Data

In the previous section, we discussed the process of identification, quantification, and valuation using the example of a medical office visit and vaccination. Suppose we wanted to obtain the cost of the hospitalization (which is what happened to the unlucky elderly file clerk whom Sandra exposed in the waiting room of the doctor's office). The first step, identifying the resources used, would be a huge task.

Micro-costing a hospitalization visit involves accounting for all the gauze pads used, all of the sheets washed, nurse time, and lab services, to name just some of the resources used. If we obtained the cost of hospitalization using a dataset, our efforts would be reduced to looking up the overall cost. This value obtained from a dataset would provide an estimate of all of the medical services used in aggregate. But what have we missed? A few things, as it turns out. For instance, one missing value is the patient's time spent in the hospital.

To measure these additional resources used (beyond the cost of the hospitalization), we need to estimate the patient time cost, which is achieved by obtaining the average length of stay (ALOS) for the hospitalization. The ALOS is an estimate of the time resources used. To assign a monetary value to this resource, we multiply the ALOS by the patient's wage. (We might value the person's leisure time at about the same price as his or her work time, so we can use just the hourly wage for all time costs. For a more detailed discussion, see Gold et al. [1996] or Neumann et al. [2016].)

PROJECT MAP

1. Think through your research question.

2. Sketch out the analysis.

3. *Collect data for your model.*

4. Adjust your data.

5. Build your model.

6. Run and test the model.

7. Conduct a sensitivity analysis.

8. Write it up.

Let's take a moment to see how this works in practice. Give the following exercises a try.

Exercises 2 and 3

2. Obtain the average 2012 hospitalization charge for influenza virus infections. To do so:
   a. Visit http://hcupnet.ahrq.gov.
   b. Click on "Create a New Analysis," and then click on "Emergency Department."
   c. Click on "Descriptive Statistics"; choose 2012 and then click "Yes" for the "Do you want data on a specific diagnosis or procedure?" question.

d. Under the "Choose how you would like to analyze data," select "Diagnosis–ICD-9-CM Codes (ICD9)."

e. You will be asked to enter an "ICD-9 Code." The code for influenza virus infection is 487.

f. After you enter the code, click on "Create Analysis." This will generate the output. However, it will not contain the average cost. Look at the left column and click on "Outcomes and Measures." Select "Hospital charges" and then click "Submit Request." What was the hospital charge for an emergency department visit for influenza in 2012?

3. Assume that the average wage for a person is $100 per day. How much wage is lost when a person is admitted for an influenza infection? (Hint: Repeat Exercise 2 to obtain mean length of stay.)

If you did Exercises 2 and 3, you may have some lingering questions. First: What did I just do? Second: Is the value that I obtained accurate? We will answer each of these questions in the next two sections. Next, we'll tackle the issue of what you just did. Then we'll tackle how to adjust costs to make sure that they are relatively accurate. For instance, we'll discuss how to adjust the data you downloaded to better reflect its opportunity cost.

Using Diagnosis Codes

If you did Exercise 2, you conducted a search for all people in the dataset who were hospitalized for influenza virus infection. To ensure that you knew exactly what you were getting, you entered a special code that refers to influenza virus infection. The software pulled all cases within the hospitalization dataset for people diagnosed with influenza virus infection and then provided the relevant information for you in tabular format.

The ICD-9 code that you entered is used universally in doctors' offices and hospitals to classify disease. Many students are familiar with these classification systems. If you are one of them, you may skip to the next section.

Diseases are categorized using a number of different systems. These systems include the International Classification for Disease (ICD), Diagnosis-Related Groups (DRGs), and the Clinical Classifications for Health Policy Research, called CCS codes (after the name of the software, the Clinical Classification Software). These codes are generally used to obtain gross cost estimates for medical visits and hospitalizations. Table 4.3 sorts out these acronyms for you.

The online dataset you used is called the Healthcare Cost and Utilization Project. As you saw in the exercise, you could have used any number of disease classification systems. The ICD system is currently in its tenth revision and is often referred to by its revision number. For example, the ninth revision is still commonly used in the United States and is referred

Table 4.3   Common Codes Used to Group Diseases

Classification System	Acronym	Description
International Classification for Disease	ICD	A comprehensive list of every disease and disease subtype
Major Diagnosis Category	MDC	Groups of ICD codes by category (e.g., "Infectious and Parasitic Diseases" or "Neoplasms")
Clinical Classifications for Health Policy Research	CCS	Groups of ICD codes by common diseases and subtypes (for example, diabetes and its various complications)
Diagnosis-Related Groups	DRGs	A list of over 700 diseases grouped by costs

to as the ICD-9 system. Currently, CMS and the rest of the United States is preparing to transition to the ICD-10 in October 1, 2015. Stay tuned for updates on our web site http://www.wiley.com/WileyCDA/WileyTitle/productCd-1119011264.html.

Costs obtained from this system are specific to a particular disease. For instance, using this system, it is possible to obtain costs for either influenza virus hospitalizations or for pneumonia secondary to influenza. In the ICD-9 system, the codes are five digits. The first three digits refer to the disease in question. For example, conduct disorders use code 312. The last two numbers refer to disease subtypes. For instance, pathological gamblers get code 31231, kleptomaniacs get code 31232, and pyromaniacs get code 31233.

Sometimes this system can be too specific. For example, diabetes mellitus can cause many different complications, each associated with its own ICD code. Examining diseases with a number of different complications takes a lot of effort to figure out which ICD codes go with which diseases. For this reason, it is sometimes preferable to use a less specific system when examining costs associated with complex diseases.

The Clinical Classifications for Health Policy Research system's CCS code system solves this problem. It groups ICD codes specific to a particular disease. For example, CCS codes can be used to examine costs for five ICD codes that are related to diabetes mellitus without complications (CCS code 49) or 38 conditions associated with complications for the disease, such as circulatory, neurological, or kidney problems (CCS code 50). They can also be used to examine each specific complication of the disease. For example, different kidney problems associated with the disease (ICD codes 25040–25043) are grouped together into diagnosis category 3.3.2.

The CCS code for influenza is 123. Take a moment and compare the charges obtained using an ICD-9 code and a CCS code using the Healthcare Cost and Utilization Project web site. You'll notice that your mean length of stay and mean charges have changed because you are capturing conditions caused by the influenza virus infection in addition to full-blown influenza infections.

While the CCS system aggregates codes for a particular illness, the DRG system aggregates diseases with similar costs. It is therefore the least disease-specific system. For example, costs related to diabetes mellitus mostly differ by the age of the patient and are listed as "Diabetes, less than age thirty-five" and "Diabetes, greater than age thirty-five." Other endocrine diseases are less common and are similar in cost, so those with an uncomplicated stay in the hospital are grouped together under the general category "Endocrine disorders without complications."

As we will see in a moment, DRGs are useful for adjusting hospital charges obtained from electronic sources.

Adjusting Costs

Costs obtained from the medical literature or electronic datasets often require adjustment before they can be included in a cost-effectiveness analysis. Suppose that you have found a good study on the cost of ambulatory care for influenza-like illness, but the study was conducted in 2000 and your other costs are from 2006. Because prices have inflated since 2000, you can't simply use the earlier cost in your analysis. Whether costs will occur in the future or have occurred in the past, they need to be adjusted to present values. (The net cost of an intervention in present terms is called the **net present value**, which will be discussed further in this chapter.)

Other forms of adjustment are also needed. Some costs, such as those you obtained in Exercise 2, might be in the correct year but might include huge profits and therefore need to be adjusted to better reflect the opportunity cost of the intervention. Hospital charges are the primary example of this type of cost distortion.

PROJECT MAP

1. Think through your research question.

2. Sketch out the analysis.

3. Collect data for your model.

4. *Adjust your data.*

5. Build your model.

6. Run and test the model.

7. Conduct a sensitivity analysis.

8. Write it up.

Hospital Charges

Data on hospitalization costs are most often obtained from hospital billing systems, which report the total bill—the **charge**—incurred by the patient. A charge is the amount that a hospital, clinic, or pharmacy bills the patient or the patient's insurance company. Some of the goods and services for which hospitals charge are inflated so that the hospital can generate profits or recover losses from investments that are unrelated to the billed admission. For instance, overbilling is one way to cover care provided to uninsured patients. (This is perhaps called "overbilling" because "overcharging" sounds too harsh.) Hospital charges are therefore almost always larger than the actual cost of the resources used. According to the 2011 Medicare Provider Analysis and Review (MEDPAR) file, actual costs are about 20 percent of the average amount charged (Centers for Medicare & Medicaid Services, 2014a).

Charges are relevant only when the free market sets the price of medical care. Thus, they apply only to largely unregulated private insurance schemes, such as those in the United States, China, and India. Private health insurance policies are increas-

> **TIPS AND TRICKS**
>
> If you are conducting research in industrialized nations other than the United States, you can skip to the "Adjusting for Inflation" section.

ingly available to private purchasers in Europe and Australia as a complement to the national health systems. Nonetheless, countries with national health systems typically report government costs in their datasets. They can therefore be used in a cost-effectiveness analysis without adjustment because they generally reflect the cost of the care that the average person uses. Since public sector programs in the United States provide services only to populations that are generally quite demographically different from the rest of the population (the poor, Native Americans, armed forces personnel, the elderly), these government costs tend not to reflect the cost of care for the average person.

This does not mean that government cost data in the United States are not useful. Although the reported Medicare costs apply only to persons over the age of 65 or those with debilitating chronic diseases, Medicare costs can be used to generate **cost-to-charge ratios**. These ratios can then be used to adjust any charge obtained from any dataset.

Medicare conducts an extensive analysis of the actual costs of hospitalizing a patient to ensure that it is paying for only the services consumed by its patients. When a Medicare patient is hospitalized, Medicare generally does not pay the hospital what the patient was charged. Rather, it pays

Table 4.4   MEDPAR Cost Data by DRG for 2011

DRG	Total Charges (1)	Covered Charges (2)	Medicare Reimbursement (3)	Number of Discharges (4)	Average Total Days (5)
1	$1,438,849,607	$1,388,494,856	$337,259,832	1,745	38.6
2	$217,693,541	$213,341,162	$45,776,248	447	19.8
...	...	...	...	...	...
178	$2,859,211,402	$2,834,639,621	$645,718,070	80,356	6.6

the hospital an amount that is roughly equal to the cost of the goods and services the hospital provides to the typical patient with a similar condition.

Medicare cost data are available through a system called Medical Provider Analysis and Review (MEDPAR) (Centers for Medicare & Medicaid Services, 2014a). In MEDPAR, each charge made to Medicare and each payment made by Medicare is listed by DRG (see Table 4.4). A list of cost-to-charge ratios generated using Medicare data can be found in Appendix D. The book's web site contains links to MEDPAR data at http://www.wiley.com/WileyCDA/WileyTitle/productCd-1119011264.html (the direct government link is horrendously long and always changing).

Notice in Table 4.4 that Medicare lists the amount it was charged (Total Charges), the amount of the charge that is covered (Covered Charges), and the amount it actually paid (Medicare Reimbursement). This last amount is the cost of the services rendered.

By forming a ratio of the reimbursements in column 3 by the charges in column 2 of Table 4.4, you can convert any ICD or CCS code to a cost that will more or less work for any age group or coding system. For instance, if we needed to convert a hospital charge of $10,000 for influenza virus infection to a cost, you might use DRG 178 (the final row in Table 4.4), which is "respiratory infections & inflammation with complicating or comorbid." A rough estimate of the opportunity cost of this $10,000 charge is:

$$\$10,000 \times \frac{\$645,718,070}{\$2,834,639,621} = \$2,278 \tag{4.1}$$

This ratio $\left(\frac{\$645,718,070}{\$2,834,639,621}\right)$ is the cost-to-charge ratio. As the name implies, it adjusts hospital charges (represented by $10,000) so that they better reflect the cost of the social resources used when a patient is hospitalized.

We can use the information contained in the MEDPAR system to estimate cost-to-charge ratios by looking for a DRG that is similar to the

ICD-9 or CCS charge we wish to use. Suppose that we wish to know the average cost of hospitalization for pneumococcal pneumonia, a specific type of bacterial pneumonia. We could pull the mean hospitalization charge for this type of pneumonia (ICD-9 code 486) from the Healthcare Cost and Utilization Project web site, and then adjust the cost according to what Medicare was charged and what it paid for cases of simple pneumonia (DRG 195). Let's give this a try.

Exercises 4 and 5

4. Calculate a cost-to-charge ratio for DRG 195 (simple pneumonia and pleurisy without complicating or comorbid condition and major complicating or comorbid condition) using Medicare's MEDPAR data (see Appendix D).

5. Calculate the average hospitalization costs for bacterial pneumonia (ICD-9 code 486) from the Healthcare Cost and Utilization Project (available at http://hcupnet.ahrq.gov/), and convert these into a cost using the cost-to-charge ratio you calculated in Exercise 4. Use 2012 data from HCUP.

Converting Other Charges

Data specific to national health systems outside the United States are usually presented in the form of costs rather than charges. When data include charges in the private sector, there is little hope of obtaining an accurate cost-to-charge ratio in many countries. Here you may need to consult with experts in insurance companies to obtain estimates of local cost-to-charge ratios. (Typically they've done the footwork to see how little they can get away with paying.)

Most researchers in the United States obtain cost data from the Medical Expenditure Panel Survey (commonly referred to as MEPS and available at http://www.meps.ahrq.gov/mepsweb/data_stats/MEPSnetHC.jsp). This dataset allows one to obtain charges *or* expenditures for medical visits and has an online tool similar to the Healthcare Cost and Utilization Project used in Exercise 2. So, can expenditures be used as a proxy for costs?

Expenditures reflect what the patient or insurance company actually paid for the billed charges. A good deal of care is charitable. Patients who received charitable care will have an expenditure of $0 for their medical visit. Conversely, some people will be "overbilled" for their treatment and pay this large amount. In these instances, the expenditures will be inflated.

TIPS AND TRICKS

The online tool for MEPS does not yet have the ability to access diseases by diagnosis code, so it is necessary to work with someone familiar with electronic data in order to obtain MEPS expenditures for specific diseases. However, a student who is determined enough can go to the MEPS web site and read through the documentation, which contains technical details for importing and cleaning the data for several statistical programming languages (e.g., SAS, STATA, and SPSS).

One examination of expenditures found that these two factors—free care and inflated charges—just about balance each other out and that expenditures in MEPS serve as a good proxy for costs (Muennig, Franks, Jia, Lubetkin, & Gold, 2005). Of course, since low-income, uninsured populations receive charitable care, they are likely to have many $0 expenditure values. Therefore, any analysis examining low-income groups alone would likely produce an underestimate of real-world expenditure values.

Adjusting for Inflation

When older cost data are used, they underestimate the cost of medical care in current terms unless they are adjusted for inflation. The methods section of most research papers states the year in which all costs were obtained, and electronic datasets always indicate the year for which the data were collected.

TIPS AND TRICKS

The examples presented here are for the United States, but students (or researchers) from any other country can follow along. A search engine should quickly get you to your relevant national consumer price index (CPI) page.

To inflate older cost data in the United States, visit the U.S. Bureau of Labor Statistics home page (http://www.bls.gov/cpi/home.htm). Under "Latest Numbers," you should see a graphic of a green dinosaur (an icon for all things old). If you click on the little green guy, you get historical cost data. Consumer prices in general (CPI-U for Consumer Price Index for Urban Consumers) are valued differently from medical prices. Medical care prices tend to go up more quickly than consumer prices, so these costs should be inflated independent of consumer costs in any cost-effectiveness analysis.

After clicking on the dinosaur icon on the Bureau of Labor Statistics web site, you should be presented with a table listing the changes in the price of medical care over the years you requested. The annual changes in medical inflation between 2004 and 2014 for the United States appear in Table 4.5.

It is important to remember that these figures might not apply to a specific treatment or disease. For example, new drugs that were introduced to the U.S. market in 1996 greatly reduced the mortality rates for HIV in developed countries but also had a large impact on the cost of care. Thus, a study on the cost-effectiveness of an intervention to treat HIV that used 1998 data would likely produce a dramatically different result than if data from two years earlier were used. Therefore, simply adjusting these costs for inflation would not suffice.

Table 4.5   Medical Component of the Consumer Price Index 2004–2014, Annual Percentage Change over Previous Year

Year	Percentage Change
2004	4.4
2005	4.2
2006	4.0
2007	4.4
2008	3.7
2009	3.2
2010	3.4
2011	3.0
2012	3.7
2013	2.5
2014	2.4

TIPS AND TRICKS

If you save tabular data from web sites with an .htm extension (regardless of your browser or operating system), you should be able to open the table in a spreadsheet program.

Exercise 6

6. You are conducting a study on a new modality to prevent heart disease but need the cost of a doctor's visit to complete your analysis. You find a study from 2011, but other data you are using are from 2014. Inflate the cost of this $100 ambulatory medical visit in 2011 to 2014 dollars using Table 4.5.

Discounting Future Costs

Medical interventions, especially preventive interventions, often result in decreased future medical costs that must be accounted for in present-day terms. Humans have a tendency to place a lower value on future events than on events that occur in the present. This phenomenon is called **discounting**. For example, if someone were to offer you $100 today or $103 a year from now, you would probably forgo the extra $3 to have the money in your pocket today.

If you wait for a payment, you may never get it. The person giving out the money might not be able to pay it in a year, or, as the receiver, you might die before you have a chance to spend it. Of course, there are other reasons that people wish to have things immediately rather than in the future, one being simple human impatience.

If you were willing to wait one year to receive an extra $3 on an investment of $100, you would earn 3 percent by waiting ($100 × 1.03 per year = $103). Imagine that you were ambivalent about whether to accept $103 a year from now or $100 today. Imagine also that you were certain that you would not be willing to accept either $99 today or $102 a year from now rather than $100 today. If $103 is the minimum amount you'll accept in one year, your time preference is said to be 3 percent (Olsen, Kvien, & Uhlig, 2012). **Time preference** refers to the discount rate that a person places on future expenditures.

If $3 is the minimum interest you'll accept, the value of $103 delivered one year into the future is equal to $100 today. This $100 is the net present value, or the value of $103 in future earnings discounted into present terms at a 3 percent rate of discount. By discounting all future costs into their present-day terms, we are accounting for the human tendency to place a lower value on future earnings. Economists call this net present value the purchasing power of the dollar at the present time. The face value of $100 will not have the same purchasing power one year from now. Therefore, adjusting for this using the discounting approach will provide us with the correct purchasing power in today's terms. Recall that in Chapter 3 we introduced the analytical (or time) horizon, which can extend beyond one year. Cost-effectiveness studies that have an analytical horizon that is greater than one year will need to discount future costs.

EXHIBIT 4.2. CAN AN ECONOMIC CRISIS REDUCE THE VALUE OF HUMAN LIFE?

The monetary value of life is determined partially by the economic contributions of those within a given society. In the United States, households were worth a lot less in 2010 than they were in 2006. Economic theory is clear that this should mean that the economic value of human life also declined in that period. Yet health economists just went ahead and kept inflating the value of QALYs during that period. Why? Well, there are at least two possible explanations. One is that it is really disruptive to the inflationary standards we have set in health economics (a discount rate of 3 percent and inflation linked to the consumer price index). Making changes would create a bit of chaos and havoc. The second possible explanation is that humans are complex critters. It is difficult for us to value human life at all (thus, the reason of existence for cost-effectiveness analysis rather than cost-benefit analysis). Devaluing human life is more difficult to accept still.

When to Use Discounting

Most cost-effectiveness analyses contain future costs. If a treatment for diabetes or high blood pressure prevents hospitalizations that occur more than one year into the future, these costs should be discounted. In fact, in cost-effectiveness analysis, all future cost and effectiveness values must be discounted into their net present value (Gold et al., 1996; Neumann et al., 2016).

The Panel on Cost-Effectiveness in Health and Medicine bases the recommended discount rate on a valuation that is roughly equal to the real rate of return on government bonds (Gold et al., 1996; Neumann et al., 2016). Because this rate varies over time and the reference case is concerned with making all cost-effectiveness analyses comparable, the panel has settled on a rate of 3 percent. Although this rate was set to be reevaluated in 2006, no action was taken in that year. One participant predicted that the 3 percent rate would not change for the foreseeable future (J. Lipscomb, personal communication, March 28, 2006).

To maintain comparability with older cost-effectiveness analyses and make sure that the results of studies conducted in the present will still be useful in the future, the Panel on Cost-Effectiveness in Health and Medicine also recommends that the study results be presented with a range of discount rates. This is a form of sensitivity analysis, which we will discuss more in Chapter 9.

Internationally, many studies use a discount rate of 5 percent (Drummond, Sculpher, Torrance, O'Brien, & Stoddart, 2005). However, standards vary from country to country.

How to Use Discounting

The general formula for discounting future costs is:

$$\text{Discounted cost} = \frac{\text{Cost of the future event}}{(1 + \text{discount rate})^{\text{years in the future}}} \qquad (4.2)$$

For example, if the hypertensive person in the preceding example were to suffer a stroke 10 years into the future and was hospitalized at a cost of $10,000, the cost of the hospitalization 10 years down the line in present-day terms at the standard discount rate of 3 percent would be:

$$\$10,000/(1.03)^{10} = \$7,441 \tag{4.3}$$

TIPS AND TRICKS

Variations in your start time will affect the estimated future value. For instance, if you find that the cost of hospitalization for tonsillitis in 2007 is $12,000, the future value will vary depending on whether the $12,000 figure was obtained January 1, 2007, or June 1, 2007. If the latter, then the discounted cost on January 1, 2008, would be $12,000/(1.03)^{0.5} = \$11,824$ rather than $12,000/(1.03)^1 = \$11,650$.

Let us give a more practical example of how this formula is used. Suppose that we find that the average elderly person with high blood pressure has a hospitalization cost of $10,000 per year. If we know that the average person in an elderly cohort will live 10 years, the total hospitalization costs and discounted hospitalization costs (at the standard 3 percent rate) might assume the form of Table 4.6.

In Table 4.6, we see that the ten-year total cost comes to around $88,000, or about $12,000 less than it would have had the figures not been discounted. As with Table 4.5, this assumes that the first

Table 4.6   Hypothetical and Discounted Costs of a Cohort of 1,000 Elderly Persons over 10 Years

Year	Time (1)	Total Cost per Person (2)	Discounted Cost (3):Col. 2 /(1.03)$^{\text{Col. 1}}$
2006	0	$10,000	$10,000
2007	1	$10,000	$9,709
2008	2	$10,000	$9,426
2009	3	$10,000	$9,151
2010	4	$10,000	$8,885
2011	5	$10,000	$8,626
2012	6	$10,000	$8,375
2013	7	$10,000	$8,131
2014	8	$10,000	$7,894
2015	9	$10,000	$7,664
Total			**$87,861**

hospitalization charge occurred at the end of the year. Had it occurred at the start of the year, we would have discounted the original $10,000 as well.

The general formula for discounting a cost over many years is:

$$\text{Present value cost} = \sum_{t}^{T} \frac{C_y}{1.03^{y-1}} \qquad (4.4)$$

where T is the mean number of years of life remaining in the cohort, and C_y is the cost for year y.

Costs Associated with Pain and Suffering

One way to think about the costs associated with pain, suffering (morbidity costs), and death (mortality costs) is that they are intangible. **Intangible costs** are perceived costs that do not have a market value. In the reference case scenario, intangible costs are captured in the HRQL score and are therefore counted in the denominator of the cost-effectiveness ratio.

Recall from Chapter 2 that these intangible costs are not actually dollar costs, but rather are measured in terms of changes in health and longevity.

One of the things that the second Panel on Cost-Effectiveness Analysis emphasizes is that health policies often have non-health impacts. If we are going to screen everyone for colorectal cancer with colonoscopy, then there may be a lot more medical waste generated than if we collectively decide not to. After all, we are asking people to go to the doctor's office and get a procedure that requires a lot of preparation gowns, gauze, gloves, and so forth. These costs should be considered when they are likely to add up to more than a rounding error in your analysis.

TIPS AND TRICKS

Some students go crazy thinking about the second Panel on Cost-Effectiveness in Health and Medicine: Why would anyone want to change a set of standards? After all, the whole point of a standard is to make analyses comparable. If you change these standards, the old analyses become worthless. Our tip for the day: "Don't think about it." The new recommendations won't affect the comparability of most analyses by too much. And they do help by creating a more standardized way of building models and of presenting information.

But what happens when the "side effects" of a policy not only impacts economic, dollar value costs, but also impact health? We might want to include these improvements in health in the denominator of our incremental cost-effectiveness ratio. When the lives of women of reproductive age are saved, it can have large impacts on the educational attainment (and thus the health) of their children. While such costs may or may not be relevant, they should at least be thought about and discussed by your research team. For example, a cost-effectiveness analysis of a cervical cancer vaccine might include improved educational attainment for the girl's future children (after she becomes a woman and a mother who would otherwise have died.) This is not as trivial as it sounds. Educational attainment can produce huge health impacts over the life course of such children.

Finally, we would like to remind you of a point made in Chapter 2. That is that earlier recommendations from the Panel on Cost-Effectiveness in Health and Medicine suggested that lost productivity and leisure time costs not be included in the numerator of the analysis. They came to this conclusion because they were worried that HRQL captures some of these costs, and including them in the numerator would amount to double counting. The second Panel on Cost-Effectiveness in Health and Medicine reversed course and suggested that they be included in the numerator. These costs can be big. One paper found that a wellness program paid for itself by increasing worker productivity (Gubler, Larken, and Pierce, 2017).

Time costs are those costs associated with the time a patient spends receiving a medical intervention or medical care. Similarly, if a caregiver or any other person must spend time away from day-to-day activities as a result of the intervention or the disease under study, the time should also be included as a cost.

Time costs are almost always determined using micro-costing techniques, usually by multiplying the time spent in treatment by the mean wage of the subjects under study.

The time in transit to a medical clinic can be found in published cost-effectiveness analyses or assumed. In industrialized nations, time in transit will be different for less serious

---

TIPS AND TRICKS

In order to find out the mean time spent with a physician based on specialty, go to the NAMCS web site at http://www.cdc.gov/nchs/ahcd/ahcd_products.htm. Select the year 2010. You will find different PDF files arranged by the year they were analyzed. Look for the 2010 NAMCS report and select NAMCS Summary Table. Download and open the summary table and find table 28, which is entitled, "Mean time spent with physician, by physician specialty: United States, 2010." You will see the mean time that patients spent with their physicians along with the standard error (SE), 25th, 50th (median), and 75th percentile. For instance, the mean time spent with a urologist in the ambulatory care setting was 18.9 minutes with an SE of 0.9 minutes.

conditions and diseases than for those requiring specialty medical care. When people in wealthy nations seek specialty care, such as care for cancer, they often want the best possible care available, so many travel long distances to well-known clinics (Secker-Walker, Vacek, Hooper, Plante, & Detsky, 1999).

In developing nations, patient time costs can be quite small because mean wages can be very low relative to the cost of the medical care they receive. Nonetheless, people who live in rural areas may have to travel for days to reach the nearest medical facility. Because data are not usually available in the developing context, costs nearly always have to be estimated. However, locals tend to have a good sense of how long the trip will take. Therefore, a qualitative assessment of travel times by the folks you are evaluating may serve as a good proxy for hard data.

The duration of physician contact by disease and physician specialty is available from the National Ambulatory Medical Care Survey (NAMCS) (http://www.cdc.gov/nchs/ahcd/ahcd_products.htm); however, this does not include an estimate of the time a patient spends waiting in the office. During the preparation of this text, the most recent NAMCS report was from 2010. According to the report, the mean contact time with a physician in an ambulatory setting was 20.8 minutes.

You calculated the average length of stay in Exercise 3. The average length of stay is, of course, a good estimator of the time a patient spends in the hospital.

Practically speaking, the wage that a person earns provides a good estimate of the opportunity cost of a patient's time or a caregiver's time. When the patient is not paid, the wage of an equivalent job may be used. For instance, an unpaid parent's time may be valued at a housekeeper's wage. (For a comprehensive list of earnings by profession, visit http://www.bls.gov/bls/wages.htm.)

Problems arise in valuing a person's time when the study focuses on women or minority populations. African Americans earn less than whites, and women earn less than men. In addition to the fact that the lower wages paid to these groups may not reflect the true opportunity cost of their labor, there is a strong ethical argument to be made that everyone's time be valued equally.

Consider, for instance, valuing the time spent receiving cancer screening. If a homemaker's wage is $8 per hour and an associate in a law firm pulls in $240 per hour, we might find that cancer screening is cost-effective only if administered to homemakers.

In theory, interventions targeted to African Americans or other minority groups or interventions targeted toward women (for example, screening mammography) should be calculated using both average wages and the wages of the group of interest. The difference in the wages between these groups can be seen as a type of systematic error in the way society values human labor, and this error can be tested in a sensitivity analysis. In practice, most researchers use the median wage for a given society and apply it to everyone.

Assessing the "Relevancy" of Cost Data

While it is important to identify all costs included in a cost-effectiveness analysis, we need only measure, valuate, and include those costs that are likely to be relevant to the analysis (Gold et al., 1996; Neumann et al., 2016). But what does *relevant* mean? In this section, we review some of the important points to consider when evaluating cost data for its relevancy.

Consider Guillain-Barré syndrome, a potentially fatal neurological complication of influenza vaccination. Approximately 1 in 1 million people who receive the vaccine may develop this condition. Of those who develop it, about 6 percent will die (Lasky et al., 1998). Although these numbers are small, it is not clear whether the cost of this condition will be relevant. This syndrome may require extended hospitalization and, in some cases, long-term care. We can estimate the impact of Guillain-Barré syndrome by using previously published studies. The estimated cost of Guillain-Barré syndrome is $194,355 (adjusted for 2013 $US), which is based on an influenza epidemic model (Meltzer, Cox, & Fukuda, 1999). Further, a study by Lavelle and colleagues reported that Guillain-Barré syndrome due to pandemic H1N1 influenza vaccination is associated with a median QALY loss of 0.0019 based on a survey evaluating community values (Lavelle, Meltzer, Gebremariam, Lamarand, Fiore, & Prosser, 2011).

The cost of Guillain-Barré in a cost-effectiveness analysis is, of course, dependent on the probability of incurring the cost. The probability of incurring the cost is 1 in 1 million. Therefore, the total cost will be $0.000001 \times \$194,355 | = \$0.19$. If the overall cost of the vaccination strategy is $10, a cost of 19 cents amounts to a rounding error. The impact on QALYs would also be quite small.

Other Cost Considerations

Sometimes it's necessary to evaluate the cost-effectiveness of the way things are done in an institution rather than conduct a simple comparison of diseases. At other times, the cost-effectiveness analysis may have such a large impact on medical care utilization nationwide that one must consider changes in the efficiency of large institutions. Finally, theoretical concerns sometimes arise when a given health intervention produces a marked increase in human life expectancy. In this section, we first discuss a framework for thinking about when costs need to be measured and then look at cost considerations that come up less frequently in cost-effectiveness analysis.

Measuring Changes in Costs

If we are measuring the cost of vaccination at IBM, we don't care what the market value of IBM is; we are concerned only with how much money will be spent on adding a vaccination program. In short, we are concerned only with costs that change as a result of the intervention. Because cost-effectiveness analyses measure changes in costs, it is important to be able to identify which costs change when an intervention is undertaken and which costs do not. In this section, you will learn how to think about the dynamic and static properties of costs.

Costs that change when a medical intervention is applied are referred to as **variable costs**. When Sandra Montero visited the company clinic, she exposed others to the influenza virus. She also took up some of the secretary's time, the medical assistant's time, and the doctor's time. Her decision to visit the company clinic therefore consumed resources that would not otherwise have been consumed, and each of the resources is an example of a variable cost.

Fixed costs are costs that do not change because of a health intervention. Whether Sandra had visited the clinic or had gone directly home, the janitors would have to clean the clinic at the end of the day, the rent would have to be paid, and so on. Administration, maintenance, medical equipment, computers, and other things that would have been bought with or without the existence of influenza patients are examples of fixed costs and should generally not be included in the analysis.

Of course, there are exceptions to this rule. Suppose that the company instituted an influenza vaccination policy that resulted in a dramatic drop in patient illnesses and visits to the clinic. The administration might choose to reduce the clinic's hours of operation to compensate for the lighter volume or even to close the clinic altogether. In this instance, the intervention (influenza vaccination) would have had a significant impact on the consumption of resources that might otherwise have been considered "fixed." If an intervention results in sufficient changes in patient volume to cause changes in staffing levels or changes in the wear and tear on medical equipment, or (conversely) merits purchasing new equipment, these changes should be accounted for if they are likely to be relevant for the analysis.

When to Use Micro-Costing

In some hospitals, when a patient comes into the emergency room with a stroke, the doctors must order medications from the hospital pharmacy.

The order is often written on the patient's chart and subsequently sent to the pharmacy for review before it is dispensed. Although this sequence of events is generally expedited in emergencies, it can still take considerable time, because the pharmacy may be located in a different part of the hospital.

It is conceivable that by the time the order is completely processed and the medication becomes available in the emergency room, the patient may have suffered serious damage from the stroke. We may therefore wish to evaluate an intervention that improves the way that emergency medications are supplied within the hospital. Since this involves shuffling around micro-costs, it is nearly impossible to conduct such an analysis using gross costing methods.

For instance, suppose that the intervention is to simply make these lifesaving medications available in the emergency room. This would greatly reduce the time required to get the medication to the patient. However, when medication dispensing is not tightly regulated and is administered emergently, dosing errors occur more often. Because the pharmacist is not overseeing the transaction, it is also possible that the wrong medication may be administered. A cost-effectiveness analysis examining this issue might assist hospital administrators in deciding whether it is better to keep these medications in the pharmacy or have them available in the emergency room. Clearly, the overall cost of a hospitalization for stroke is going to do very little to help us out with this analysis.

Micro-costing should be used when the cost-effectiveness analysis is centered on changes in the way the resource is delivered. Micro-costing is also useful when a particular cost is not available in the medical literature or electronic data. For example, in our influenza study, we won't have an estimate of the cost of side effects to vaccination, so we will need to micro-cost these events. Micro-costing may also more closely estimate the opportunity cost of medical goods and services (Gold et al., 1996; Neumann et al., 2016).

The major disadvantages of micro-costing are that it requires a lot of work, costs can be missed, and the costs you do get often lack **external validity**. External validity refers to the extent to which the results of a study are generalizable to settings other than the one in which the data were collected. For instance, if we obtained the cost of a vaccine from New York City, it might not reflect the cost of a vaccine in Tulsa, Oklahoma. This is especially a problem in analyses using data across developing countries, where the cost of a drug, laboratory test, or medical services can vary by tenfold from one country to another. (Recall from Chapter 3 the variation in medical and hospital prices by country based on the report from the International Federation of Health Plans [2013].)

Micro-costing is also resource intensive, especially when applied to complex costs, such as the cost of hospitalization. Unless one uses administrative systems designed to measure resource consumption, it is also easy to miss important costs.

Friction Costs and Transfer Payments

Within the context of cost-effectiveness analysis, *friction costs* are incurred when an intervention increases administrative expenses. One example is when absenteeism or unemployment rates increase because of illness. Such costs can usually be excluded from a cost-effectiveness analysis because they tend to be very small relative to other costs. In those rare instances in which an intervention is expected to have a very large impact on administrative costs at a worksite or in a government agency, researchers should consider including friction costs in their analysis (Gold et al., 1996; Neumann et al., 2016).

Transfer payments are payments made from one entity to another as part of a social contract, such as social security payments. For instance, workers pay into the social security system with the expectation that the money will be returned to them when they retire. In this instance, the money is transferred from workers' paychecks to the government and is then transferred back from the government to the worker at a later date. The only resources consumed when transfer payments are made are the friction costs of administering such programs. Therefore, only the friction costs associated with transfer payments need to be included in a cost-effectiveness analysis. And even then, they need to be included only if they will be sufficiently large to merit their inclusion.

Savings Associated with Premature Death

While future medical costs can be reduced by a successful health intervention, they can also be lowered as a result of a premature death. If an intervention is effective at reducing the severity of a disease, then future ambulatory care, hospitalization, and medication costs will all likely be lower among those who received the intervention. However, future medical costs will also be lower if someone dies prematurely from an accident or some other unfortunate event.

Typically, such costs are lower than wages, so death is often economically undesirable if it happens to a young person. But if we count savings in future medical costs for someone who dies around the age of retirement, it can seem as if death is desirable from an economic standpoint (Gold et al., 1996; Neumann et al., 2016; Economist Group, 2003). For example, one study found that smokers actually save society money because they tend to die at a relatively young age, while nonsmokers tend to develop chronic diseases later in life and rack up huge medical bills (Barendregt,

Bonneux, & van der Maas, 1997). Moreover, the SARS outbreak of 2003 did not create widespread economic panic in part because it disproportionately affects the elderly (Economist Group, 2003). This then raises the question: If premature death is associated with a reduction in future medical costs, should these savings be included in a cost-effectiveness analysis?

The Panel on Cost-Effectiveness in Health and Medicine decided to put its theoretical concerns aside and allow researchers to exclude these future medical costs among survivors from the analysis. However, if future medical costs are likely to have a large impact on the analysis, the panel recommends that these costs be tested in a sensitivity analysis. This way, the analysis can be compared with studies that do not include such costs. Future medical costs are available using electronic data sources, such as MEPS.

Summary

Cost is an essential variable for cost-effectiveness analysis. Without it, you can't perform any economic research. Identifying the costs you need is based on what type of analysis you perform (CEA or CBA) and the perspective you take (payer or societal). A CEA does not include the cost of lives lost, but a CBA does. A payer level includes only the cost of medical care itself and other social and clinical services (ranging from the cost of the ambulance to the cost of time in a rehabilitation center), because that is all the payers have to pay for. The societal perspective, which is recommended as the primary perspective for CEA, includes all costs.

To sort out costs, the student must think about what happens to people who have a particular disease. Those with a heart attack tend to come into the hospital by ambulance. The emergency department visit and the hospital visit will include all of the medical costs while the person is in the hospital. But it won't include all of the time that the poor guy loses from work and leisure. Once out of the hospital, the person may undergo rehabilitation. While all of the drug costs incurred as an inpatient are included in the hospital billing data (for example, DRG codes are associated with diagnosis and can be found in the CMS MEDPAR database), they are not included in the outpatient data. So you need to add these costs separately.

Different sources of data present costs in different ways. As a general rule, you want to make sure that you are comfortable with using a source that you are familiar with or can trust. Certain data contain charges to the patients rather than the actual cost of delivering care. In order to figure out the costs, you will need to apply a cost-to-charge ratio factor to the charges. For instance, if you are interested in the cost-effectiveness of an intervention for a payer, the cost is more relevant than the charge to the patient. Therefore, you will need to use a cost-to-charge ratio factor to estimate the cost to the payer.

Once you have your costs, then you will need to think about the effects of time such as discounting and inflation. Future costs will need to be discounted because the value of a dollar today is greater than a year from now. Conversely, the value of a dollar a year ago needs to be inflated to the present value of the dollar today. Making these adjustments gives decision makers an idea of the net present value of the interventions.

Further Readings

Students interested in further discussions on how productivity costs are calculated for use in cost-effectiveness analysis are encouraged to read papers by Brouwer and Koopmanschap (2005) and van den Hout (2010).

Curtiss and colleagues (Curtiss, Lettrich, & Fairman, 2010) wrote a great article about the different pharmaceutical drug price benchmarks available. In it, they provide a short history of legal issues surrounding AWP and the aftermath of the settlement. Students can also browse the CMS web site for the NADAC, which contains the costs files for prescription drugs (http://www.wiley.com/WileyCDA/WileyTitle/productCd-1119011264.html).

Students are also encouraged to explore the Bureau of Labor and Statistics (BLS) web site to find out the salaries of different health professionals (http://www.bls.gov/bls/blswage.htm). Students will also find the calculator for adjusting for inflation on the BLS web site useful for their work (http://data.bls.gov/cgi-bin/cpicalc.pl).

References

Barendregt, J. J., L. Bonneux, and P. J. van der Maas. (1997). The Health Care Costs of Smoking. *New England Journal of Medicine* 337(15): 1052–1057. http://doi.org/10.1056/NEJM199710093371506.

Brouwer, W. B. F., and M. A. Koopmanschap. (2005). The Friction-Cost Method: Replacement for Nothing and Leisure for Free? *PharmacoEconomics* 23(2): 105–111.

Centers for Medicare & Medicaid Services. (2014a, October 30). Medicare Fee for Service for Parts A & B. Retrieved March 23, 2015, from http://www.cms.gov/Research-Statistics-Data-and-Systems/Statistics-Trends-and-Reports/MedicareFeeforSvcPartsAB/.

Centers for Medicare & Medicaid Services. (2014b, December 8). The Medicare Part B Drug and Biological Average Sales Price Quarterly Payment Files (2014). Retrieved January 11, 2015, from http://www.cms.gov/Medicare/Medicare-Fee-for-Service-Part-B-Drugs/McrPartBDrugAvgSalesPrice/2014ASPFiles.html.

Centers for Medicare & Medicaid Services. (2015). Pharmacy Drug Pricing. Retrieved March 24, 2015, from http://www.medicaid.gov/Medicaid-CHIP-Program-Information/By-Topics/Benefits/Prescription-Drugs/Pharmacy-Pricing.html.

Curtiss, F. R., P. Lettrich, and K. A. Fairman. (2010). What Is the Price Benchmark to Replace Average Wholesale Price (AWP)? *Journal of Managed Care Pharmacy* 16(7): 492–501.

Drummond, M. F., M. J. Sculpher, G. W. Torrance, B. J. O'Brien, and G. L. Stoddart. (2005). *Methods for the Economic Evaluation of Health Care Programmes,* 3rd ed. New York: Oxford University Press.

Economist Group. (2003, April 10). Epidemics and Economics. *The Economist.* Retrieved from http://www.economist.com/node/1698814.

Gold, M. R., J. E. Siegel, L. B. Russell, and M. C. Weinstein. (1996). *Cost-Effectiveness in Health and Medicine.* New York: Oxford University Press.

Gubler, T., I. Larken, and L. Pierce. Doing Well by Making Well: The Impact of Corporate Wellness Programs on Employee Productivity. Available online at: https://papers.ssrn.com/sol3/papers.cfm?abstract_id=2811785. Accessed 8/21/17.

Horsman, J., W. Furlong, D. Feeny, and G. Torrance. (2003). The Health Utilities Index (HUI®): Concepts, Measurement Properties and Applications. *Health and Quality of Life Outcomes* 1, 54. http://doi.org/10.1186/1477-7525-1-54.

Kolata, G. (2001). Medical Fees Are Often Higher for Patients Without Insurance. *New York Times on the Web,* A1, A13.

Lasky, T., G. J. Terracciano, L. Magder, C. L. Koski, M. Ballesteros, D. Nash, . . . R. T. Chen. (1998). The Guillain-Barré Syndrome and the 1992–1993 and 1993–1994 Influenza Vaccines. *New England Journal of Medicine* 339(25): 1797–1802. http://doi.org/10.1056/NEJM199812173392501.

Lavelle, T. A., M. I. Meltzer, A. Gebremariam, K. Lamarand, A. E. Fiore, and L. A. Prosser. (2011). Community-Based Values for 2009 Pandemic Influenza A H1N1 Illnesses and Vaccination-Related Adverse Events. *PLoS ONE* 6(12): e27777. http://doi.org/10.1371/journal.pone.0027777.

Meltzer, M. I., N. J. Cox, and K. Fukuda. (1999). The Economic Impact of Pandemic Influenza in the United States: Priorities for Intervention. *Emerging Infectious Diseases* 5(5): 659–671. http://doi.org/10.3201/eid0505.990507.

Muennig, P., P. Franks, H. Jia, E. Lubetkin, and M. R. Gold. (2005). The Income-Associated Burden of Disease in the United States. *Social Science & Medicine* 61(9): 2018–2026. http://doi.org/10.1016/j.socscimed.2005.04.005.

Neumann, P. J., G. D. Sanders, L. B. Russell, J. E. Siegel, and T. G. Ganiats. (2016). *Cost-Effectiveness in Health and Medicine.* New York: Oxford University Press.

Olsen, I. C., T. K. Kvien, and T. Uhlig. (2012). Consequences of Handling Missing Data for Treatment Response in Osteoarthritis: A Simulation Study. *Osteoarthritis and Cartilage/OARS, Osteoarthritis Research Society* 20(8): 822–828. http://doi.org/10.1016/j.joca.2012.03.005.

Secker-Walker, R. H., P. M. Vacek, G. J. Hooper, D. A. Plante, and A. S. Detsky. (1999). Screening for Breast Cancer: Time, Travel, and Out-of-Pocket Expenses. *Journal of the National Cancer Institute* 91(8): 702–708.

Van den Hout, W. B. (2010). The Value of Productivity: Human-Capital Versus Friction-Cost Method. *Annals of the Rheumatic Diseases* 69(Suppl. 1): 189–191. http://doi.org/10.1136/ard.2009.117150.

CHAPTER 5

PROBABILITIES AND DECISION ANALYSIS MODELS

Overview

If cost-effectiveness analysis were a building, probabilities would be its scaffolding. Probabilities indicate how likely subjects are to become ill, how likely subjects are to see a doctor, and so on. Therefore, they provide a framework for deciding how much an intervention will cost and how effective it will be.

A decision analysis model is essentially a series of values (such as costs or HRQL scores) bound together by a series of probabilities. In this chapter, you will get a general overview of probabilities and then begin the process of learning how they tie together to form a decision analysis model.

The Idea Behind Decision Analysis

Imagine that you have $100,000 to invest. You've always wanted to study public health, but you've also dreamed about writing a novel. If you write a novel, you reason, you can simply invest the money in a mutual fund and earn interest, making small withdrawals as needed. Since you are undecided between the two options, you examine which will be the better option financially. Decision analysis is a tool for making decisions using statistical probabilities.

Decision analysis is based on a concept called **expected value,** in which the value of an uncertain event (such as making $10,000 in the stock market) is weighed against the chances that the event will occur. For example, if you know that the historical average increase in a particular mutual fund is 10 percent per year, then the expected value of the

LEARNING OBJECTIVES

- Define the term *expected value.*

- Contrast the expected payoffs with the expected value.

- Describe how probabilities work in decision analysis models.

- List the basic components of a decision analysis model.

- Calculate the expected value for a treatment strategy.

- Determine, based on the expected costs and expected probabilities, what the most cost-effective strategy is.

return on your $100,000 investment is 0.1 × $100,000 = $10,000 over one year.

In decision models, the expected value is calculated for each chance node and compared to a competing chance node. This provides us with a comparison of the expected value for two different strategies. Later in this chapter we will show you how to calculate the expected value for two different strategies: Vaccinated and Not Vaccinated (Supportive Care).

For now, let's return to the previous example of writing a book or attending a public health school. You set your sights five years down the road and assume that if you go to a public health school, all of the $100,000 would be spent on your education after living expenses are taken into account, but you would be able to earn about $50,000 per year working in public health after graduation. After taxes and living expenses, you estimate that you would save about $10,000 over the three years after graduation (this is your payoff for choosing to go to a public health school).

If you decide to write a novel, you will have spent your $100,000, along with the interest on the mutual fund, on living expenses over the five-year period. If you publish the novel, you could earn an additional $30,000 (payoff). Your college English professor advises you that there is about a 1 percent chance that you will be published. Therefore, the "invest and write" option will produce a return (or expected payoff) of $30,000 × 0.01 = $300. The expected payoff is the average weighted payoff for a specific event pathway of a particular strategy. The **expected value** is the sum of the expected payoffs for a particular strategy. In this example, the expected value for writing a novel is $300 ($300 + $0). Figure 5.1 illustrates a decision tree model based on this scenario.

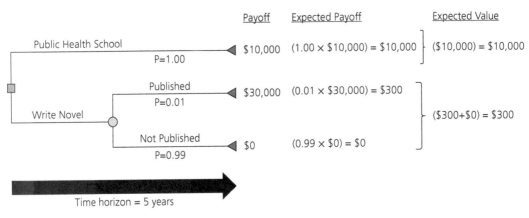

Figure 5.1   Decision Tree for Whether to Pursue Public Health School or Write a Novel

Since $10,000 is more than $300, you might go for the career in public health. However, you might not be satisfied with your calculations. There is a chance that the mutual fund could do very well, but there is also a chance that you could lose money. If it does well, you could end up with leftover money from your mutual fund investment at the end of five years. So if you write the book, you might make money even if you don't publish. But if the mutual fund loses money, you might not be able to finish your novel, which would be quite depressing.

There is also a chance that you will not find a job right out of public health school (Figure 5.2). Using a decision analysis model, you can estimate the ranges of possible earnings (or expected values) associated with each decision at the end of the five-year period. Ideally, you would want a rough idea not only of the average earnings associated with each decision, but also the chance that you will end up in the gutter with a bottle of wine if you choose one over the other. This way, not only will you have a better idea of which decision is riskier, but you'll also know the chances of a very bad outcome.

In Figure 5.2, the probability of finding a job is reduced to 50 percent. However, the expected value for going to a public health school is $5,000 ($5,000 + $0), which is still larger than the expected value of writing a book ($300). Therefore, based on these probabilities, it would be a wise decision to enroll in a public health school rather than write a book.

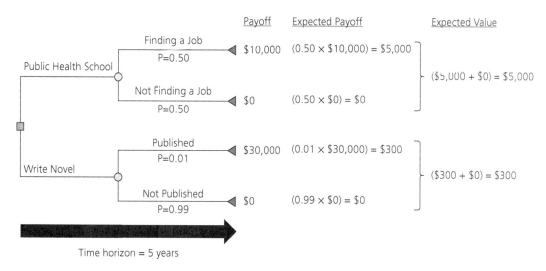

Figure 5.2   Decision Tree with the Potential for Not Finding a Job After Public Health School

So far, we've managed to develop our research question and have created a basic chart outlining what we need to do to finish our analysis. We've also taken the first step toward understanding cost data, so we now have a rough understanding of how to work with the costs that go into each box in an event pathway.

Now, let's imagine that we've dug through the medical literature and datasets and found the probabilities and costs needed to estimate the expected value for each strategy outlined in the vaccination model discussed earlier. In this chapter, we'll see how to combine costs and probabilities and how to build a decision analysis model that actually tests these strategies to see which one is the most cost-effective.

Decision analysis models are powerful tools to influence policy decisions and clinical recommendations. They can assist policymakers on making recommendations in the face of little to no available evidence. However, they are also subject to the same level of scrutiny as a randomized clinical trial or similar study. In this chapter, you will learn how to develop a decision model and analyze its components in order to critique other models when making a decision about the cost-effectiveness of a particular treatment strategy.

As you prepare to develop your own decision model, you will need to understand some of the concepts of probability. Don't worry if you've never had a course in probability. We will provide a brief introduction to the tools you'll need to successfully navigate and build your own decision models.

WHEN SHOULD MAMMOGRAPHY BE PERFORMED?

Recall the mammography example at the beginning of Chapter 1. In the 1980s, there was a lot of uncertainty about the benefit and harm of performing mammography in young women, especially those less than 50 years old. Mammography is an X-ray of the chest for the purpose of detecting breast cancer.

When a mammography is performed, there is a chance that false positive results may occur. Just as important, there is unnecessary radiation exposure and increased costs to the patient and healthcare system. On the other hand, mammography comes with a lot of potential benefits. These include early detection of breast cancer, reduced treatment costs, less morbidity, and decreased mortality from breast cancer. But the evidence for performing mammography in women less than 50 years old was limited and conflicting.

In order to address this problem, researchers used a mathematical model and integrated the evidence available at the time (Eddy, Hasselblad, McGivney, & Hendee, 1988). Mathematical models have been used in determining the probability of expected benefits (efficacy) and costs associated with a treatment decision. In this case, the decision was whether or not to start mammography on women who were 50 years old or less. In their conclusion, the authors recommended that women with average risk of breast cancer would benefit from clinical breast examination (but not mammography) annually starting at age 40 and mammography every one to two years starting at age 50. Women with high risk of breast cancer should have annual mammography starting at age 40.

The U.S. Preventive Services Task Force (USPSTF) made recommendations that reflected these findings; however, there were debates and concerns that these recommendations would miss detection of early breast cancer in women with average risk who were less than 50 years old. In 2009, the USPSTF updated their recommendation to no longer recommend annual mammography in women between 40 and 49 years old. They also recommended biennial mammography in women between 50 and 74 years. They felt that, among women age 75 years and older, the evidence on the benefits of biennial mammography is insufficient. The USPSTF came to these conclusions through a combination of a systematic review of the existing evidence and by using mathematical models.

Other organizations such as the American Cancer Society, National Cancer Institute, and the American College of Obstetricians and Gynecologists had similar recommendations for women 50 years or older. But they differed in when mammography should be started in women less than 50 years old. As a result, different recommendations have been provided by these different organizations. To this day, the USPSTF and other medical organizations continue to debate this issue.

Probabilities

Probability is the chance that a certain outcome will occur. It ranges between the values of 0 and 1. Zero indicates a 0 percent chance that something will occur, and 1 indicates a 100 percent chance that something will occur. How certain are we that an event will occur 100 percent of the time? We know that the sun will rise in the morning 100 percent of the time (ignoring the cosmic life span of the galaxy). So the probability of the sun rising tomorrow morning is almost 100 percent (and if it doesn't rise, this exercise doesn't matter anyway, so let's say 100 percent). However, we also know that the probability of winning the lotto is almost 0 percent (actually, if this were the California Lotto, the probability of winning is $1/175,223,510$ or 6×10^{-9}).

Probability is useful for describing uncertainty. In everyday life, we wrestle with an abundance of uncertainty. For example, what is the probability that the Los Angeles Dodgers will win the pennant this season?

Or what is the probability that you'll get a ticket for speeding? In an ideal world, we make decisions based on the probability that we believe to be true. In the case of the Dodgers winning the pennant, you may place a bet on them to win; or in the case of speeding, you may decide to speed if your chance of getting a ticket is very low. Probability has a funny way of determining how we behave and, ultimately, what kind of decisions we make.

In health care, there are large amounts of uncertainty with treatment decisions. Even though we profess to use evidence-based medicine for our decisions, the number of available (or unavailable) studies introduces varying degrees of uncertainty. In decision analysis, this uncertainty would be the probability of survival or death, cured or not cured, diseased or not diseased. Probabilities are generated through observations or studies. Sometimes, probabilities are derived through little more than beliefs.

Some Basic Rules of Probability

There are several important concepts you must remember when using probability in decision analysis models. The first is that events in a model branch must be *mutually exclusive* and *independent*. When two events are *mutually exclusive*, it means that one event cannot occur at the same time as the other event. For example, we have two events, survive or die. These two events are *mutually exclusive* because a person cannot be both at the same time (even if you are Schrödinger's cat). Another example of a *mutually exclusive event* is cured or not cured. These two events are *mutually exclusive* because they cannot possibly occur simultaneously in a single person. Figure 5.3 provides an illustration of two events that are mutually exclusive of one another. Notice that the two events do not overlap. After being treated with a Vaccine, the patient either Remains Well or Becomes Ill.

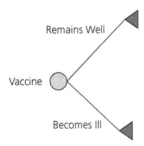

Figure 5.3   Example of Two *Mutually Exclusive* Events

BASIC COMPONENTS OF A DECISION ANALYSIS MODEL

Basic decision analysis models have four components: (1) a decision node (usually represented as a square), (2) branches (lines), (3) chance nodes (circles), and (4) terminal nodes (triangles). The decision node indicates which choices we wish to evaluate, the chance node indicates the probabilities of two or more possible events, and the terminal node indicates the end points we wish to evaluate.

Two events (Remains Well and Becomes Ill) are *independent* of one another if the probability of one event happening does not influence the probability of another event happening.

Suppose you are given a chance to select a random number from a hat (you cannot see what number you are selecting). The first time you reach inside the hat, you draw a number 5. You are instructed to return the number back into the hat and redraw a different number. You select 5 again. The probability of drawing a 5 the first time is the same as drawing a 5 again the second time. This is possible because you returned the number back into the hat; therefore, each time you draw a number, the probability of getting a number is *independent* of the first time you drew the number. (Unless you believe in psychic phenomena.)

If you were instructed not to return the number 5 back into the hat, then you would not be able to draw a 5 again (unless there was another 5 in the hat). This would mean that the probability of drawing a 5 after you already drew a 5 is 0 percent. Your probability of selecting 5 again is *dependent* on your drawing it in the first attempt. This is an example of an event being dependent on another event.

The concept of *mutually exclusive* and *independent* events will continue to be reintroduced in probability theory and decision analysis modeling. We will see more examples throughout the chapter.

Another important concept is the complement rule. If two events are *mutually exclusive, independent,* and result in only two outcomes, then the complement rule states that the probability of one event occurring and not occurring must sum up to 1. For example, a person can be Cured or Not Cured. Keep in mind that the sum of the probabilities must be 1 (or 100 percent). Therefore, if the probability of Cured is denoted by P, then the probability of Not Cured is denoted by $1 - P$. In other words, if the probability of Cured was 70 percent, then the probability of Not Cured must be 30 percent.

Another important rule of probability is the multiplicative rule of independent events. Under the multiplicative rule, the probability that two events will occur is the product of the probabilities of the individual events. For instance, if we were interested in the probability of both Event A and Event B occurring, we would multiply them together. This can also be described as P(A and B) = P(A) × P(B). In decision modeling, we use the probabilities of independent events as inputs in our model. Because of this, we will use the multiplicative rule of independent events to get the probability of each event pathway.

Applying the Rules

You are now ready to tackle some of the probabilities used in decision models. Don't worry if you are not familiar with all the rules. It's okay. We believe that there is a "high probability" that you will be comfortable with them after reading this chapter. For the purpose of this chapter, we will focus on only the ones presented above.

An event (or treatment) pathway is the cumulative experience that a patient or population goes through after a decision is made. In other words, it is the cumulative consequences that result after a decision is made. In Figure 5.3, the pathways a patient experiences after receiving a Vaccine can result in two different outcomes: Remains Well or Becomes Ill. However, that's not the end of the pathway. In Figure 5.4, the treatment pathway continues if a patient Becomes Ill. Patients can also Recover or See Doctor, indicating that the treatment pathway has consequences if the Vaccine intervention does not work. These event pathways have different probabilities.

In Figure 5.4, a patient is given a treatment intervention (Vaccine), which leads to one of the following two events: Remains Well or Becomes Ill.

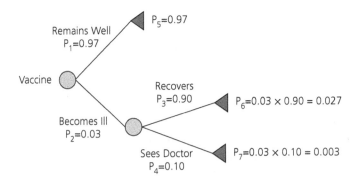

Figure 5.4   Probabilities of Outcomes for Patients Receiving the Vaccine Intervention

Suppose that the Vaccine had a probability of Remains Well that was 0.97 (or 97 percent). By the complement rule, the probability of Becomes Ill is 0.03 (or 3 percent). Suppose further that the probability that a patient Recovers is 0.90 (or 90 percent). We use the complement rule again to find the probability of Sees Doctor, which is 0.10 (or 10 percent).

Now we can calculate the probabilities for the different terminal nodes at P_6 and P_7. The probability that a patient who receives a Vaccine and Becomes Ill and Recovers is 2.7 percent ($0.03 \times 0.90 = 0.027$), which can also be written as $P_2 \times P_3 = P_6$. Similarly, the probability that a patient who receives a Vaccine and Becomes Ill and Sees Doctor is 0.3 percent ($0.03 \times 0.10 = 0.003$), which can also be written as $P_2 \times P_4 = P_7$.

Notice that all the probabilities of the treatment pathways sum up to 1 ($P_5 + P_6 + P_7 = 1$). This is a very useful and important check to make sure that you did your calculations correctly.

Congratulations! You now know how to calculate probabilities for terminal nodes. This is an important concept because future examples will use this to estimate the probabilities of multiple event pathways in a decision analysis model.

We will continue with our discussion of probability by providing you with an example to work through. Consider the vaccination example that has already been introduced. We will expand on this and include a different decision strategy whereby people are not vaccinated (Not Vaccinated). Then we will compare the two strategies using a decision tree model.

PROJECT MAP

1. Think through your research question.

2. Sketch out the analysis.

3. Collect data for your model.

4. Adjust your data.

5. *Build your model.*

6. Run and test the model.

7. Conduct a sensitivity analysis.

8. Write it up.

Decision Analysis Models

Imagine that you have captured the string of probabilities and outcomes possible for those who are vaccinated. For instance, the product of the chance of getting influenza and the cost of getting influenza is one in a string of costs and probabilities leading to the overall cost of influenza. The weighted mean value of all of those events added together is called an **event pathway**. An alternative way of representing an event pathway is with a **decision analysis model**. Decision analysis models are used to represent a visual, simplified version of the event pathway. It is considered simplified because the disease is broken down to its important components such as potential outcomes and consequences of treatment or intervention. A decision analysis model calculates the costs and QALYs associated with events in an event pathway at the same time.

The purpose of a decision model is to provide a simplified framework to answer the question "What treatment strategy is cost-effective?" But recall that we must also ask "For whom is this cost-effective?" Patients who are concerned about cost-effectiveness may be worried about the out-of-pocket cost for buying medications that were prescribed to them, transportation fees, opportunity costs of disease, and decreased quality of life. A healthcare payer may be more interested in the medical costs of the disease (of course, some payers would be more interested in their patients dying rather than remaining sick and racking up costs). Therefore, they would be interested in seeing which treatment strategy would result in the least amount of resources used but yield a high efficacy or benefit. Providers may be more interested in individual patient improvement rather than in monitoring costs. Therefore, providers are likely to prescribe and select treatment strategies that they believe are the best for their patients despite the costs (to the insurance company's dismay).

Recently, the Good Research Practices in Modeling Task Force, a collaboration between the International Society for Pharmacoeconomics and Outcomes Research (ISPOR) and the Society for Medical Decision Making (SMDM), created guidelines for the construction and assessment of decision analysis models.

We will highlight important elements of the guidelines by introducing them to you in this chapter. For readers who are interested in reading more about the guidelines, you can find them at the following web sites: http://www.ispor.org/taskforces/GRPModelingTf.asp or http://mdm .sagepub.com/content/32/5.toc.

A SHORT SUMMARY OF THE ISPOR/SMDM GOOD RESEARCH PRACTICES IN MODELING TASK FORCE REPORT

This is a condensed summary of the original version.

1. An important first step in developing a decision model is conceptualizing the problem. This step requires the investigator to consider the opinions of subject-matter experts and stakeholders to appropriately identify the problem.

2. The next step requires the investigators to identify the target population of interest, the time horizon (time when the appropriate benefits and costs should be measured), and the perspective of the analysis. The task force on Cost-Effectiveness in Health and Medicine recommends that the problem be based on societal perspective. However, if another perspective is used, then the investigators should disclose what benefits and costs were eliminated as a result.

3. Investigators should design the decision model based on the conceptualization of the problem and not by the available data. It is tempting to design a decision model based on the data at your disposal; however, you may miss important gaps or events that are critical to the study question of interest. Therefore, a balance between building a model based on the disease problem and the available data is needed in order to develop a model that is valid. This will be a challenge since head-to-head studies between several treatment strategies are often not readily available because they have not been performed.

4. Recall from Chapter 3 the importance of time. The *time horizon* for decision analysis models should be long enough to capture relevant events and outcomes but must also be based on the disease problem. The *time horizon* is the time that the model will run for and includes the point at which the treatment strategy was initiated through the time when the outcome of interest is measured. For example, if the decision model evaluated the cost-effectiveness of influenza vaccine efficacy, then the time horizon should be long enough to capture the influenza events and short enough to prevent other issues from creeping into the analysis. Influenza is seasonal, and a long time horizon (greater than one year) will not be very relevant because there are different influenza strains from year to year that affect the exposure-disease relationship. Therefore, an appropriate time horizon to study the effects of influenza vaccine is one year.

5. A sensitivity analysis should be performed to test the robustness of the model. Constructing a model will result in some uncertainty about the structure and parameters. Methods to test the effects of uncertainty on the results are presented in Chapter 9.

6. Transparency and validation of the model are necessary for other researchers to be able to replicate your findings. A technical appendix or supplement that contains details about

Let's return to our example from the beginning of this chapter. We have two competing strategies: Vaccinated or Not Vaccinated (Supportive Care). We want to know which strategy is cost-effective at preventing influenza in patients who are vaccinated or not vaccinated in a typical influenza season. Since a typical influenza season lasts one year, the time horizon of the decision analysis model will be set for one year. Let's assume that we are interested in the perspective of the healthcare payer. This means that the person who has to decide where to invest limited resources is interested in the treatment strategy that will provide the most "bang for the buck." In other words, which treatment strategy would be the most cost-effective in preventing influenza?

In Figure 5.5, we see a magnified view of the natural course of events for people who were not vaccinated (the Not Vaccinated arm in the diagram) at the start of influenza season. First, we need to know the probability that someone will become ill. Second, we need to know the probability that someone with the flu will stay at home rather than see a doctor. In Chapters 2 and 4, we mentioned that *not* seeing a doctor could be associated with costs (because the patient ends up getting sick and is hospitalized, or because the patient ends up infecting others) or savings (because the patient avoids the cost of the doctor's visit). For now, let's assume that staying at home does not cost or save any money.

In Figure 5.6 we see the vaccination side of the event pathway (Vaccine). The probabilities in this event pathway need to be specific to those who have received a vaccination. The vaccine not only alters the chance of becoming ill but also alters the chance of seeing a doctor or being hospitalized if the patient does become ill. (Recall that some people get a mild illness when exposed to the virus even though they were vaccinated.)

Now let's turn to costs. Let's assume that the cost of a doctor's visit or a hospitalization is similar between those who have and those who have not received a vaccination. Let's also assume that the cost of illness and hospitalization will be similar. The main difference is that everyone in the Vaccine arm gets a vaccination that costs $10, and the probability of getting

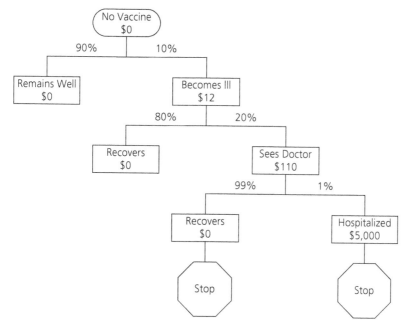

Figure 5.5   Course of Events During an Influenza Season Among Those Receiving Supportive Care Alone

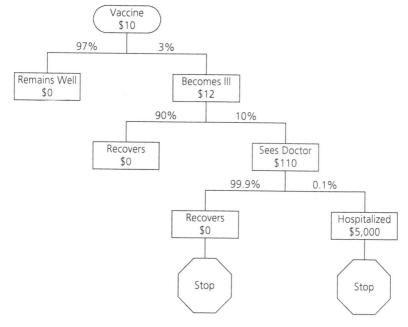

Figure 5.6   Course of Events During an Influenza Season Among Those Receiving a Vaccination

Table 5.1   Probabilities and Costs for Vaccinated and Not Vaccinated (Supportive Care) Strategies

	Vaccination		No Vaccination (Supportive Care)	
Parameter	Probability	Cost	Probability	Cost
Remains Well	0.97	$0	0.70	$0
Becomes Ill (includes OTC remedies)	0.03	$12	0.30	$12
Recovers	0.90	$0	0.80	$0
Sees Doctor	0.10	$110	0.20	$110
Recovers (after seeing doctor)	0.999	$0	0.99	$0
Hospitalization	0.001	$5,000	0.01	$5,000

sick is lower (3 percent versus 30 percent). So in Figures 5.5 and 5.6, we see that we have to collect information on (1) the cost of the vaccine, (2) the cost of illness in general (for example, the cost of over-the-counter flu remedies), (3) the cost of the doctor's visit, and (4) the cost of hospitalization. We can also list our probabilities and costs in a table (see Table 5.1).

Glancing at Figures 5.5 and 5.6, it seems that vaccination is associated with a lower chance of getting sick (0.97 versus 0.70), seeing a doctor (0.10 versus 0.20), and getting hospitalized (0.001 versus 0.01) among those who have been vaccinated compared to those not vaccinated. In fact, as we'll see in a minute, the total cost of illness among those who have received a vaccine is approximately $10.71, while those who have not will, on average, rack up an average total cost of $13.20. We will show you how these costs were calculated later in this chapter.

But one element is important in these calculations: Everyone in the Vaccine pathway will incur a $10 vaccine cost (top of Figure 5.6). If no one gets ill, then everyone in the Vaccine arm will still incur the $10 vaccine cost even though they would not have otherwise incurred any costs; if everyone gets a vaccination at the beginning of the season but there was no outbreak of influenza, the money spent on vaccination would have been wasted. But if everyone is exposed to the virus, the group getting the vaccine is probably going to have lower total costs. Therefore, we also assume that everyone (that is, 100 percent of the population) is exposed to the influenza virus.

Exercise 1

1. Let's assume that if you do not receive a vaccine and then get sick, the cost of illness is $84. However, when you get vaccinated, the cost of illness is only $38. What is the cost of the supportive care and vaccination strategies if the incidence rate of influenza virus infection is just 1 percent?

We have introduced some of the fundamental components of a decision analysis model. So far, we have looked at the event pathways for Vaccinated and Not Vaccinated separately. However, we are interested in determining which strategy is the most cost-effective. This can get a little tricky to answer with the diagrams we have. Fortunately, there is a helpful shortcut to performing calculations within the event pathway sketches. This shortcut is called a *decision tree* model. Figure 5.7 is called a simple *decision tree* and is essentially the event pathway flipped on its side.

In Figure 5.7, both competing alternatives (vaccination and supportive care) are fused together, and this is denoted as a square box. This box is called a *decision node*. The decision node represents the point in the decision tree where the provider or policymaker chooses treatment intervention for the subject or population. Think of the decision node as a referee holding the competing alternatives apart as they set out to do battle. Following this square, you'll see a circle. The circle is called a *chance node*. A chance node is followed by two or more possible outcomes. In this case, the outcomes are Remains Well and Becomes Ill. The stop signs in Figures 5.5 and 5.6 are

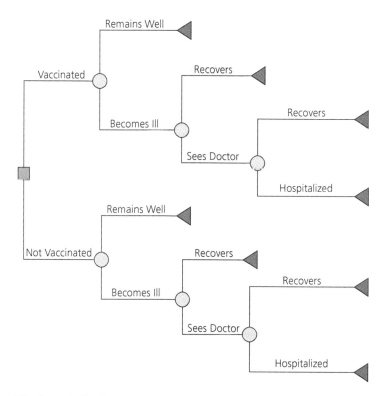

Figure 5.7   Supportive Care Versus Vaccination Decision (Figures 5.5 and 5.6) Represented as a Decision Analysis Tree

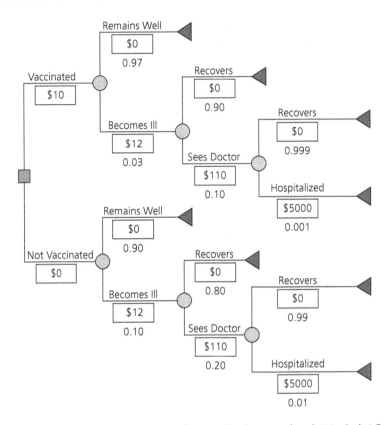

Figure 5.8   Event Pathway for Vaccination Versus Supportive Care Represented as a Decision Analysis Tree

represented in a decision analysis model as a triangle at the very end of the model. Triangles in decision models are also called *terminal nodes.*

In Figure 5.8, each box beneath the branches of the decision tree displays the cost associated with that event pathway. For instance, everyone who receives a vaccination incurs a cost of $10 for the vaccine. The probabilities in Figure 5.8 are located just below the cost. For example, patients who receive a vaccine have a probability of 0.97 of remaining well. In the next couple of sections, we'll see how the probabilities and costs are calculated for each event pathway.

Calculating the Probability of Each Strategy

An important element in a decision tree is the probability that an outcome will occur. The probabilities at each chance node contribute to the terminal probabilities. For instance, the probability of a patient who was vaccinated, Becomes Ill, and Recovers is the product of the probabilities associated with that event pathway. Thus, to calculate the probability for each terminal node, we will need to apply the multiplicative rule for independent events. In other words, the probability of the above event pathway is the probability of Becomes Ill (0.03) multiplied by the probability of Recovers (0.90). Therefore, the probability of a patient who was vaccinated, Becomes Ill, and Recovers is 0.027 (0.03 × 0.90). Each terminal node is calculated using this multiplicative rule for independent events. The final value that you obtain at the terminal node is called the *expected probability*.

Figure 5.9 illustrates the expected probability for each terminal node. Notice that the sum of the probabilities for the Vaccination strategy is 1. Similarly, the sum of the probabilities for the Supportive Care strategy is 1. This is an application of the second rule of probability. You should make sure that the probabilities of the terminal nodes sum up to 1 for each treatment strategy to ensure that you did your calculations correctly. If the sum of the terminal nodes does not equal 1, then there is an error in the model or the calculation. Review your numbers and make sure that you carefully perform these calculations.

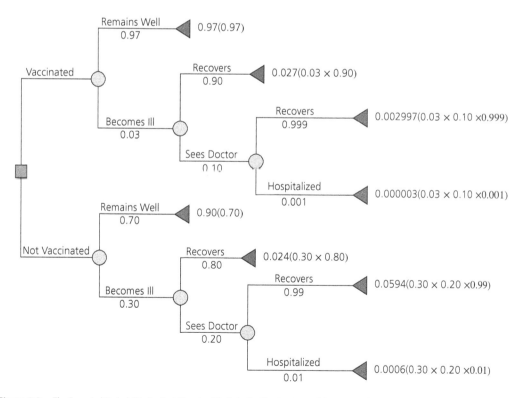

Figure 5.9   The Expected Probability for Each Terminal Node in the Vaccination and Supportive Care Decision Tree

Exercise 2

2. What is the expected probability for a patient who receives Supportive Care, Becomes, Ill, Sees a Doctor, and is Hospitalized?

Calculating the Cost of Each Strategy

Previously, you were asked to take it on faith that the cost of care for Not Vaccinated (or Supportive Care) for infected people is $13.20 and the cost of care for vaccinated persons who become ill anyway is $10.71. Now we'll see how to get these numbers.

We will need to calculate the *total cost* for each terminal node in the decision tree. The total cost for an event pathway is the cumulative cost associated with all branches of the pathway that precedes the terminal node. For example, for a patient who receives vaccination and Remains Well, the total cost for that event pathway is $10 [$10 (for the vaccine) + $0 (Remains Well)]. In addition, the total cost for a person who received a vaccine ($10 for the vaccine), Becomes Ill ($12 for aspirin and flu medications), Sees a Doctor ($110 for the office visit), and Recovers ($0) is $132 ($10 + $12 + $110 + $0). Figure 5.10 calculates the total cost for each terminal node.

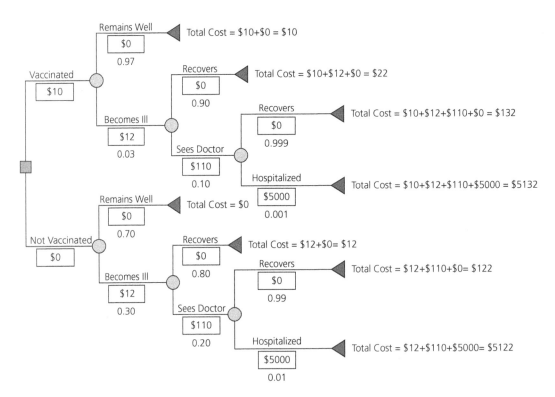

Figure 5.10   The Total Cost for Each Terminal Node in the Vaccination and Supportive Care Decision Tree

Exercise 3

3. What is the total value of the Cost variable for a subject in the Supportive Care arm who sees a doctor and is subsequently hospitalized?

Putting It All Together

Imagine that you were evaluating 100 subjects at the beginning of influenza season and that the flowchart in Figures 5.5 and 5.6 is a giant funnel. If you poured the subjects into the top of the flowchart, they would trickle through it, some going one way and others going the other way.

Subjects who trickle through a given node incur that cost. So a subject who becomes ill in the Supportive Care arm incurs a cost of $12 for over-the-counter medications. If he then sees a doctor, he adds $110 to this cost and has now accumulated a total cost of $122. If he then recovers, his total cost is $122 (because the cost of recovery is $0).

In Figure 5.10, the costs have been added up at the end of each terminal node. However, the costs calculated at the end of the terminal node only give us the total cost associated with that event pathway. It does not incorporate the probabilities of falling into that pathway, as our example of a giant funnel illustrates for us. The cost for each terminal node is based on the mean probability of falling into a particular event pathway. When we multiply each cost by each probability in a pathway and then add those costs together, we get what is called the **expected cost** of a pathway. In order for us to see the *expected* cost for each terminal node, we need to weigh the total costs of each terminal node with the probability of falling into that terminal node. Fortunately, we have already shown you how to calculate the probability at each terminal node and presented them in Figure 5.7.

Figure 5.11 provides the expected costs for each terminal node. The expected cost is calculated by multiplying the probability with the total cost for each terminal node. For example, the expected cost for a person who received Supportive Care, Becomes Ill, and is Hospitalized after seeing a doctor is $3.07 [$(0.30 \times 0.20 \times 0.010) \times (\$5,122)$]. You can calculate the expected costs for a person who receives vaccination, Becomes Ill, and is Hospitalized after seeing a doctor as $0.02 [$(0.03 \times 0.10 \times 0.001) \times (\$5,132)$].

Exercise 4

4. What is the expected cost of a person who received a vaccine and remains well?

After calculating the expected costs for each terminal node, you can sum them up for each treatment strategy (Vaccinated or Not Vaccinated). For Vaccinated, the total expected cost is $10.71, and for Supportive Care,

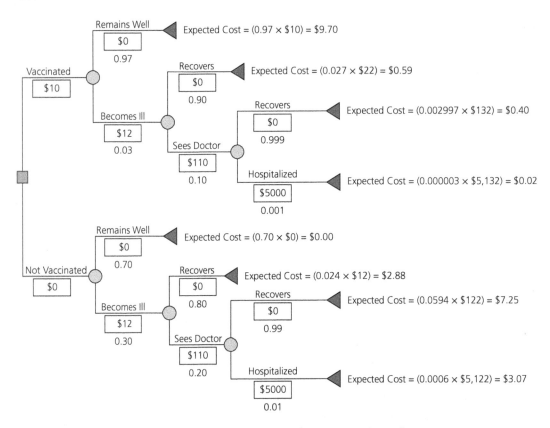

Figure 5.11   Expected Costs for Each Terminal Node in the Vaccination and Supportive Care Decision Tree

it is $13.20. Table 5.2 summarizes the calculations for the expected costs for each terminal node. The expected cost for the Vaccinated strategy is $10.71 ($9.70 + $0.59 + $0.40 + $0.02). The expected cost for the Supportive Care strategy is $13.20 ($0.00 + $2.88 + $7.25 + $3.07).

Now we can put these results together into our decision tree. Figure 5.12 provides the total cost and probability for all the terminal nodes. Each terminal node has the total cost followed by the probability of the outcome of that event pathway. For instance, the total cost for a patient who is Vaccinated, Becomes Ill, and Recovers is $22, and the probability of that outcome is 0.027.

In some texts these terminal node values are called *payoffs*. Because this is a decision tree on cost-effectiveness, there are two payoffs of interest: cost and efficacy. The *cost* is the amount of resources used for each event; the *efficacy* is the outcome of interest defined by the researcher. In our example, defining the efficacy is important in determining how to interpret whether

Table 5.2   Calculation of Expected Cost for Each Event Pathway for Vaccination and Supportive Care Strategies

Vaccination Arm	Probability	Total Cost	Calculation	Expected Costs
Terminal 1	0.97	$10	(0.97 x $10)	$9.70
Terminal 2	0.027	$22	(0.027 x $22)	$0.59
Terminal 3	0.002997	$132	(0.002997 x $132)	$0.40
Terminal 4	0.000003	$5,132	(0.000003 x $5,132)	$0.02
Total	1.00			$10.71
Supportive Care Arm				
Terminal 1	0.70	$0	(0.70 x $0)	$0.00
Terminal 2	0.240	$12	(0.240 x $12)	$2.88
Terminal 3	0.0594	$122	(0.0594 x $122)	$7.25
Terminal 4	0.0006	$5,122	(0.0006 x $5,122)	$3.07
Total	1.00			$13.20

one strategy is cost-effective relative to another. A widely used method to determine whether a strategy is cost-effective is the *rollback* method. We will introduce and discuss this method in the next sections.

Rollback Method (Thinking Inside the Tree)

A common method used to identify the most cost-effective strategy is the *rollback* method. Rollback calculates the pathway with the greatest payoffs. It provides a decision maker with the strategy and pathway that will yield the greatest return. It involves working backward from the terminal nodes to the beginning of the decision tree model. For instance, if we want to calculate the total cost and probability of the Sees Doctor node in the Supportive Care arm of the node (see Figure 5.13), we need to know the total costs and probability for the terminal nodes that follow it. In this case, these terminal nodes include Recover and Hospitalization.

The expected cost and outcome for each chance node are calculated by taking the probability of the branches of the decision tree associated with the event pathway and multiplying it by the costs and probabilities of that pathway. For instance, we are interested in the expected costs and probability for a person who sees a doctor after receiving supportive care. There are two event pathways that can occur at this chance node: Recovers and Hospitalized. The probability of falling into the Recovers pathway is

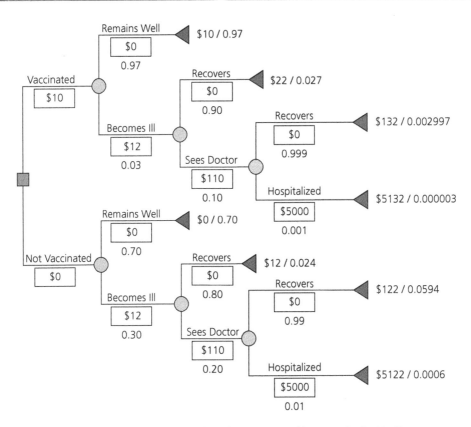

Figure 5.12   Total Cost and Probability for All Terminal Nodes in the Vaccination and Supportive Care Decision Tree

0.99. The cost of the Recovers pathway is $122 and the probability is 0.0594. Multiplying the cost and probability of the Recovers pathway by 0.99 yields an expected cost and outcome of $120.78 (0.99 × $122) and 0.0588 (0.99 × 0.0594), respectively.

But this is only half the story. Notice that another complementary event occurs: Hospitalized. We need to calculate the expected cost and outcome for this event pathway using the same methods. Therefore, the expected cost and outcome are $51.22 (0.01 × $5,122) and 0.000006 (0.01 × 0.0006), respectively. Combining these results in their respective categories we get the expected cost and outcome for a person who receives supportive care, becomes ill, and is hospitalized as $172 ($120.78 + 51.22) and 0.0588 (0.0588 + 0.000006), respectively. Figure 5.14 illustrates how the expected cost and outcome are calculated for the chance node where a patient receives Supportive Care, Becomes Ill, and Sees Doctor.

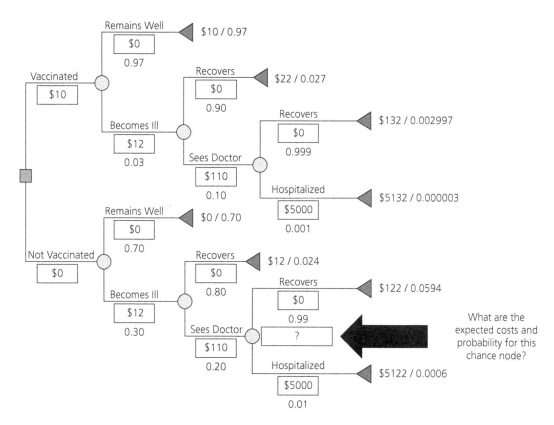

Figure 5.13   Expected Cost and Outcomes for Each Chance Node in the Vaccinated and Supportive Care Decision Tree

Note: The arrow indicates the chance node of interest.

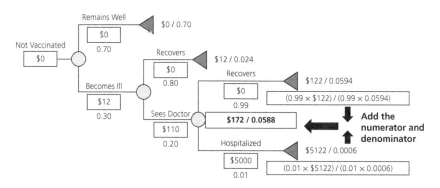

Figure 5.14   Calculation for the Expected Cost and Probability for a Patient Who Receives Supportive Care, Becomes Ill, and Sees Doctor

Exercises 5 to 7

(Use Figure 5.15 to answer the following questions.)

5. What are the expected costs and probabilities for a person who is Vaccinated (chance node A)?

6. What are the expected costs and probabilities for a person who is not Vaccinated (or Supportive Care) (chance node B)?

7. Compare cost and probabilities between the two strategies (A versus B). Which one is the most cost-effective?

Thus, if we believe the figures we've entered so far, the overall cost of the Vaccinated strategy ($10.71) is about $2.49 lower than the cost of the Supportive Care strategy ($13.20), which is exactly what we found in the previous section when we calculated the values by hand. In the next few chapters, we'll see what happens when we test these values using sensitivity analysis. Before going down that path, though, let's apply what you have already learned about decision analysis models.

TIPS AND TRICKS

At this point, you might be wondering why everything is rounded off to the nearest dollar. That's to get you used to rounding, which is the general rule in cost-effectiveness analysis. Cost-effectiveness researchers are a bit more honest than others in that they admit that the estimates are rough. In many scientific studies, you'll see estimates rounded to two decimal places. For instance, it's not uncommon to see a risk ratio of 1.22 or 3.54. Sure, that was the estimate for that group of people at that particular time in those particular circumstances. But if you do the study again, you'll probably not get a number that's even in the confidence interval of the original estimate. In cost-effectiveness analysis, it's not uncommon to give the reader a little wink and a nudge with a number like $12,000 per QALY gained when the number the researcher obtained is $12,431 per QALY gained. As long as the calculation method is transparent for another researcher to replicate, rounding to the nearest dollar is considered appropriate.

FOR EXAMPLE: WHY YOU'LL NEVER CATCH A DECISION ANALYST IN A CASINO

Gambling casinos, like decision analysis models, use the concept of **expected value** to ensure that they will profit off gamblers. For the casino to make a profit, earnings at tables and slot machines must, on average, be greater than the casino's expenses. Casinos tend to employ a large staff and have spectacular displays of opulence, such as re-creations of downtown Manhattan in miniature. Thus, the probability that the client will lose must be significantly greater than the probability of winning if the casino wishes to keep its doors open. Although the occasional winner will surface from a wild night of gambling, the average person can expect to lose money.

Recall that technical types call the various options that you are deciding between *competing alternatives*. Decision analysis can thus be described as the process of making an optimal choice among competing alternatives under conditions of uncertainty. In the case of cost-effectiveness analysis, the competing alternatives are the different medical interventions we are studying (e.g., Vaccinated versus Not Vaccinated).

In the past, researchers performing a cost-effectiveness analysis had to write a computer program that would calculate the cost and effectiveness of different medical interventions, or attempt to calculate all of the costs

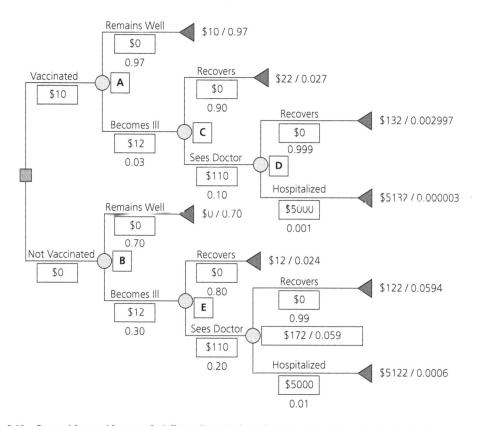

Figure 5.15 Expected Costs and Outcomes for Different Chance Nodes in the Vaccinated and Supportive Care Decision Tree

and probabilities on a spreadsheet. Today, most cost-effectiveness analyses can be easily assembled using decision analysis software (e.g., TreeAge and Crystal Ball).

You have already learned the basics of building a decision analysis model. The basic functions of all decision analysis software packages are more or less similar. If you choose to follow the examples provided here using decision analysis software, you will get a better understanding of the concepts behind decision analysis. Tips on using different software packages are also provided throughout this book. A list of software packages with online links and evaluations is provided at http://www.wiley.com/WileyCDA/WileyTitle/productCd-1119011264.html. Many of these companies offer free trial versions of their software.

Types of Decision Analysis Models

There are a number of types of decision analysis models. The most basic is a **simple decision analysis tree**, which we used in our examples in this chapter. Simple decision trees are usually employed to examine events that will occur in the near future. They are therefore best suited to evaluate interventions to prevent or treat illnesses of a short duration, such as acute infectious diseases. They may also be used to evaluate chronic diseases that may be cured (for example, by surgical intervention). When these trees are used to evaluate diseases that change over time, they sometimes become too unruly to be useful.

For chronic or complex diseases, it is best to use a **state transition model**. This type of model allows researchers to incorporate changes in health states over time into the analysis. For example, if a person has cancer, there is a chance that the person will recover within a year and then relapse. There is also a chance that the person will remain sick for some time or will die soon. With every passing month (or year), the chance of survival, recovery, or deterioration changes. These models, which are also called **Markov models**, allow researchers to track changes in the quality of life and the cost of a disease over time when different health interventions are applied. We will discuss Markov models in more detail in Chapter 6. In fact, we will spend most of our time on these types of models because they are by far the most common in cost-effectiveness analysis.

Another type of model is the discrete event simulation or agent-based simulation. Agent-based models take into account the interactions that individual cases have with one another. This way, it is possible to watch a disease spread within day-to-day interactions between participants. They can also account for human nature. For instance, people who are healthy may want to avoid being next to a person who is sick, thereby reducing their chance of being ill. Agent-based models are considered advanced modeling techniques that go beyond the scope of this book. We mention them here because they are very important if you are evaluating something that prevents an infectious disease. Certain behaviors can also spread through social networks, such as smoking. Some people believe that conditions such as obesity might even spread through social networks. (For a good image of this, visit http://www.nejm.org/doi/full/10.1056/NEJMsa066082 and view the animation.) Like Markov models, these models also take time into consideration. The difference is that we are worried about how long it takes one person to come into contact with another rather than a fixed period of time, such as a year.

Finally, complex systems models can evaluate a simulation in real time rather than time to event, like an agent-based model, or a fixed transition time, like a Markov model. We ended Chapter 1 by introducing you to complex system dynamics. Recall that these models consider how different variables influence one another over time. These models help us understand the "big picture," or how something that you plan on can cause many things that you didn't plan on to happen. They are especially useful when designing policy models.

One classic example resides in transportation policy. As cities built smooth roads, more people purchased cars, and the roads became congested. In response, cities widened the roads and built more of them. This created an incentive for driving, thereby again increasing the number of cars until the roads were again congested. As this cycle repeated itself, people moved farther and farther away from city centers (because they could purchase cheaper land and build big houses on it). This led to urban sprawl, massive amounts of air pollution, many deaths from automobile crashes, pedestrians getting hit, bicyclists getting hit, noise pollution, and a sedentary lifestyle that contributed to the obesity and heart disease epidemic. The cycle repeated itself until about 2007, when people started to resist cars and the number miles driven started to fall in the United States. These problems could have been foreseen with a complex system dynamics model.

While such models are beyond the scope of an introductory textbook, we recommend that any students who wish to model policies at least consider adding a complex systems component to their analysis.

Summary

In this chapter, you learned to incorporate probability into a decision analysis tree. You also learned some basic probability rules. Like costs, probabilities are an essential part of the decision analysis framework. Each event pathway follows a decision and its consequences, which is associated with some cost. You determined what this expected cost is and used it to determine whether the intervention was cost-effective.

You also learned about the elements of a decision analysis model and its role in cost-effectiveness analysis. The construction of a decision analysis model depends on the nature of the disease and the expected outcomes. However, it should reflect the reality that is relevant to the economic question you have. The rollback method allows you to determine, from a decision analysis viewpoint, which strategy is the most cost-effective.

Finally, we introduced some advanced models that can simulate the path of the disease more realistically. Later in the book, we'll put Markov models to the test, and use them to estimate changes in life expectancy associated with a given intervention.

Further Reading

For an in-depth discussion of probability theory, we recommend reading *Probability in Medicine* by Edmond A. Murphy (1979). Students interested in a detailed discussion regarding decision models should refer to *Decision Modelling for Health Economic Evaluation* (Briggs, Claxton, & Sculpher, 2006). For an introduction to agent-based models, please refer to Karnon and colleagues (Karnon, Stahl, Breanna, Caro, Mar, & Möller, 2012).

Vensim®, Systems Thinking for Education and Research (STELLA), and Powerism® are software packages that can build and analyze dynamic system models. Curious students are encouraged to explore these other models. Vensim offers an excellent page on complex system dynamics models, which can be found at http://vensim.com/resources/.

Another helpful text that provides a general introduction is *Essentials of Pharmacoeconomics*, 2nd edition, by Karen Rascati (2014). Finally, for those who wish to venture into complex system dynamics, check out *Business Dynamics* by John D. Sterman (2000). Or if you prefer, you may contact us, and we will do our best to help you.

References

Briggs, A., K. Claxton, and M. Sculpher. (2006). *Decision Modelling for Health Economic Evaluation*. New York: Oxford University Press.

Eddy, D. M., V. Hasselblad, W. McGivney, and W. Hendee. (1988). The Value of Mammography Screening in Women Under Age 50 Years. *Journal of the American Medical Association* 259(10): 1512–1519.

Karnon, J., J. Stahl, A. Brennan, J. J. Caro, J. Mar, and J. Möller. (2012). Modeling Using Discrete Event Simulation: A Report of the ISPOR-SMDM Modeling Good Research Practices Task Force-4. *Medical Decision Making* 32(5): 701–711. http://doi.org/10.1177/0272989X12455462.

Murphy, E. A. (1979). *Probability in Medicine.* Baltimore: Johns Hopkins University Press.

Rascati, K. (2014). *Essentials of Pharmacoeconomics,* 2nd ed. Philadelphia: Lippincott Williams & Wilkins.

Sterman, J. D. (2000). *Business Dynamics: Systems Thinking and Modeling for a Complex World.* New York: McGraw-Hill Irwin.

CHAPTER 6

CALCULATING LIFE EXPECTANCY

Overview

So far, you've learned how to work with costs and how to enter them into a decision analysis model. You now know that the probabilistically weighted cost of each competing alternative is called the expected value of that strategy. Costs, though, are just one component of the expected value. The expected value of QALYs—the quantity and quality of life among people receiving each strategy—is the most important component of a cost-effectiveness analysis.

In this chapter, we first take a quick look at how to calculate changes in life-years gained when an intervention is administered using a hand calculator or spreadsheet program. Then we see how this is done using a Markov model. In Chapter 7, you will learn about health-related quality-of-life (also known by the acronym HRQL) scores. You will learn how to adjust life expectancy for health-related quality of life to calculate QALYs in Chapter 8.

Hand-Calculating Years Gained

If we are studying vaccination against the influenza virus, we'll first want to know how many deaths would have occurred without vaccination. These data can be obtained from death certificate records, prospective studies, or national health surveys that have been linked to mortality data. (Data sources are covered in detail in Chapter 12.) In this example, we'll use hypothetical data to simplify things a bit.

Suppose our hypothetical cohort consists of healthy people aged 15 to 65. Our research question might assume the form: "Is vaccination more cost-effective than

LEARNING OBJECTIVES

- Given a life table, calculate life-years gained or lost due to an intervention (or no intervention).

- Recognize when to use a half-cycle correction to calculate life-years gained or lost with interval age ranges.

- Sketch a simple Markov model to calculate average life expectancy or loss.

- Use age-specific mortality rates to estimate the total number of deaths for each age cohort.

- Given the rollback results of a Markov model, identify and explain the values at each node.

supportive care among healthy people aged 15 to 65 in the United States?" We'll define the supportive care as "Do not vaccinate people, and treat the flu symptoms if they become ill." Let's say that we are evaluating a work- and school-based vaccination strategy, in which just about everyone has to get vaccinated.

WHOM ARE WE STUDYING?

One perpetual problem in cost-effectiveness analysis is matching the demographic characteristics of the cohort in the datasets or research papers we are using to the demographic characteristics of the cohort in our research question. If we found an article on influenza-related deaths that used older wealthy white people as subjects, the mortality rate might be very different from the rate we wish to use in a study looking at a younger representative sample of the U.S. population.

One way to conduct the analysis is to look at the age at which unvaccinated people died of influenza (Table 6.1). If we knew their average life expectancy at the age that each subject actually died, we could then add all of the life-years lost across all subjects. For instance, if the average 20-year-old has a life expectancy of 78.5 years, then an influenza death at age 20 results in the total loss of 78.5 years − 20 years = 58.5 years.

The remaining life expectancy for people of any given age can be obtained from a life table. U.S. life tables are available from the National Center for Health Statistics (http://www.cdc.gov/nchs). Links to life tables from other countries can be found using a search engine. The Organization for Economic Cooperation and Development (http://www.oecd.org/) is a good source for developed countries and the World Health Organization for industrializing nations (http://www.who.int/gho/mortality_burden_disease/life_tables/life_tables/en/).

Life tables for the United States in 2011 are provided in Appendix B. (For some reason, these publications are always 5 years behind.) Check out

Table 6.1   Number of Deaths due to Influenza Virus Infection, by Age Group

Age	Annual Number of Deaths
15 to 24 years	6
25 to 34 years	11
35 to 44 years	24
45 to 54 years	54
55 to 64 years	69

this appendix now so that you can see where we are getting our data. In Appendix B, the final column of the first table contains the information we are looking for: the remaining life expectancy for each age group. Most life tables you encounter will be similar. Appendix B also has life expectancy at a given age by race and gender in the United States.

GROWING OLDER, LIVING LONGER

Some students may wonder why you need a life table to figure out the mean age of death for people from a given age group if you already know what human life expectancy is. After all, if life expectancy is 78 years in your country and a person dies at age 40, you could just assume that he lost $78 - 40 = 38$ years of life. The bad news is that people in different age groups have ever-expanding life expectancies, so you always have to look up the life expectancy at any given age. The good news is that *your* life expectancy is longer than you might think. (So you are wasting fewer precious moments of life reading this book than you first imagined.)

As it turns out, human life expectancy at birth in the United States is somewhere around 78 years. But as we grow older, our life expectancy grows with us. For instance, 70-year-olds can expect to live a full additional 15 years, to age 85. The reason is that those who make it past birth trauma have gotten a good deal of risk behind them. Those with serious illness or risk factors for premature mortality such as smoking tend to die younger, too. Thus, the healthiest people make it to age 70, and, because they are healthier, they have more life to look forward to. The other bit of good news is that life expectancy at birth also tends to increase from one year to the next in most countries, thanks in part to the appropriate use of health interventions. In fact, life expectancy in the United States was just 47.3 years at the turn of the twentieth century (Arias, 2014).

Table 6.2 lists deaths, the mean age of death due to the flu, and life expectancy (had the subject survived the influenza infection) by age group for our hypothetical cohort of 15- to 65-year-olds. One important part of this table is the midpoint of each age interval. Assuming that someone who is 15 years old is just about as likely to die as someone who is 25, the average age of death among 15- to 25-year-olds will be about (15 years of age + 25 years of age)/2= 20 years of age. (In Table 6.2, the 15-to-24 age interval represents everyone who just turned 15 to everyone who is 24 years and 364 days and 23 hours old, so the midpoint is 20 years.)

In the influenza study, we are interested only in subjects aged 15 to 65. Nonetheless, someone who dies at age 64 still loses around 20 years of life. Therefore, a death even at this age counts for a lot of lost life expectancy.

Table 6.2   Deaths, Mean Age of Death due to Influenza Virus Infection, and Life Expectancy for Persons Aged 15 to 65

Age	Deaths due to Influenza (1)	Midpoint Age in Interval (2)	Life Expectancy at Midpoint (3)
15 to 24 years	6	20	78.5
25 to 34 years	11	30	79
35 to 44 years	24	40	79.6
45 to 54 years	54	50	80.6
55 to 64 years	69	60	82.3

From the information in Table 6.2, we can easily calculate the total years of life lost to influenza infection in the cohort (see Table 6.3). This is just equal to the life expectancy at that age (column 3 of Table 6.3) minus the mean age of death due to influenza virus infection (column 2). The total years of life lost among all people in each age interval is the number of deaths (column 1) times the average number of years of life lost per person (column 4).

To obtain the total years of life lost due to influenza virus infections, add across the age groups. At the bottom of Table 6.3, we thus see that just over 5,000 years of life are lost annually in the United States due to influenza virus infection among otherwise healthy 15- to 65-year-olds. This is the total quantity of life we would expect to lose in the supportive care arm of our analysis.

So how many additional life-years would we get from vaccination? In the research question posed here, we are evaluating a scenario in which nearly everyone gets vaccinated. One estimate is that because the efficacy

Table 6.3   Calculating Total Years of Life Lost due to Influenza Virus Infection in the United States

Age	Deaths Due to Influenza (1)	Midpoint Age (2)	Life Expectancy at Age (from Life Table) (3)	Years of Life Lost per Person (Col. 3 – Col. 2) (4)	Total Years of Life Lost (Col. 1 × Col. 4) (5)
15 to 24 years	6	20	78.5	58.5	351
25 to 34 years	11	30	79	49	539
35 to 44 years	24	40	79.6	39.6	950
45 to 54 years	54	50	80.6	30.6	1,652
55 to 64 years	69	60	82.3	22.3	1,539
Total	164				5,032

of the vaccine is 70 percent, we could prevent 70 percent of all deaths, and therefore 70 percent of all years of life that would otherwise have been lost. Thus, we might estimate that we can prevent 5,000 years of life × 0.7 = 3,500 years of life that would otherwise have been lost.

However, some students of public health may be familiar with the concept of *herd immunity*. Herd immunity occurs when the level of vaccination is so high that the virus fizzles out altogether, and no cases of disease remain. If we believe that we can achieve herd immunity, we would prevent all 5,000 years of life lost. (This is one example of the difference between efficacy and effectiveness.)

TIPS AND TRICKS

We can round values for expected life-years saved because we are interested in getting an estimate. Therefore, rather than use 5,032 years of life × 0.7 = 3,522 years of life that would have been lost, we rounded to the nearest hundredth to make our presentation easier to read.

Stop here for a moment and think about the implications of this. This is 164 (total deaths due to influenza) × 0.7 (efficacy of vaccine) = 115 lives saved. Among those people, there are about 3,500 total extra years of life enjoyed by these 115 people. These are mothers, fathers, children, and spouses who would still be alive at the end of the influenza season if the government followed your recommendations to provide vaccination to everyone in the United States (that is, in this hypothetical example). But if you found that vaccination was costly relative to other things done in health, you could be saving more lives by directing needed resources to more important lifesaving interventions.

HOW TO SAVE LIVES THROUGH INACTION

You learned earlier in the book that if you have a fixed amount of funding for health care, cost-effectiveness analysis will tell you how to maximize the total number of lives you are saving with those scarce resources. But what if you don't have a fixed amount to spend, such as occurs in private sector health systems? In the United States, clinicians often order loads of medical tests when the patient comes to see them, many of which are known to be cost-ineffective. There is also a tendency to use the newest and most expensive therapies. All of this is justified on the grounds that it just might save a life. After all, a clinician might reason, what is money relative to precious life? In reality, all of this unnecessary care probably raises insurance premiums. This increased cost forces many employers to drop insurance carriers. It also pushes those who pay for insurance on their own out of the insurance market.

Given that insurance itself is probably lifesaving and is a fairly efficient medical expenditure (Muennig, Franks, Jia, Lubetkin, & Gold, 2005), forcing people out of the insurance market can increase overall mortality. Therefore, clinicians who mistakenly believe that they are helping their patients with excessive testing and treatment may in fact be killing unseen people.

Calculating Life-Years Lost Using Markov Models

Let's take a look at how our influenza analysis might progress had we used year-to-year data rather than age intervals. Suppose that instead of the deaths in Table 6.3, we followed a cohort of 1 million unvaccinated 15-year-olds from the ages of 15 through 100. (This requires a leap of faith, but humor us for a little bit.)

Any one of these 1 million folks can survive to the next age, die of influenza, or die of something else. In Table 6.4, column 2 represents deaths due to influenza, column 1 represents deaths due to all causes, and column 3 the total number of people surviving each year of life. (Note that there are no deaths due to influenza virus infection recorded after the age of 65 because we are interested only in deaths due to influenza among people between the ages of 15 and 65.) Table 6.4 has been truncated so that it fits in the book.

TIPS AND TRICKS

Over 100 years of education research, dating back to the great John Dewey, has shown that students learn best by doing. From this point on, we highly recommend that students with access to a computer follow along on a spreadsheet using the examples in the book. You will find full tables and free spreadsheet software at http://www.wiley.com/WileyCDA/WileyTitle/productCd-1119011264.html.

In Table 6.4, we start with 1 million 15-year-olds (column 3), but 407 die in the first year (column 1). This leaves 1,000,000 − 407 = 999,593 survivors at age 16.

Suppose that we wish to calculate the total number of years lived by this cohort of 1 million 15-year-olds. You might be thinking that this is just the sum total of column 3 values in Table 6.4. After all, each interval is one year in length, and those are the total number of people alive each year. That's true, but remember that people who die don't all die on January 1. On average, the 407 15-year-olds dying in row 1, column 1 of Table 6.4 will die about six months into the year (in June). All those dying will therefore have lived about half a year on average, and we need to count this additional

Table 6.4   Total Deaths, Deaths due to Influenza Virus Infection, and Total Survivors in a Cohort of 1 Million 15-Year-Olds

Age	Deaths Due to Any Cause (1)	Died from Influenza (2)	Total Surviving (3)
15	407	1	1, 000, 000
16	575	0	999, 593
17	683	0	999, 018
18	728	2	998, 335
19	734	0	997, 607
20	898	0	996, 873
. . .	. . .	. . .	. . .
95	11, 589	0	29, 011
96	8, 754	0	17, 422
97	3, 989	0	8, 668
98	1, 234	0	4, 679
99	2, 038	0	3, 445
100	664	0	1, 407

life. Because the 407 people who died between the ages of 15 and 16 lived a half-year of life on average, we subtract $\left(\frac{407}{2}\right)$ or 203.5 rather than all 407 years of life for that year. Researchers call this a **half-cycle correction**, which is a correction factor to account for midcycle transitions (Naimark, Bott, & Krahn, 2008).

As shown in Table 6.5, this half-cycle correction is calculated as column 1 − column 2 × 0.5. The number of years of life lived by a group of people is referred to as *person-years*. Thus, there were 997,797 person-years lived between the ages of 15 and 16. If we sum all person-years together, we find that this cohort lived 63,670,217 person-years between the ages of 15 and 100 years.

We can also calculate the number of years lived by the average person in the cohort. To obtain this average, we would simply divide the total number of years lived (person-years) between the ages of 15 and 100 years by the total number of people at the start of the study. The average number of years lived by the average 15-year-old is also known as the life expectancy at age 15. In this case, it would be 63,670,217 person-years/1,000,000 persons = 63.67 years. This is precisely how life expectancy was calculated in the life table in Appendix B by the professionals at the National Center for Health Statistics.

TIPS AND TRICKS

To generate Table 6.5 using the electronic version of Table 6.4, simply add a column after the Total Surviving column, name it "Person-Years," and perform the calculations. To enter the formula, type "= D2 – B2 * 0.5" (without the quotes). Next, click on the cell in which you just entered the formula (cell E2). The cell will appear highlighted. Grab the lower right-hand side of the cell. It should turn into a plus sign. Now drag it all the way down to the final age group. The spreadsheet program should have done all of the calculations for you, so that you don't have to reenter the formula in each cell. If it doesn't work on the first try, try again. You'll get the hang of it eventually.

TIPS AND TRICKS

If we divide the number of deaths by the number of survivors in Table 6.6, we obtain the mortality rate. The mortality rate at any given age in this example is equal to the probability of death at that age. Most often we will know the mortality rate in the cohort, but not the total number of deaths. So how do we re-create it? The number of deaths at any age is equal to the product of the total number of survivors at any given age and the mortality rate for persons of that age or in that age group (see Table 6.7).

Now we have the total person-years and life expectancy of people in this cohort of 1 million unvaccinated 15-year-olds (regardless of whether they died of the flu). How do we get the incremental gain in person-years or life expectancy among those who have received the influenza vaccination? To make things simple, let's say that the influenza vaccine is 100 percent effective. Now we repeat this process with and without the deaths due to influenza virus infection (see Table 6.6).

As you can see from Table 6.6, the gain in person-years is 63,678,453 – 63,670,217 = 8,236 person-years. Note that we stopped exposing the subjects to influenza once they hit age 65. Thus, the total number of deaths in the age groups 65 through 100 is identical. As a result, there are fewer survivors going forward into the unvaccinated group.

It may not be a surprise to most of you that this whole process can be modeled in a way that is quick and versatile. What will be surprising is how easy it is to become a super modeler using standard software.

Alternatively, this could be presented graphically with a series of health states. In Figure 6.1, we represent the preceding analysis as a simple state transition diagram. The

Table 6.5 Total Person-Years Lived by the Cohort of 1 Million 15-Year-Olds

Age	Alive (1)	All Deaths (2)	Person-Years (Col. 1 − Col. 2 × 0.5) (3)
15	1, 000, 000	407	999, 797
16	999, 593	575	999, 306
17	999, 018	683	998, 677
18	998, 335	728	997, 971
19	997, 607	734	997, 240
20	996, 873	898	996, 424
. . .	. . .	. . .	. . .
95	29, 011	11, 589	23, 217
96	17, 422	8, 754	13, 045
97	8, 668	3, 989	6, 674
98	4, 679	1, 234	4, 062
99	3, 445	2, 038	2, 426
100	1, 407	664	1, 075
Total	64, 169, 845		63, 670, 217

Alive health state has two arrows going outward. One reenters the Alive health state, and the other arrow goes toward the Dead health state (also known as the *absorbing state,* since one cannot resurrect themselves after dying). Each arrow is associated with a transition probability that must sum to a total probability of 1. You will have more hands-on experience with Markov models in Chapter 13.

Principles of Markov Modeling

Most interventions have some component of time to them. For instance, to model screening mammography, we must have some way to measure the progress of breast cancer over time when left untreated. We must also account for changes over time among women who are treated for the disease but not cured. Moreover, we don't provide screening mammography just once. We might provide it every six months or once every five years.

To model events that unfold over time, we want some sort of recursive component in our model. A **recursive event** is one that repeats over and over. For example, if we were evaluating screening for high blood pressure, we might want to capture the cost of diagnosing and treating high blood pressure in year 1 and then include the cost of ongoing treatment in years

Table 6.6   Person-Years Lived Among the Cohort of 15-Year-Olds, Including and Excluding Deaths due to Influenza Virus Infection

Age	All Deaths			All Deaths but Influenza-Related Deaths		
	All Deaths (Unvaccinated)	Total Surviving	Person-Years	Total Deaths Less Influenza Deaths	Total Surviving	Person-Years Less Influenza
15	407	1,000,000	999,797	406	1,000,000	999,797
16	575	999,593	999,306	575	999,594	999,307
17	683	999,018	998,677	683	999,019	998,678
18	728	998,335	997,971	726	998,336	997,973
19	734	997,607	997,240	734	997,610	997,243
20	898	996,873	996,424	898	996,876	996,427
...	...	...	...	...	...	...
95	11,589	29,011	23,217	11,589	29,175	23,381
96	8,754	17,422	13,045	8,754	17,586	13,209
97	3,989	8,668	6,674	3,989	8,832	6,838
98	1,234	4,679	4,062	1,234	4,843	4,226
99	2,038	3,445	2,426	2,038	3,609	2,590
100	664	1,407	1,075	664	1,571	1,239
Total			63,670,217			63,678,453

Table 6.7   Age-Specific Mortality Rates, Survivors, and Number of Deaths in the Cohort of 1 Million 15-Year-Old Subjects

Age	Mortality Rate (1)	Alive (2)	All Deaths (Col. 1 × Col. 2) (3)
15	0.0004	1,000,000	407
16	0.0006	999,593	575
17	0.0007	999,018	683
18	0.0007	998,335	728
19	0.0007	997,607	734
20	0.0009	996,873	898
...	...	...	...
95	0.3995	29,011	11,589
96	0.5025	17,422	8,754
97	0.4602	8,668	3,989
98	0.2637	4,679	1,234
99	0.5915	3,445	2,038
100	0.4718	1,407	664

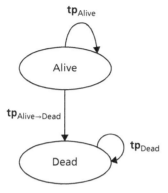

In this example, all patients begin in the Alive health state. The transition probability of remaining alive is denoted as tp_{Alive}. The transition probability of going from Alive to Dead is denoted by $tp_{Alive \rightarrow Dead}$. Those that are in the Dead health state remain there, which is denoted by tp_{Dead}.

Figure 6.1   Markov Model for Influenza Mortality in 15-Year-Olds

2, 3, 4, and so on, until the patient dies. (We never cure high blood pressure; we just provide symptomatic treatment.)

Recall from Chapter 5 that a model that contains some component of time in it is called a state transition model or Markov model (Figure 6.2). Figure 6.2 can be thought of as a machine for shuffling people through time. The bent fork in the road represents the chance that any given subject will die in a particular year. Subjects are cycled through once per year. With each passing year, the number of subjects in the dead fork increases. The rate at which the number of subjects collect at the dead node is equal to the age-specific mortality rate.

Now you will see why we took you through the whole exercise of calculating person-years.

We have opted to describe Markov models in a way that is easy to understand. The actual way that the computer performs these calculations differs somewhat from what is described here.

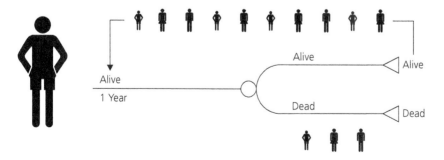

Figure 6.2   Basic Concept of a Markov Model

Note: Subjects start at time zero (the large figure). They are then exposed to a chance of death. Survivors gain one year and return to the start of the model, where they are again exposed to a chance of death. Those who die exit the model. This process is repeated until all subjects die. The mean number of times a subject passes through the model is equal to the life expectancy of the cohort.

Subjects who are alive at the end of the first cycle of the model are assigned one person-year, and those who die are assigned no person-years. Suppose that subjects die at the same age-specific mortality rate that they did in Table 6.5. If we start at age 15 and send 1 million subjects through 85 cycles to age 100 years, there will be 63,670,217 total person-years gained, and the average subject will have accrued 63.67 years. Said another way: The average number of times survivors rotate through the model is equal to the average number of person-years lived by that cohort. The average number of rotations is therefore equal to the life expectancy of the cohort.

TIPS AND TRICKS

You would be well served to take the time now to build your own Markov model. The online component of this book, Program in Cost-Effectiveness and Out-comes, contains a downloadable laboratory manual with links to demo software and step-by-step exercises for building your own Markov models. See http://www .wiley.com/WileyCDA/WileyTitle/ productCd-1119011264.html.

Using a Markov model, we can count more than the years that accrue as the model completes cycles. We can also count medical costs, living costs, health-related quality-of-life scores, or whatever else might be relevant for our analysis. For instance, suppose we are interested in calculating the lifelong cost associated with breast cancer in patients who have been diagnosed using a screening mammogram. We would start the model using the average age of onset of breast cancer. The number of survivors would be determined using the probability of death specific to women who have been diagnosed with breast

Table 6.8 Progression of a Cohort of 10 Women with Breast Cancer over a Six-Year Period

Year	Women Surviving	Discounted Years Lived[a]	Cost of Treating Breast Cancer[b]	Discounted Cost[a]
1	10	9.7	$100,000	$97,087
2	9	9.0	$90,000	$84,834
3	8	7.8	$80,000	$73,211
4	7	6.7	$70,000	$62,194
5	6	5.6	$60,000	$51,757
6	5	4.6	$50,000	$41,874
Total		**43.4**	**$450,000**	**$410,957**

[a] Beginning in January of the reference year at a 3 percent rate of discount.
[b] Costs in this column have not been half-cycle corrected for simplicity of presentation. In an actual analysis, it would be important to base the figures on person-years rather than on the number of deaths.

cancer using screening mammography. Each patient who is still living at the end of the year gains one year of additional life (one person-year). But she can also be assigned medical costs, home healthcare costs, transportation costs, and so forth. Women who die do not accrue such costs, so these women neither gain a year of life nor accrue costs.

Thus, if the average annual cost of living with breast cancer were $10,000, a group of 10 women would incur a cost of 10 × $10,000 = $100,000 in year 1. Now imagine that by year 2, one woman died. Year 2 costs would then be 9 × $10,000 = $90,000. If we continued this process until the last subject died, we would not only have the average number of life-years lived, but the total cost incurred by these women over that time period. (See Table 6.8.)

Markov Models in Practice

Let's take a moment to see how a Markov model works using TreeAge Pro software (Figure 6.3). For a moment, we'll return to the influenza example so that you can see how Markov modeling works in its most basic form.

The first thing that you come across in Figure 6.3 is a box that says "Markov Information" followed by "Term: _stage > 103." The "Term" in this case stands for "Termination," and tells the program how many one-year loops it is going to make before it stops. In this case, it will loop 103 times (or until all of the subjects are dead). The odd notation "_stage" is a function used by TreeAge Pro to keep track of how many cycles have been completed. In this model, one cycle is one year; thus, when _stage is equal to 10, ten years have passed.

TIPS AND TRICKS

Software is always changing. Therefore, we have used the latest version of TreeAge Pro (2015) throughout this book. However, future versions of TreeAge Pro may change the interface, which can create inconsistencies in the examples. If you see an inconsistency, please refer to the book's web site for updates http://www.wiley.com/WileyCDA/WileyTitle/productCd-1119011264.html.

In Figure 6.3 there is an initial Alive/Dead branch followed by another Alive/Dead branch. The first Alive/Dead branch (top) also contains a box called "Markov Information." This is followed by various reward ("Rwd") terms. For now, just consider the "Incr Rwd." This stands for incremental reward and tells the program what to add up every time a subject passes through the Alive branch. The incremental reward can be anything. For instance, it can be an annual medical bill for someone with breast cancer.

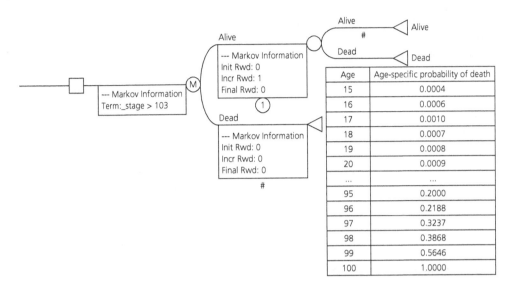

Age	Age-specific probability of death
15	0.0004
16	0.0006
17	0.0010
18	0.0007
19	0.0008
20	0.0009
...	...
95	0.2000
96	0.2188
97	0.3237
98	0.3868
99	0.5646
100	1.0000

Figure 6.3   Complete Decision Analysis Tree for Calculating Life Expectancy Using TreeAge Pro

For now let's count the incremental reward in years. In this figure, the incremental reward is set to 1 for the Alive branch and 0 for the Dead branch. Thus, every time a subject passes through the Alive branch, the running total reward is increased by 1, representing one year of life. Every subject who dies gets a reward of 0 (zero; no additional years of life) and exits the model. (If this is all terribly depressing to you, just remember that these are hypothetical subjects.)

Note that below the "Markov Information" box on the Alive branch, you'll also find the number 1 (circled in Figure 6.3). This number indicates that at time 0 (before the first loop), there is a 100 percent chance of being alive and moving forward into the model. This is followed by a circle (a chance node) and another Alive/Dead option (recall from Chapter 5 that squares are decision nodes, circles are chance nodes, and triangles are terminal nodes). At this point, there is a chance of dying. In Figure 6.3, the chance of dying at any age is presented as a table.

For instance, following the previous example, it tells the program that when the subject is 15 years old, he has a 0.0004 chance of dying. To reiterate, there are two Alive/Dead branches, but only the second determines who lives and who dies. The first branch is used to either absorb the subjects who die or pass the subjects who survive back into the tree. For this reason, the first dead node is called the *absorbing state*.

Let's call the table in Figure 6.3 "tDead2003[age]." This reflects the age-specific probability of death in the United States in 2003. Again, every time a subject passes through the Dead branch, no points are given, and the subject exits the model. Thus, when subjects are 20 years old, 0.0009 will die and accrue no points, but $1 - 0.0009 = 0.9991$ will live and accrue a reward equal to one year of life. When subjects are 95 years old, 0.2 (20 percent) will die, and 0.8 will live to see age 96.

If there is no chance of death (the values in tDead2003 are all equal to 0), the incremental reward will be 103 years because we have told the model to stop cycling after 103 turns. Other things can cause the model to stop cycling as well. Most important, the model will stop looping once the total proportion of subjects remaining alive reaches 0.

Once the model stops looping, it presents the mean value of the incremental reward. In the previous section, you learned that if you add up the total number of survivors in a cohort, you end up with the total person-years in that cohort. You also learned that if you divide the sum of all person-years across age groups by the total number of people at the start of the cohort, you end up with the cohort's life expectancy. This is the expected value of the number of years lived by the average person in the cohort.

TIPS AND TRICKS

Recall that all future values, whether costs or years of life, must be discounted at a rate of 3 percent. Fortunately, TreeAge Pro has a function built in that allows all values to be discounted at a specified rate. Chapter 13 walks students through the process of entering the discounting function into TreeAge Pro. In short, any value entered in the "Incremental" box must be discounted.

This expected value is obtained by **rolling back** the model. Figure 6.4 is the rolled-back version of a Markov model that uses the age-specific probability of death for the general population. The 77.9 years is the life expectancy of the cohort, and "P = 1" following the expected value

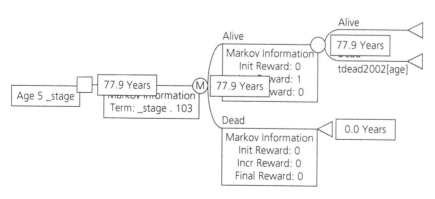

Figure 6.4   A Rolled-Back Model Using the Probability of Death for the General U.S. Population

indicates that the probability of achieving this value is 1.0. At the Dead branch, you'll see "0.0 Years," which indicates that all subjects have died. The "0.0 Years" notation indicates that the sum of incremental reward values for all subjects who have passed through this branch is 0.

In the Alive branch, the final proportion of subjects in this branch of the tree is 0, and the total incremental value is 77.9 years.

Soon, we will see how to assign costs (e.g., cost of hospitalization, cost of a medical visit) to each year a subject survives. We'll also see how to enter health-related quality-of-life (HRQL) scores to calculate QALYs. First, though, we'll take a break from modeling and look at HRQL measures in more detail.

Exercises 1 to 3

1. Imagine that you were interested in the life expectancy of patients who received the influenza vaccination. You decided to build a Markov model with four states: Healthy, Sick, Recovered, and Dead. Suppose the vaccine effectiveness was 75 percent and mortality due to illness was 5 percent. Patients who get sick have a 95 percent probability of recovering, and remain in this state as a healthy patient. Sketch the Markov model including the transition probabilities.

2. For this exercise, use a spreadsheet program to construct your Markov model. Assume a time horizon of 10 weeks with a 1-week cycle. Also assume that the efficacy and mortality rate are constant over 10 weeks. Start with a hypothetical cohort of 1,000 patients who received the influenza vaccine and are alive and in the healthy state. How many patients would be Healthy after 10 weeks of the influenza season?

3. Try building this same Markov model using TreeAge Pro. Use the rollback method. What differences do you notice?

Summary

Life-years is an important outcome for cost-effectiveness analysis. In this chapter, you've learned how to calculate life-years lost using a spreadsheet. In addition, you've also learned to calculate mortality with the same methods. We introduced a unique tool called a Markov model to help estimate the life-years lost and mortality using powerful software called TreeAge Pro. Using a Markov model allows you to simulate the life expectancy using transition probabilities that you can generate from a life table. However, Markov models are not limited to calculating life expectancy. In fact, they have many other uses in cost-effectiveness that you will learn about with a worked example in Chapter 13. So stay tuned.

Further Readings

Students interested in learning more about herd immunity should read the short manuscript titled "'Heard Immunity': A Rough Guide" by Paul Fine and colleagues (Fine, Eames, & Heymann, 2011).

A free trial of TreeAge Pro 2015 can be downloaded from the web site https://www.treeage.com/. Students are encouraged to review the tutorial videos that are available on YouTube on the TreeAgePro channel.

References

Arias, E. (2014). United States Life Tables, 2009. *National Vital Statistics Reports* 62(7). Hyattsville, MD: National Center for Health Statistics.

Fine, P., K. Eames, and D. L. Heymann. (2011). "Herd Immunity": A Rough Guide. *Clinical Infectious Diseases* 52(7): 911–916. http://doi.org/10.1093/cid/cir007.

Muennig, P., P. Franks, H. Jia, E. Lubetkin, and M. R. Gold. (2005). The Income-Associated Burden of Disease in the United States. *Social Science & Medicine* 61(9): 2018–2026. http://doi.org/10.1016/j.socscimed.2005.04.005.

Naimark, D. M. J., M. Bott, and M. Krahn. (2008). The Half-Cycle Correction Explained: Two Alternative Pedagogical Approaches. *Medical Decision Making* 28(5): 706–712. http://doi.org/10.1177/0272989X08315241.

CHAPTER 7

WORKING WITH HEALTH-RELATED QUALITY-OF-LIFE MEASURES

Overview

Recall that a quality-adjusted life-year (QALY) may be thought of as a year of life that is lived in perfect health. In Chapter 2, we learned that HRQL scores assume a value between 0 and 1. This ratio may be simply thought of as a continuum of values ranging from perfect health to death. Thus, if a medical intervention adds 10 years of life and each of these years is associated with an HRQL of 0.7, the medical intervention would have resulted in a gain of 0.7×10 years $= 7$ years of perfect health (7 QALYs).

In this chapter, we take the first step toward calculating QALYs as we learn the basic theory behind HRQL scores, learn how to obtain HRQL scores for cost-effectiveness analyses, and learn how to use HRQL scores using worked examples.

LEARNING OBJECTIVES

- Distinguish between the different methods for generating preference scores.

- Explain why preference-weighted generic instruments are useful in generating utility scores.

- Identify the attributes or domains of the EuroQol instrument (EQ-5D).

- Use the EQ-5D Crosswalk Index Value Calculator to determine the index value for a given dimension score.

This section is implemented with a crescendo-like teaching technique in which information is broken into small parts and then reassembled into a workable whole. This may seem somewhat repetitive to some students, but it forces most people to learn the material more naturally and effectively.

Framework

In this section, we briefly discuss the formal methods used to translate a person's perception of the quality of life in various health states into an HRQL score. It provides some definitions, a basic outline of how HRQL scores are generated, and, finally, a more detailed description of how these scores are collected and used. This will allow you to follow along with a clear understanding of how this process works. Keep in mind that these measures were designed with consistency, rather than specificity, as a primary objective (Gold, Franks, McCoy, & Fryback, 1998; Sullivan & Ghushchyan, 2006; Sullivan, Lawrence, & Ghushchyan, 2005).

First, the definitions.

A **preference score** is a number between 0 and 1, where 0 represents "I'd just as soon be dead," and 1 represents perfect health. For instance, a preference score of 0.7 represents 70 percent of the way between "I'd just as soon be dead" and "I'm in perfect health." Take this on faith for a moment.

Recall from Chapter 1 that health state reflects how well or how badly people are doing with respect to a given aspect of a particular disease or condition. For instance, not being able to get out of bed is a health state. So are moderate depression and having some pain. One's health status is the collection of health states.

Whereas a preference score refers to a single health state, an HRQL score is essentially an overall preference score for multiple health states. (Some experts will quibble with this, but it's confusing to think of an HRQL score in any other way.)

Second, this essentially is how HRQL scores are generated:

1. Preference scores for a set number of health states are obtained from a large sample of people. For instance, people will be asked to assign a preference score to "some mobility limitations" or "in severe pain."

2. Statistical analyses are conducted on these preference scores such that we know what a given health state is worth to the average person in the sample. For instance, we'll know that "some mobility limitations" has a preference score of 0.7.

3. These values are translated into a type of score sheet that requires the user to check off broad categories of health states. For instance, the score sheet might contain a category called "Mobility." The user is then required to check off one of three states: "No problems getting around," "Some problems getting around," and "Immobilized." It might also contain a category called "Pain" that contains "No pain," "Moderate pain," and "Severe pain."

4. It translates these health states into an overall HRQL score. If the user checks "Some problems getting around" and "Severe pain," the score sheet provides an overall HRQL score of, say, 0.3.

Now we'll examine these steps in detail. Obviously, the steps just given provide a very basic outline. Immediate questions should pop into mind such as "How does this translation happen?" Now all your questions will be answered.

Preference Scores

Preference scores are taken directly from a sample of subjects from the general population that is subjected to a series of exercises based on expected utility theory. Expected utility theory is little more than a way of turning health states such as level of pain into a number (the preference score).

The "utility" part of expected utility theory is the preference score for a given health state (for example, being unable to walk) when a person is otherwise in perfect health. For instance, given that the utility of perfect health is 1 and the utility of death is 0, a fellow in perfect health who cannot walk because of a war injury might have a preference score of 0.6. This indicates that to the average person who cannot walk but is in otherwise perfect health, each moment of life is worth 60 percent of that of a person who can fully walk.

The "expected" part of "expected utility theory" implies that these utilities are derived by calculating expected values, as you would with a decision analysis model. How might such a decision analysis model look? Consider the **standard gamble** technique.

Suppose you had an illness that required you to remain in bed for the rest of your life, and an evil magician appeared at your bedside. This magician told you that you could either remain as you are for the rest of your life or play a potentially deadly game. If you won this game, you would regain perfect health, but if you lost, you would die. To make an informed decision, you would want to know the chances of winning the game. The standard gamble technique is designed to estimate the risk of death that a patient would be willing to accept in a gamble for perfect health (Gafni, 1994; Torrance, 1976; Torrance, Thomas, & Sackett, 1972).

In this technique, subjects must choose between a health state (such as remaining in bed) and a gamble in which there is a chance of perfect health or death (see Figure 7.1). The chance of death is changed until the decision between the health state and the gamble is perceived to be about equally desirable to the subject. This process is akin to bargaining, but bargaining for perfect health. The probability decided on (p in Figure 7.1) is the utility for that health state.

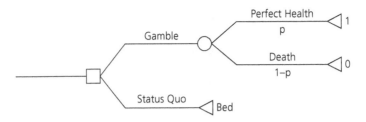

Figure 7.1   Trade-off Between the Status Quo Health State and a Gamble

For example, suppose the subject is certain that she would be willing to risk a 40 percent chance of death in exchange for the opportunity to recover from her illness but would definitely not be willing to accept a 60 percent chance of death. In other words, if the chance of death were 60 percent, she would choose the health state. The researcher would scale the probability of death up from 40 percent until the patient is ambivalent about whether to take the gamble or remain in bed. Suppose that she finally landed on a probability of 0.55, or a 55 percent chance that she would survive. She values each year of life she lives at about 0.55 year of perfect health. The standard gamble method is based on the fundamental axioms of the von Neumann and Morgenstern utility theory, which gives it credibility in generating utility scores (von Neumann & Morgenstern, 1953).

Another technique that uses expected utility theory is called the **time trade-off** method (Mehrez & Gafni, 1990; Torrance, 1976; Torrance et al., 1972). Here, the patient is asked how much time in poor health she would be willing to trade for perfect health. Thus, the patient has to forgo future years of life in poor health in exchange for fewer years of life in perfect health. Once the subject has decided how much time she would be willing to sacrifice for better health, the HRQL score is obtained by dividing the life expectancy in the state of illness by life expectancy in perfect health.

Note: There has been some concern that the time trade-off method is not grounded in behavioral theory, which limits its use as a tool to estimate utility scores (Mehrez & Gafni, 1990). Regardless, the time trade-off method has an advantage over the standard gamble by being easy to use.

A final, rather primitive method involves the use of a rating scale (Torrance, 1976). The subject is asked to rate the health state on a scale of 1 to 100, where 0 is the worst imaginable and 100 is the best imaginable. Rating scales are easy to administer and inexpensive; however, they do not capture individuals' true preferences regarding their trade-offs, so they can't be used in the reference case. But it comes up at cost-effectiveness cocktail parties, so we mention it here to keep you from staring listlessly at your martini olive.

In the expected utility theory, preference scores are captured before the event. This is also known as *decision utility* (Dolan & Kahneman, 2008; Nord, Daniels, & Kamlet, 2009). On the other hand, a preference score captured after experiencing the event is known as *experienced utility*. How would the preference score change if the same individual were evaluated after the event occurred? This can result in a change in health status ranking, which would have an impact on how we allocate our resources.

Exercise 1

1. List the three preference scoring methods that are available for direct measurement. Which would you prefer to use?

Who Should Valuate HRQL?

The Panel on Cost-Effectiveness in Health and Medicine recommends that HRQL scores be determined using preference-weighted instruments that are based on a representative sample of people within society (Gold, Siegel, Russell, & Weinstein, 1996; Neumann, Sanders, Russell, Siegel, & Ganiats, 2016). Others believe that these scores should be obtained from people who have the disease under study. People with a disease, it is argued, know what life is like with that disease and would thus be better at valuing the corresponding quality of life than the average person would.

The problem with deriving HRQL scores from people with the disease under study is that such scores are not consistent with the societal perspective. Remember that we are interested in valuing all inputs into our cost-effectiveness analysis from the perspective of everyone in society. Deriving HRQL scores using only people with a particular disease betrays this principle. Instead, the scores should be representative of the value that the average person would assign to a particular health state (Gold et al., 1996; Neumann et al., 2016).

How does a healthy person know what it is like to have a particular disease? To generate HRQL scores for health states, a sample of people go through a formal exercise in which they study different aspects of a health state. Once the person has an idea of what life might be like with the disease, the subject undergoes one of the expected utility exercises (similar to those described here) to generate an HRQL score.

When the scores are derived from a representative sample of people in a community, they are referred to as **community-derived preferences**. Again, the word *preference* refers to a person's perception of what life is like in a given health state. (This perception is coaxed out with the standard gamble or time trade-off technique.)

By sampling a large group of people, we can be relatively certain to obtain the average impact of the disease, but we cannot apply these scores to individuals. Consider a study that evaluates a medication used to treat arthritis. While eccentric old writers who sit around scrawling notes in smoky cafés all day would probably prefer arthritis in their knees, runners would probably prefer to have arthritis in their hands. Moreover, both writers and runners would be affected by the arthritis in different ways. For instance, a writer earning a living from writing may see arthritis as a more severe disease than the runner would because it could lead to financial instability. Often the term *preference score* is used interchangeably with the word *utility* in cost-effectiveness analysis.

Deriving HRQL Scores

Much as a computer hides all of the complicated programming code behind a point-and-click interface, **preference-weighted generic instruments**— the score sheets used to generate HRQL scores—hide this methodology behind a simple survey form. One such instrument, the EQ-5D, is presented in Appendix C and in Exhibit 7.1 (EuroQol Group, 1990). In the past, the EQ-5D had three levels for each attribute (no problems, some problems, and extreme problems). However, recent testing demonstrated that increasing the number of levels from three to five improves the reliability and sensitivity while retaining the benefits of the EQ-5D. The EQ-5D now has five levels for each attribute and is now referred to as the EQ-5D-5L (the older instrument is now referred to as the EQ-5D-3L).

EXHIBIT 7.1. EQ-5D-5L HEALTH DOMAINS

MOBILITY

I have no problems in walking about

I have slight problems in walking about

I have moderate problems in walking about

I have severe problems in walking about

I am unable to walk about

SELF-CARE

I have no problems washing or dressing myself

I have slight problems washing or dressing myself

I have moderate problems washing or dressing myself

I have severe problems washing or dressing myself

I am unable to wash or dress myself

USUAL ACTIVITIES (*e.g., work, study, housework, family, or leisure activities*)

I have no problems doing my usual activities

I have slight problems doing my usual activities

I have moderate problems doing my usual activities

I have severe problems doing my usual activities

I am unable to do my usual activities

PAIN/DISCOMFORT

I have no pain or discomfort

I have slight pain or discomfort

I have moderate pain or discomfort

I have severe pain or discomfort

I have extreme pain or discomfort

ANXIETY/DEPRESSION

I am not anxious or depressed

I am slightly anxious or depressed

I am moderately anxious or depressed

I am severely anxious or depressed

I am extremely anxious or depressed

These preference-weighted generic instruments may be completed using information from the medical literature. Generic HRQL instruments can also be completed by people familiar with the disease you are studying, such as patients with the disease or the doctors who are familiar with treating them (Gold et al., 1996; Neumann et al., 2016). Such a range of people can fill them out and get comparable scores because the categories are quite broad. Most people would agree that someone with a cold has some discomfort but not severe discomfort. For this reason, too, it's not necessary to obtain a large sample of people to fill these out. Three doctors or three patients ought to do if the condition you are evaluating is relatively straightforward.

Once the instrument is completed, the researcher inputs the responses into a simple formula that produces an HRQL score suitable for use in a reference case cost-effectiveness analysis. This is discussed in the next section.

In the following sections, we examine how to obtain scores using preference-weighted generic instruments, how to use scores derived from published lists, and how to use HRQL scores in nonreference case measures, such as the disability-adjusted life-year (DALY). Very large research efforts sometimes also generate scores by taking a sample of subjects through a series of exercises based on expected utility theory (e.g., the standard gamble or time trade-off) so that they can generate HRQL scores from scratch.

Using Preference-Weighted Generic Instruments

Preference-weighted generic instruments (or HRQL instruments) are often used in cost-effectiveness analysis because the process of determining community-derived HRQL scores is costly and time-consuming (Gold et al., 1996; Neumann et al., 2016). Each preference-weighted generic instrument has its strengths and weaknesses. Examples are the Quality of Well-Being (QWB) scale, the Health Utility Index (HUI), the SF-6D, the Quality of Life and Health Questionnaire, and the EQ-5D-5L.

Recall that these instruments may be used to convert responses from physicians or patients who have experience with the disease under study into HRQL scores that estimate preferences derived from a representative community sample. Alternatively, researchers can sometimes obtain information about the disease from the medical literature and then use this information to fill in the blanks of a preference-weighted generic instrument. In other words, preference-weighted generic instruments are essentially tools that translate survey responses into HRQL scores derived from a large, representative community sample of people who have gone through exercises grounded in expected utility theory.

TIPS AND TRICKS

Researchers who never consider that their work will be used for cost-effectiveness analyses often use a measure called the SF-36 to get a sense of how a participant is doing on a very wide array of measures of mental health, physical health, and other measures of functioning. This mammoth instrument is much more precise than any of the instruments that are used in cost-effectiveness analyses. The problem is that it does not return a score between 0 and 1. And, anyway, it is not compatible with the reference case. Oftentimes, though, you will find that you have a lot of information about the health-related quality of life of a study participant but, frustratingly, won't have a usable HRQL score. Enter the SF-6D, which pulls measures from the SF-36 that can be used to generate a QALY-compatible score between 0 and 1. To learn more about this great instrument, see https://www.qualitymetric.com/Portals/0/Uploads/Documents/Public/SF-6D.pdf.

Again, to reiterate, each of these scores derived from the community sample is associated with a particular aspect of a given health state (as in Exhibit 7.1). Each of these responses is referred to as a **dimension** (also known as an **attribute** or **domain**). One example of a dimension is "depressed versus happy." Another is whether someone can get around. The dimensions are broken into levels (for example, "no problem," "some problem," or "severe problems"). Preference-weighted generic instruments are therefore more generally called **multiattribute health status classification systems**, because they combine different levels of many different attributes of a given disease into a single HRQL score (Drummond, Sculpher, Torrance, O'Brien, & Stoddart, 2005).

So what's the difference between these and a health state? *Health state* is a more general term. For instance, being able to walk is a health state, but so is just being alive. We wouldn't typically speak of being alive as a health dimension.

The dimensions captured by an instrument can represent aspects of a disease beyond the biological symptoms the disease causes. For instance, diabetes can cause blindness or the inability to walk. These conditions may in turn affect the person's ability to function in society and may place strains on his or her relationships with others. Blindness, the inability to walk, a person's ability to function in society, a person's ability to relate to others, and a person's ability to work are all examples of health dimensions.

Let's see how this might play out in one example. Consider the man with moderately severe diabetes. He has numbness in the feet and some problems walking but can still take care of himself. He has intermittent pain and moderate discomfort from intestinal manifestations of the disease. Because he is not

TIPS AND TRICKS

Culture influences the way that we think about health states and therefore affects the results of exercises such as the time trade-off or standard gamble. For this reason, the preference scores used in preference-weighted generic instruments vary from country to country. The EQ-5D-5L contains preference weights from a number of countries, so translating scores requires the application of a different scoring formula. Currently, the EQ-5D-5L is still in the process of generating these adjustments for all countries. In the meantime, adjustments are made using mapping methods to the EQ-5D-3L.

dependent on others, the disease has not greatly affected his autonomy, and he does not feel anxious or depressed as a result. Knowing this, filling out the instrument (Exhibit 7.1) becomes merely a matter of checking off the boxes.

In this instance, the man has some trouble walking about, so we might check the second box in Exhibit 7.1 under "Mobility." He does not have any problems with self-care, so we might check the first box there. We weren't given any information about his ability to perform his usual activities. If his usual activities involve sitting in front of the television set, then we might check the first box. But most people would be sufficiently hampered by the foot numbness and intermittent pain to limit usual activities, so we might check the second box. On the Pain/Discomfort scale, you would probably give him a moderate rating. The rating for Anxiety/Depression is tricky. Some folks become depressed by the onset of chronic disease, while others shrug it off. Most adapt fairly well over time, though, so we might want to check the "I am not anxious or depressed" box.

Probably most students provided with this information would check off a similar pattern of boxes, even though the information about usual activities was incomplete. Again, this is the beauty of these instruments; they allow enough leeway that there is a low likelihood that two people would generate radically different scores when given a particular scenario.

Let's now score that man's HRQL using U.S. weights (see Appendix C for the weights). In Figure 7.2, we provide you with a hypothetical EQ-5D-5L sheet that has been filled out by a patient. To obtain the HRQL score for him using the EQ-5D-5L, take a look at the scores for this poor guy in Figure 7.2. (Recall that each area is a domain and each score is a dimension.) His scores are 1, 2, 3, 4, and 5, which means that there are no problems with mobility, slight problems with self-care, moderate problems with usual activities, severe problems with pain/discomfort, and extreme problems with anxiety/depression. Once we have identified the dimension scores, we need to download the EQ-5D-5L Crosswalk Index Value Calculator from the EuroQol web site http://euroqol2015.org.s1.rodekiwi .nl/news-list/article/interim-scoring-for-the-eq-5d-5l-eq-5d-5l-crosswalk-index-value-calculator.html. If the link doesn't work, you can download the Interim scoring from our online resources (link: http://www.wiley.com/ WileyCDA/WileyTitle/productCd-1119011264.html). You should be able to download the calculator, which is a spreadsheet. Locate the dimension score 12345 on the column labeled "5L profile" in the "EQ-5D-5L Value Set" worksheet. Then locate the country of interest (we want to look at the United States). The index value is 0.370 for the U.S. patient with a dimension score of 12345. Ouch!

What if you don't have a tidy case scenario like this one? In most cases, we will have a decision analysis model that looks something like the one in Figure 7.3. Suppose that we wish to model the effects of a diabetes treatment on modulating the severity of the disease. In this model, subjects with diabetes are classified into three states: mild, moderate, and severe.

MOBILITY

I have no problems in walking about ☑

I have slight problems in walking about ☐

I have moderate problems in walking about ☐

I have severe problems in walking about ☐

I am unable to walk about ☐

SELF-CARE

I have no problems washing or dressing myself ☐

I have slight problems washing or dressing myself ☑

I have moderate problems washing or dressing myself ☐

I have severe problems washing or dressing myself ☐

I am unable to wash or dress myself ☐

USUAL ACTIVITIES (e.g., work, study, housework, family, or leisure activities)

I have no problems doing my usual activities ☐

I have slight problems doing my usual activities ☐

I have moderate problems doing my usual activities ☑

I have severe problems doing my usual activities ☐

I am unable to do my usual activities ☐

PAIN/DISCOMFORT

I have no pain or discomfort ☐

I have slight pain or discomfort ☐

I have moderate pain or discomfort ☐

I have severe pain or discomfort ☑

I have extreme pain or discomfort ☐

ANXIETY/DEPRESSION

I am not anxious or depressed ☐

I am slightly anxious or depressed ☐

I am moderately anxious or depressed ☐

I am severely anxious or depressed ☐

I am extremely anxious or depressed ☑

Figure 7.2   EQ-5D-5L Form Filled Out by a Patient

Source: USA (English) © 2009 EuroQol Group EQ-5D™ is a trademark of the EuroQol Group.

At the end of the year, subjects in the Mild branch are returned to the Alive branch, where they are exposed to a risk of death, remaining in the Mild category, or progressing to the Moderate or Severe category.

Were we to assign HRQL scores to this model, we would need three scores: (1) asymptomatic, (2) moderate diabetes, and (3) severe diabetes.

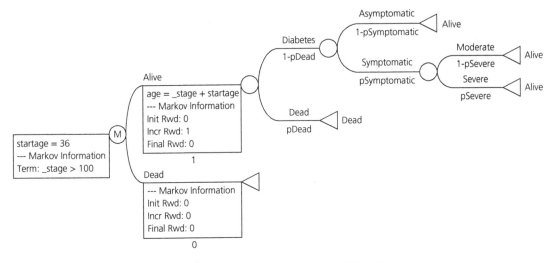

Figure 7.3   Diabetes Markov Model Depicting Three Health States: Mild, Moderate, and Severe Diabetes

We have to decide what asymptomatic/mild, moderate, and severe diabetes look like. To estimate the HRQL of each severity level of diabetes using the EQ-5D-5L, we could turn to an endocrinologist who sees the disease all the time. Most endocrinologists would check the top box for each dimension of mild diabetes because it does not produce any symptoms. There might be some disagreement as to what moderate or severe diabetes looks like, but if we asked five or six endocrinologists, we would probably get a good idea of what the HRQL score for these health states looks like as well.

TIPS AND TRICKS

By now you should have a rough idea of how many professionals you might need to consult to obtain your HRQL score. If the disease is straightforward, a few will do. If it is not, you'll need a few more. If three professionals come up with the same score, you are probably good to go. But if the scores differ, you'll probably need a larger sample. This isn't a problem if the researcher is able to obtain information on health states from the medical literature.

You probably sense that using the EQ-5D-5L to score this disease will provide a rough or shotgun approach to deriving a score. Since diabetes mostly affects self-care, mobility, and ability to perform usual activities while potentially causing anxiety and depression, this is probably a good instrument for scoring this disease. However, if we wanted to derive the HRQL of someone with kleptomania, we probably wouldn't get very far with the EQ-5D-5L; we would have only a gauge of how much anxiety the condition was causing the average kleptomaniac. For this reason, it is a good idea to think about the dimensions of one's HRQL that are affected by the disease under study and try to match it to the instruments available as best as one can (Gold et al., 1996; Neumann et al., 2016).

Let us consider another example. The Quality of Well-Being (QWB) scale measures mobility, physical activity, social activity, and the effect of various symptoms such as fatigue on HRQL (Kaplan & Anderson, 1988). If we were to use the QWB to obtain an HRQL score for diabetes, we would capture the impact diabetes might have on the subject's social life, but the instrument would still miss his depressed mood.

Fortunately, instruments such as the EQ-5D-5L and QWB are based on a representative sample of people's preferences for disease states, meaning that these tools have undergone rigorous testing for reliability and validity. We can trust that these instruments are capturing the necessary HRQL elements that are of interest to us. Because preferences reflect many people's subjective perception of what life would be like with a disease, it is not absolutely necessary to capture all dimensions of a disease in any given instrument.

Why? Consider the example of the runner and the writer with arthritis. Even if you didn't have a questionnaire that included mobility limitations, the plight of each of these folks would be partially captured in (1) ability to perform daily activities, (2) anxiety and depression, and (3) pain and discomfort. Obviously, you will be able to get a better-specified score with mobility in the instrument, but you'll still get some idea of the person's HRQL score with these other three dimensions.

Exercises 2 and 3

2. What are the attributes or domains of the EuroQol instrument (EQ-5D)? Explain why having a multiattribute health status classification system is useful in generating utility scores.

3. Suppose you have an EQ-5D-5L dimension score of 14213. What is the index value for a U.S. patient? For a U.K. patient?

Generating HRQL for Acute Conditions

In the previous example, we saw how we might score diabetes using a case scenario or the input of an endocrinologist. In that example, we saw that a subject's HRQL was determined by the severity of disease from one year to the next. Now let's look at how the EQ-5D-5L might be used to generate an HRQL score for influenza (a condition that lasts for only five

Table 7.1 Example of How an HRQL Score for Influenza Illness May Be Derived Using the EQ-5D

	Day 1 (No Symptoms)	Day 2 (Symptoms Begin)	Day 3 (Most Severe)	Day 4 (Improving)	Day 5 (Feels Better)
Mobility	1	5	5	1	1
Self-care	1	1	3	1	1
Usual activity	1	5	5	5	1
Pain	1	1	1	1	1
Anxiety/depression	1	1	1	1	1
Score for day	1.000	0.242	0.138	0.556	1.000

Note: The severity rating for each day and each dimension in the EQ-5D-5L is presented for each state. For instance, on day 2, influenza is given a dimension score of 51511, which corresponds with an index value of 0.242 for a U.K. patient.

days) using data from the medical literature. Note that these instruments are not intended for estimating HRQL scores for a single day, but since we are examining an acute infectious disease, we have no choice.

This example uses rounded data from Keech, Scott, and Ryan (1998), who estimate that subjects with the flu are confined to bed for two days, require one day of caregiver support, and miss three days of work on average (Keech, Scott, & Ryan, 1998). Now let us assume that on days 1, 4, and 5, most patients with influenza-like illness are able to get around, but they are confined to bed on days 2 through 3. Let us assume that people generally have some self-care difficulties on day 3 and miss work on days 2 through 4. We'll pretend that this is an English patient and apply U.K. weights.

To obtain an HRQL score for any given day, determine the dimension score for each day. For instance, we see that on day 2, the person's dimension score is 51511, which corresponds with an index score of 0.242 for a U.K. patient. (Preference-based values can also mean preference weights, utility scores, and index values. These terms can be used interchangeably.)

TIPS AND TRICKS

Here we applied HRQL scores to an acute illness: influenza virus infection. We got creative by averaging the scores across various days of illness. This serves to illustrate how HRQL can change throughout the course of illness. However, in reality, HRQL scores are not designed to be applied to acute infectious diseases. Unfortunately, there is no alternative system for acute illness, so we have to make do with these scores.

The mean HRQL over the five days spent with the flu is calculated by averaging across all days (adding up all of the values and dividing by 5), yielding a score of 0.587.

HRQL Scores Generated from Other Health Surveys

It is also possible to use large national health surveys that contain questions similar to those in preference-weighted generic instruments to generate complete lists of HRQL scores for different diseases. This is especially useful for estimating the average HRQL for people with and without a disease because it provides a national average. It also comes in handy when estimating the overall HRQL associated with a risk factor for multiple diseases. For instance, the Medical Expenditure Panel Survey (MEPS) has been used to estimate the HRQL of people with and without health insurance and the HRQL of people with varying levels of income (Muennig, Franks, & Gold, 2005; Muennig, Franks, Jia, Lubetkin, & Gold, 2005). From 2000 to 2003, MEPS has included the SF-12 and EQ-5D to capture patient health status and health preference (Fleishman, 2005). However, starting in 2004, MEPS continued to capture the SF-12 and added the Kessler Index and Patient Health Questionnaire.

TIPS AND TRICKS

In an earlier Tips and Tricks, we mentioned how to convert SF-36 scores into SF-6D scores. What if you don't have a full SF-36? Another method for generating HRQL scores is from a health status survey (e.g., SF-12). In this case, we do not have all of the components of the SF-6D that we need to obtain an HRQL score. Converting from a health status score to a preference-based score is a lot trickier if you don't have all of the study data that you need. The methods that are used involve a lot of advanced statistics such as probability mapping based on Bayesian theory, so we won't be covering much of this in the text. (You already have a lot to worry about!) Instead, we just want you to be aware of the possibility to convert health status scores into preference-based scores that can be used as utility scores for cost-utility analysis. For example, you can convert the scores from the SF-12 to the EQ-5D in order to generate QALYs for a cost-utility analysis (Le, 2014; Le & Doctor, 2011; Sullivan, 2006).

How does this work? The mean responses from the national survey in question are essentially matched to responses on the generic instrument. The MEPS even contains a variable with each subject's HRQL score, so there is no need to do all of the matching yourself. Of course, using a national dataset to calculate an HRQL score requires familiarity with the use of datasets and a statistical software package.

Other Considerations and Reminders

When beginning cost-effectiveness researchers first roll up their sleeves and get to work on a cost-effectiveness analysis, they often derive their HRQL score without really considering what it means. In this section, we briefly review a few of the most commonly overlooked contributors to HRQL.

Effect of Age on HRQL

In general, younger people tend to think about health very differently from older people. An elderly person may not place a high value on sexual function, for example, but a younger person almost certainly will. Moreover, because younger people are on average in better health than older people, they tend to have higher average HRQL scores and tend to place very different values on different health states. Table 7.2 provides a description of the average EQ-5D preference scores by age categories. As the average person gets older, the EQ-5D preference scores are lower.

Table 7.2 EQ-5D Preference Score Variation Among Age Categories

Age Category (Years)	EQ-5D Preference
18-24	0.90
25-34	0.88
35-44	0.85
45-54	0.81
55-64	0.79
65-74	0.76
75 and greater	0.66

Source: Center for Financing, Access, and Cost Trends, Agency for Healthcare Research and Quality. Medical Expenditure Panel Survey, Household Component, 2000 Full-Year File.

Effect of Disease Stage on HRQL

It is important to obtain HRQL scores specific to different stages of a disease. For instance, adult-onset diabetes is usually asymptomatic in its early stages; however, various aspects of a diabetic's health tend to deteriorate over time. These changes include the loss of sensation in limbs, loss of vision, repeated hospitalizations, and a number of other problems. These conditions also tend to develop concurrent with one another, complicating the person's overall health status. For example, in a longitudinal study conducted by the U.S. Study to Help Improve Early Evaluation and Management of Risk Factors Leading to Diabetes (SHIELD) study group, the average EQ-5D scores decreased for patients with diabetes from 0.798 in 2004 to 0.767 in 2009 (Grandy, Fox, & SHIELD Study Group, 2012). This decrease makes sense because diabetes is a progressive degenerative disease. Given enough time, the average patient will have a decrease in the HRQL.

Effect of an Intervention on HRQL

If diabetes is appropriately managed, the likelihood of developing future complications is reduced; thus, the general health status of treated persons will be improved relative to those who are untreated. However, the treatment itself can be associated with side effects that can have an impact on a person's health.

Because a cost-effectiveness analysis must evaluate the differences between people who have and have not received a particular intervention, such as medications used to treat diabetes mellitus, scores must be estimated for subjects in the intervention and nonintervention groups. The trick thus becomes deciding how to measure how much the treatment slows the progression of the disease relative to no treatment and how much harm the treatment is itself causing. Clearly this kind of nuanced analysis must be conducted with the input of endocrinologists and guided by the medical literature. For example, newly diagnosed diabetics who received a lifestyle intervention had a slower reduction in their EQ-5D

TIPS AND TRICKS

When there is a lower utility score because of an intervention's side effect we call this a "disutility." In cost-utility analysis, significant disutility scores should be applied in the adjustment of QALYs. For instance, patients who received glyburide are concerned about weight gain and hypoglycemia (Sinha, Rajan, Hoerger, & Pogach, 2010). Therefore, the QALYs should be adjusted with this disutility in mind.

scores over time compared to those without any intervention (Irvine, Barton, Gasper, Murray, Clark, Scarpello, & Sampson, 2011). However, this is not always the case. Drugs that are used for diabetes may treat some of the problems, but side effects can have a negative impact on the EQ-5D scores (Boye, Matza, Walter, Van Brunt, Palsgrove, & Tynan, 2011; Matza, Boye, Yurgin, Brewster-Jordan, Mannix, Shorr, & Barber, 2007). If the side effects are really bad (e.g., decreased libido, kidney failure, or death), then the utility score for the intervention may actually be lower compared to no treatment. Knowing this kind of relationship will help you better understand the impact of the intervention on QALYs.

Use of HRQL Scores in Diverse Populations

Health-related quality-of-life scores for a disease may be different for men and women, persons of different social classes, and other groups. Some care should be taken when applying HRQL scores to a group that differs demographically from the general population. For example, blacks who have worse health than whites (measured by premature mortality) nevertheless have higher HRQL scores (Lubetkin, Jia, Franks, & Gold, 2005). However, after adjustment for age, gender, income, education, and conditions, blacks had higher HRQL scores compared to whites. Be aware that there is a rich and complex dynamic between socioeconomic statuses that may not always be captured with HRQL scores.

Keep in mind that the population you are studying may not be the same as another population. Having the correct HRQL score will help in making your results generalizable to the population that you are targeting.

Disease-Specific HRQL Instruments

So far, we have been focusing on generic HRQL instruments. We call them "generic" because they reflect the health preference scores for a patient's overall general health. If you were interested in the utility score for a specific disease (e.g., diabetes), there are disease-specific HRQL instruments available (Guyatt, Feeny, & Patrick, 1993). For example, the Diabetes-39 (D-39) is a disease-specific HRQL instrument designed to measure the quality of life for patients with diabetes (Boyer & Earp, 1997). Disease-specific HRQL instruments are great at being responsive to changes in specific treatment for a certain disease. However, there may be some issues when using the utility scores to compare other diseases. We want you to be aware that these disease-specific instruments are available and may be an option if you are interested in the effects of just one disease.

Fees Associated with HRQL Instruments

These HRQL instruments are a culmination of hard work and repeated experimental studies to test for reliability and validity. Consequently, it is reasonable to expect that there be a licensing fee to use them. Researchers who plan to use these HRQL instruments need to acquire the survey and manual. The manual will have the instructions for scoring and handling issues that may come up, such as missing data. Therefore, it is important to make sure that you consider the cost of licensing these instruments and include them in your budget (or grants). For example, the HUI cost starts out at approximately $5,000 (http://www.healthutilities.com/). The cost of the EQ-5D-5L is dependent on the type and size of study you plan to do. Fees for the EQ-5D-5L are provided once you contact the EuroQol Executive Office with a prepared proposal (http://www.euroqol.org/eq-5d-products/how-to-obtain-eq-5d.html). (Since this is economics, we shouldn't be too surprised that the inventors of these instruments are behaving according to a free-market economy.)

Using Disability-Adjusted Life-Years

One additional method that should be mentioned is the practice of deriving preference scores from experts rather than a representative community sample. The scores associated with the DALY were derived using experts in part because it was necessary to generate scores for many conditions and in part because the scores were to be applied to people in distinct geographical regions of the world (Lopez, Mathers, Ezzati, Jamison, & Murray, 2006).

The disability-adjusted life-year is a QALY in reverse: It measures the years of healthy life lost to disease rather than the years of healthy life gained by an intervention. Because of this, the HRQL scores associated with the DALY vary on a scale where 0 is equal to perfect health and 1 is equal to death (the opposite of HRQL scores associated with QALYs). To convert a DALY score into a standard HRQL score, the score must be subtracted from 1.0.

Recall that generic preference-weighted instruments are based on community-generated preference weights. If a physician fills out the instrument, therefore, the physician's responses are translated into community weights. In the DALY, health professionals generate the weights themselves. This presents a number of problems (Gold et al., 1996; Neumann et al., 2016). For example, physicians may be likely to overrate the physical aspects of an illness but underrate the psychological aspects. These scores are therefore not technically QALY compatible—and for good reason: The

DALY can actually change the ranking of some diseases in a league table relative to QALY-compatible measures (Gold & Muennig, 2002).

The DALY is the preferred measure of the World Health Organization (WHO) (World Health Organization, 2015). The WHO uses the DALY to quantify the burden of disease from morbidity and mortality for global comparisons. The Institute for Health Metrics and Evaluation (IHME) also uses DALYs to measure the global burden of diseases (Institute for Health Metrics and Evaluation, 2015). The WHO and IHME can use the DALYs to rank disease of importance for individual countries or regions, which is especially useful for global health studies. For instance, road injury was ranked as the fourth leading cause of increased DALYs in the United States in 1990. By 2010, road injury had dropped to the ninth leading cause of increased DALYs, probably due to improvements in vehicle safety and regulations. You can verify this by going to the IHME web site (http://www .healthdata.org), clicking on Results, and then Data Visualizations. Scroll down to GDB Arrow Diagram and click on it. After you click on it, change the "Global" selection to the United States. Keep the default metric as DALYs. Compare the road injury rank from 1990 to 2010. You will find that road injury improved from 1990 to 2010.

As we will see in Chapter 8, cost-effectiveness analyses that do use the DALY must modify the methods used slightly because this measure was designed for burden-of-disease analysis rather than cost-effectiveness analysis.

Summary

HRQL is a multidimensional construct that encompasses the physical, social, and mental functioning of people. You have learned that these preferences were derived from expected utility theory and can be applied to cost-effectiveness analysis. In addition, you now have some experience with using HRQL instruments (e.g., EQ-5D) to capture preference scores. Preference-weighted generic HRQL instruments can be used to capture the many different attributes of a given disease into a single score. However, disease-specific HRQL instruments are better at capturing changes in HRQL scores due to an intervention.

Although most of our discussion has centered around QALYs, the DALYs have been used by the WHO and IHME when measuring the global burden of diseases. DALYs have been used to rank the global morbidity and mortality of each country to each other as a common metric for comparison. For those of you who decide to work in global health, the DALYs might be a metric you will use in cost-effectiveness analysis.

Further Readings

Developing an HRQL instrument involves a lot of work and research. A good overview of this can be found in *Reliability and Validity of Data Sources for Outcomes Research & Disease and Health Management Programs*, edited by Dominick Esposito (2013).

Students interested in learning more about the Medical Expenditure Panel Survey (MEPS) are encouraged to visit their web site (Agency for Healthcare Research and Quality, 2009).

A more detailed description of disease-specific instruments for diabetes is provided in a review paper by El Achhab and colleagues (2008).

The EuroQol web site has very good information regarding the history and origins of the EQ-5D, licensing, and scoring, that the interested student should explore at http://www.euroqol.org. In addition, students should also explore the Health Utility Index web site at http://www.healthutilities.com.

Students interested in learning more about the global burden of disease and DALYs should visit the IHME's web site (http://www.healthdata.org) (Institute for Health Metrics and Evaluation, 2015). The IHME's web site has some great data visualization tools that you can fiddle with to generate some interesting statistics about global health.

References

Agency for Healthcare Research and Quality. (2009, August 21.) Medical Expenditure Panel Survey (MEPS). Retrieved January 5, 2015, from http://meps.ahrq.gov/mepsweb/about_meps/survey_back.jsp.

Boye, K. S., L. S. Matza, K. N. Walter, K. Van Brunt, A. C. Palsgrove, and A. Tynan. (2011). Utilities and Disutilities for Attributes of Injectable Treatments for Type 2 Diabetes. *European Journal of Health Economics: Health Economics in Prevention and Care (HEPAC)* 12(3): 219–230. http://doi.org/10.1007/s10198-010-0224-8.

Boyer, J. G., and J. A. Earp. (1997). The Development of an Instrument for Assessing the Quality of Life of People with Diabetes. Diabetes-39. *Medical Care* 35(5): 440–453.

Dolan, P., and D. Kahneman. (2008). Interpretations of Utility and Their Implications for the Valuation of Health. *Economic Journal* 118(525): 215–234. http://doi.org/10.1111/j.1468-0297.2007.02110.x.

Drummond, M. F., M. J. Sculpher, G. W. Torrance, B. J. O'Brien, and G. L. Stoddart. (2005). *Methods for the Economic Evaluation of Health Care Programmes*, 3rd ed. New York: Oxford University Press.

El Achhab, Y., C. Nejjari, M. Chikri, and B. Lyoussi. (2008). Disease-Specific Health-Related Quality of Life Instruments Among Adults Diabetic: A Systematic

Review. *Diabetes Research and Clinical Practice* 80(2): 171–184. http://doi.org/10.1016/j.diabres.2007.12.020.

Esposito, D. (Ed.) (2013). *Reliability and Validity of Data Sources for Outcomes Research and Disease and Health Management Programs.* Lawrenceville, NJ: ISPOR.

EuroQol Group. (1990). EuroQol—A New Facility for the Measurement of Health-Related Quality of Life. *Health Policy* (Amsterdam, Netherlands) 16(3): 199–208.

Fleishman, J. A. (2005). *Methodology Report No. 15: Demographic and Clinical Variations in Health Status.* (AHRQ Pub. No. 05-0022.) Rockville, MD: Agency for Healthcare Research and Quality. Retrieved from http://www.meps.ahrq.gov/data_files/publications/mr15/mr15.shtml.

Gafni, A. (1994). The Standard Gamble Method: What Is Being Measured and How It Is Interpreted. *Health Services Research* 29(2): 207.

Gold, M. R., P. Franks, K. I. McCoy, and D. G. Fryback. (1998). Toward Consistency in Cost-Utility Analyses: Using National Measures to Create Condition-Specific Values. *Medical Care* 36(6): 778–792.

Gold, M. R., and P. Muennig. (2002). Measure-Dependent Variation in Burden of Disease Estimates: Implications for Policy. *Medical Care* 40(3): 260–266.

Gold, M. R., J. E. Siegel, L. B. Russell, and M. C. Weinstein. (1996). *Cost-Effectiveness in Health and Medicine.* New York: Oxford University Press.

Grandy, S., K. M. Fox, and SHIELD Study Group. (2012). Change in Health Status (EQ-5D) over 5 Years Among Individuals With and Without Type 2 Diabetes Mellitus in the SHIELD Longitudinal Study. *Health and Quality of Life Outcomes* 10: 99. http://doi.org/10.1186/1477-7525-10-99.

Guyatt, G. H., D. H. Feeny, and D. L. Patrick. (1993). Measuring Health-Related Quality of Life. *Annals of Internal Medicine* 118(8): 622–629.

Institute for Health Metrics and Evaluation. (2015). Global Burden of Disease (GBD). Retrieved March 27, 2015, from http://www.healthdata.org/gbd.

Irvine, L., G. R. Barton, A. V. Gasper, N. Murray, A. Clark, T. Scarpello, and M. Sampson. (2011). Cost-Effectiveness of a Lifestyle Intervention in Preventing Type 2 Diabetes. *International Journal of Technology Assessment in Health Care* 27(4): 275–282. http://doi.org/10.1017/S0266462311000365.

Kaplan, R. M., and J. P. Anderson. (1988). A General Health Policy Model: Update and Applications. *Health Services Research* 23(2): 203–235.

Keech, M., A. J. Scott, and P. J. Ryan. (1998). The Impact of Influenza and Influenza-Like Illness on Productivity and Healthcare Resource Utilization in a Working Population. *Occupational Medicine* (Oxford, England), 48(2): 85–90.

Le, Q. A. (2014). Probabilistic Mapping of the Health Status Measure SF-12 onto the Health Utility Measure EQ-5D Using the US-Population-Based Scoring Models. *Quality of Life Research* 23(2): 459–466. http://doi.org/10.1007/s11136-013-0517-3.

Le, Q. A., and J. N. Doctor. (2011). Probabilistic Mapping of Descriptive Health Status Responses onto Health State Utilities Using Bayesian Networks: An Empirical Analysis Converting SF-12 into EQ-5D Utility Index in a National US Sample. *Medical Care* 49(5): 451–460. http://doi.org/10.1097/MLR.0b013e318207e9a8.

Lopez, A. D., C. D. Mathers, M. Ezzati, D. T. Jamison, and C. J. Murray. (2006). *Global Burden of Disease and Risk Factors*. New York: Oxford University Press.

Lubetkin, E. I., H. Jia, P. Franks, and M. R. Gold. (2005). Relationship Among Sociodemographic Factors, Clinical Conditions, and Health-Related Quality of Life: Examining the EQ-5D in the U.S. General Population. *Quality of Life Research* 14(10): 2187–2196. http://doi.org/10.1007/s11136-005-8028-5.

Matza, L. S., K. S. Boye, N. Yurgin, J. Brewster-Jordan, S. Mannix, J. M. Shorr, and B. L. Barber. (2007). Utilities and Disutilities for Type 2 Diabetes Treatment-Related Attributes. *Quality of Life Research* 16(7): 1251–1265. http://doi.org/10.1007/s11136-007-9226-0.

Mehrez, A., and A. Gafni. (1990). Evaluating Health Related Quality of Life: An Indifference Curve Interpretation for the Time Trade-off Technique. *Social Science & Medicine* 31(11): 1281–1283.

Muennig, P., P. Franks, and M. Gold. (2005). The Cost Effectiveness of Health Insurance. *American Journal of Preventive Medicine* 28(1): 59–64. http://doi.org/10.1016/j.amepre.2004.09.005.

Muennig, P., P. Franks, H. Jia, E. Lubetkin, and M. R. Gold. (2005). The Income-Associated Burden of Disease in the United States. *Social Science & Medicine* 61(9): 2018–2026. http://doi.org/10.1016/j.socscimed.2005.04.005.

Neumann, P. J., G. D. Sanders, L. B. Russell, J. E. Siegel, and T. G. Ganiats. (2016). *Cost-Effectiveness in Health and Medicine*. New York: Oxford University Press.

Nord, E., N. Daniels, and M. Kamlet. (2009). QALYs: Some Challenges. *Value in Health* 12: S10–S15. http://doi.org/10.1111/j.1524-4733.2009.00516.x.

Sinha, A., M. Rajan, T. Hoerger, and L. Pogach. (2010). Costs and Consequences Associated with Newer Medications for Glycemic Control in Type 2 Diabetes. *Diabetes Care* 33(4): 695–700. http://doi.org/10.2337/dc09-1488.

Sullivan, P. W. (2006). Mapping the EQ-5D Index from the SF-12: US General Population Preferences in a Nationally Representative Sample. *Medical Decision Making* 26(4): 401–409. http://doi.org/10.1177/0272989X06290496.

Sullivan, P. W., and V. Ghushchyan. (2006). Preference-Based EQ-5D Index Scores for Chronic Conditions in the United States. *Medical Decision Making* 26(4): 410–420. http://doi.org/10.1177/0272989X06290495.

Sullivan, P. W., W. F. Lawrence, and V. Ghushchyan. (2005). A National Catalog of Preference-Based Scores for Chronic Conditions in the United States. *Medical Care* 43(7): 736–749.

Torrance, G. W. (1976). Social Preferences for Health States: An Empirical Evaluation of Three Measurement Techniques. *Socio-Economic Planning Sciences* 10(3): 129–136. http://doi.org/10.1016/0038-0121(76)90036-7.

Torrance, G. W., W. H. Thomas, and D. L. Sackett. (1972). A Utility Maximization Model for Evaluation of Health Care Programs. *Health Services Research* 7(2): 118.

Von Neumann, J., and O. Morgenstern. (1953). *Theory of Games and Economic Behavior*. Princeton, NJ: Princeton University Press.

World Health Organization. (2015). Metrics: Disability-Adjusted Life Year (DALY). Retrieved March 27, 2015, from http://www.who.int/healthinfo/global_burden_disease/metrics_daly/en/.

CHAPTER 8

CALCULATING QALYS

Overview

This chapter demonstrates various approaches to calculating QALYs. Each approach provides a unique perspective on what QALYs are, how they are used, and how they are calculated. We call these methods (1) the life table method, (2) the Markov method, and (3) the summation method.

In the life table method, a spreadsheet is used to calculate the number of deaths and person-years remaining in a hypothetical cohort, as we did in Chapter 6. These person-years are then adjusted for HRQL to obtain the total QALYs lived (Erickson, Wilson, & Shannon, 1995; Muennig & Gold, 2001). In the Markov method, subjects in a hypothetical cohort gain 1 QALY for each year they remain alive. We also saw in Chapter 6 how this worked but used life-years rather than QALYs. The summation method is used when we have concrete information on the changes in life-years and HRQL associated with an intervention already on hand (Drummond, Sculpher, Torrance, O'Brien, & Stoddart, 2005).

We also discuss the disability-adjusted life year (DALY), which is often used in studies within developing countries or studies comparing the burden of disease among nations. While a QALY is a year of perfect health gained, a DALY is a year of perfect health lost to disease (Lopez, Mathers, Ezzati, Jamison, & Murray, 2006; Murray & Lopez, 1997). Those who use DALYs are not simply a bunch of pessimistic health economists. Rather, this inverted definition arises from how DALYs are used (typically, to capture the burden of disease) and how they are calculated.

LEARNING OBJECTIVES

- Calculate the QALYs using the different methods introduced in this chapter.

- Construct a life table based on the probability of survival for a hypothetical cohort.

- Derive the quality-adjusted life expectancy given a life table.

- Calculate the total QALYs over a given amount of time using discounting.

- Describe the usefulness of DALYs in comparisons across different countries.

We begin by exploring how to calculate the incremental number of QALYs gained by summation. We demonstrate how to calculate QALYs using the life table method and then move on to a worked example using Markov models. The last bit will be dedicated to the DALY.

Using the Summation Method

Let's go a few months into the future. You have finished reading this book, and a researcher wants to hire you to help her team perform a cost-effectiveness analysis of a new treatment for a tropical disease, leishmaniasis, in sub-Saharan Africa.

They've provided you with five years of follow-up data from a randomized controlled trial. You've calculated the change in costs, but you need to figure out how this treatment has changed the quality and quantity of life for these subjects over this five-year period.

The summation method is most often used when gains in life expectancy and HRQL are more or less identifiable. This situation is sometimes encountered in economic evaluations conducted in developing countries. It's also quite useful for illustrating the basic concepts behind QALYs (Drummond et al., 2005).

Suppose that the new treatment for leishmaniasis has an unknown impact on the overall quality of life but improves life expectancy by one year over the five-year span of the study and that the average person with the disease has a three-year life expectancy. We consult the literature and find that the average HRQL of people with leishmaniasis is 0.5 and the average untreated life expectancy is three years. Thus, each year that the subjects are alive, they gain 0.5 QALYs. Assuming that the treatment prolongs life but produces no improvement in HRQL, the two interventions (treatment versus no treatment) would accrue the following QALYs:

$$\text{Treatment: } 0.5 + 0.5 + 0.5 + 0.5 = 2 \text{ QALYs}$$

$$\text{No treatment: } 0.5 + 0.5 + 0.5 + 0 = 1.5 \text{ QALYs} \tag{8.1}$$

The total number of QALYs gained by treatment is 2 QALYs − 1.5 QALYs = 0.5 QALYs. Had we not adjusted for HRQL, the gain would have been 4 years − 3 years = 1 year.

Now suppose that we estimate the impact of the treatment on various health states and calculate changes in HRQL using a preference-weighted instrument. If we know that the mean HRQL of treated people is 0.6 and the mean HRQL of untreated people is 0.5, then we can also account for the ability of the drug to improve one's quality of life:

$$\text{Treatment: } 0.6 + 0.6 + 0.6 + 0.6 = 2.4 \text{ QALYs}$$

$$\text{No treatment: } 0.5 + 0.5 + 0.5 + 0 = 1.5 \text{ QALYs} \qquad (8.2)$$

The total number of QALYs gained by treatment is $2.4 - 1.5 = 0.9$.

Now let us go one step further and consider the lifetime health pathway for people with this disease. Suppose that a different group of researchers managed to obtain year-to-year data on the subjects' specific HRQL with this disease. They also intervened at an earlier stage of disease, so the cohort lived longer, and followed them over many years. The researchers manage to plot the health status in the number of deaths over time of subjects in their cohort (Figure 8.1). The light-shaded curve in the figure represents their quality-adjusted life expectancy (QALE) if untreated, and the dark-shaded curve represents their average QALE if treated. In this case, the incremental gain in QALYs is equal to the area under the dark-shaded curve minus the area under the light-shaded curve. Said another way, it is equal to $\text{QALE}_{Treated} - \text{QALE}_{Untreated}$.

We see, too, that the average treated person on this graph lived 12 years and the average untreated person 13 years. However, the total QALYs gained differs substantially because the treated group has a higher HRQL. Keep this image in your head; it will come in handy to understand how more complex methods work.

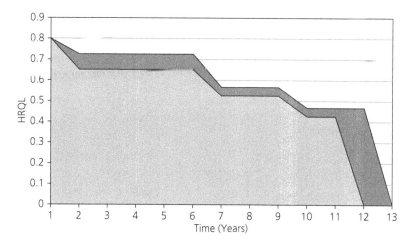

Figure 8.1   Year-to-Year Progress of Treated and Untreated Subjects with Leishmaniasis

Note: The light area represents untreated patients and the dark area treated patients. The incremental gain in QALYs is the difference between the dark area and light area.

Using the Life Table Method

Life expectancy may be calculated using a **standard life table** or an **abridged life table** (Anderson, 2000). A standard life table calculates life expectancy for a group of people based on the mortality rate over one-year age intervals, and an abridged life table uses five-year (or longer) age intervals. Thus, although an abridged life table provides information across a wider age range, a standard life table is slightly more accurate. Appendix B contains abridged life tables and quality-adjusted life tables for the U.S. population for 2011.

TIPS AND TRICKS

Actually, abridged life tables can be difficult to calculate because there are several adjustments that are done (Anderson, 2000; Hsieh, 1991; Reed & Merrell, 1995). These adjustments are not always intuitive and transparent. For example, the abridged life table for the United States in 2011 uses a different type of adjustment to estimate person-years lived for each year and may not be reproducible. For our purpose, we focus on how to use the life tables to estimate quality-adjusted life expectancy.

Pull up the spreadsheet we used in Chapter 6 containing person-years. (If you are following along without the spreadsheet, Table 6.5 is renamed Table 8.1 and presented as follows.)

Let's begin by calculating life expectancy at each age in Table 8.1. To do this, first sum up the total person-years lived in the cohort starting with the first cell at the bottom of column 3. Thus, we add the number of person-years lived by 100-year-olds (1,075) to the number lived by 99-year-olds (2,426) in the age 99 cell of column 3 to obtain the cumulative total person-years by age 99 (1,075 + 2,426 = 3,501). We then repeat this process across all ages as in column 4 of Table 8.2. (The values in column 4 may be slightly higher due to rounding in column 3.)

TIPS AND TRICKS

Notice that we applied the midpoint correction here. For the completed exercise, see Table 8.1 at http://www.wiley.com/WileyCDA/WileyTitle/productCd-1119011264.html.

Finally, to calculate life expectancy at each age, we divide the number of subjects alive at the start of any given age interval (column 1) by the cumulative total person-years (column 4) up to that age (see Table 8.3). Recall that by dividing the total number of years lived by the total number of people who lived them yields the mean number of years lived per person.

Table 8.1   Total Person-Years Lived by the Cohort of 1 Million 15-Year-Olds

Age	Alive (1)	All Deaths (2)	Person-Years (Col. 1 − Col. 2 × 0.5) (3)
15	1,000,000	407	999,797
16	999,593	575	999,306
17	999,018	683	998,677
18	998,335	728	997,971
19	997,607	734	997,240
20	996,873	898	996,424
...	...	...	...
95	29,011	11,589	23,217
96	17,422	8,754	13,045
97	8,668	3,989	6,674
98	4,679	1,234	4,062
99	3,445	2,038	2,426
100	1,407	664	1,075
Total	64,169,845	999,257	63,670,217

Table 8.2   Sum of Person-Years Across Age Groups for the Cohort of 1 Million 15-Year-Olds

Column	1	2	3	4
Age	Alive	All Deaths	Person-Years Col. 1 − Col. 2 × 0.5	Cumulative Person-Years Sum of Col. 3 Values from Bottom
15	1,000,000	407	999,797	63,670,217
16	999,593	575	999,306	62,670,421
17	999,018	683	998,677	61,671,115
18	998,335	728	997,971	60,672,439
19	997,607	734	997,240	59,674,468
20	996,873	898	996,424	58,677,228
...	...	...	...	...
95	29,011	11,589	23,217	50,500
96	17,422	8,754	13,045	27,283
97	8,668	3,989	6,674	14,238
98	4,679	1,234	4,062	7,564
99	3,445	2,038	2,426	3,501 ⇐ 1,075 + 2,426
100	1,407	664	1,075	1,075

Table 8.3   Calculating Life Expectancy at a Given Age

Age	Alive (1)	All Deaths (2)	Person-Years (Col. 1 – Col. 2 × 0.5) (3)	Cumulative Person-Years (Sum of Col. 3 Values from Bottom) (4)	Life Expectancy (Col. 4/Col. 1) (5)
15	1,000,000	407	999,797	63,670,217	63.67
16	999,593	575	999,306	62,670,421	62.70
17	999,018	683	998,677	61,671,115	61.73
18	998,335	728	997,971	60,672,439	60.77
19	997,607	734	997,240	59,674,468	59.82
20	996,873	898	996,424	58,677,228	58.86
...	...	...	...	...	...
95	29,011	11,589	23,217	50,500	1.74
96	17,422	8,754	13,045	27,283	1.57
97	8,668	3,989	6,674	14,238	1.64
98	4,679	1,234	4,062	7,564	1.62
99	3,445	2,038	2,426	3,501	1.02
100	1,407	664	1,075	1,075	0.76

Note: Life expectancy at any age is calculated by the total years alive at that age by the cumulative person-years lived at that age. For patients who are 100 years old, the life expectancy is calculated as the person-years divided by the number alive $\left(\frac{1,075}{1,407} \right)$.

You just learned how to build a life table. In the first part of Chapter 6, you learned how to work with abridged data. In the second part, you learned how to calculate the total person-years and the life expectancy using year-to-year data. Here, we combine these two concepts. Table 8.4 is an abridged life table for 2011, the latest table available for our 2015 publication deadline.

In this table, we begin with the probability of dying within any age group, which is essentially the mortality rate for that age group (column 1). This rate is obtained using national mortality data (Hoyert & Xu, 2012). We then apply this mortality rate to a hypothetical cohort of 100,000 newborn babies (column 2) to obtain the total number of deaths in each age interval (column 3). (In other words, column 3 is column 1 times column 2.) Total person-years in the interval are estimated by multiplying the difference between column 2 – column 3 × 0.5 by the number of years in the interval. (Therefore, column 4 = 5 × (column 2 – column 3 × 0.5).) The calculation of column 4 for year 0–1 involves using a separate factor of 0.128 (column 4 (age interval 0–1) = 0.128 × 100,000 + (1 – 0.128) × 99,394). (Separation

Table 8.4   Abridged Life Table for 2011

Age (Years)	Probability of Dying Between Ages X and $X+N$ (1)[a]	Number Surviving to Age X (2)	Numberc Dying Between Ages X and $X+N$ (Col. 1 x Col. 2) (3)	Person-Years Lived Between Ages X and $X+N$ (4)	Total Number of Person-Years Lived Above Age X (Sum of Col. 4 Values) (5)	Expectancy of Life at Age X (Col.5/Col. 2) (6)
0–1	0.006058	100,000	606	99,472	7,969,412	79.7
1–5	0.001054	99,394	105	496,709	7,869,940	79.2
5–10	0.000603	99,289	60	496,298	7,373,231	74.3
10–15	0.000709	99,230	70	495,972	6,876,934	69.3
15–20	0.002438	99,159	242	495,192	6,380,962	64.4
20–25	0.004296	98,917	425	493,525	5,885,770	59.5
25–30	0.004824	98,493	475	491,275	5,392,245	54.7
30–35	0.005638	98,017	553	488,705	4,900,970	50.0
35–40	0.006985	97,465	681	485,622	4,412,265	45.3
40–45	0.010006	96,784	968	481,499	3,926,643	40.6
45–50	0.016018	95,816	1,535	475,241	3,445,144	36.0
50–55	0.024459	94,281	2,306	465,639	2,969,904	31.5
55–60	0.035105	91,975	3,229	451,802	2,504,265	27.2
60–65	0.049332	88,746	4,378	432,785	2,052,463	23.1
65–70	0.07331	84,368	6,185	406,377	1,619,678	19.2
70–75	0.110896	78,183	8,670	369,239	1,213,301	15.5
75–80	0.172915	69,513	12,020	317,514	844,061	12.1
80–85	0.274093	57,493	15,758	248,069	526,547	9.2
85–90	0.429792	41,735	17,937	163,830	278,478	6.7
90–95	0.617599	23,797	14,697	82,244	114,648	4.8
95–100	0.787828	9,100	7,169	27,577	32,404	3.6
100 and over	1.000000	1,931	1,931	4,827	4,827	2.5

[a]Values were derived from U.S. Life Tables 2011. Calculations for these values require further adjustments that are beyond the scope of this text. For now, just focus on how these numbers are important in determining QALYs.

factors change with each U.S. Life Table, which can be found with each publication.)

Note: This is not the exact value you will see in the U.S. Life Table because we did not apply any of the nuanced adjustments. You do not need to worry about it for this chapter.

Summing column 4 data by age interval, we obtain the total person-years lived by the cohort up to that age. And, finally, the total person-years in the cohort divided by the number of subjects at the start (in this case 100,000 persons) is equal to the life expectancy of the cohort (column 5).

Quality-Adjusted Life Expectancy

Quality-adjusted life expectancy (QALE) is the number of years of perfect health one can expect to live at birth. You get this number by multiplying the total person-years within an age interval by the age-specific HRQL score for that age interval (see Table 8.5).

In Table 8.5, we see that the people in the first year had an HRQL of 0.95 (this was obtained from the Medical Expenditure Panel Survey). The product of the HRQL score and the person-years in the age interval yields the total QALYs lived by the cohort in that age interval. If we sum the total QALYs lived in each age interval across all intervals, we get the total QALYs lived by the cohort. Once again, we divide by the 100,000 people at the start of the cohort to get QALE.

TIPS AND TRICKS

To follow along, download Example 8.2 from http://www.wiley.com/WileyCDA/WileyTitle/productCd-1119011264.html.

Of course, a person's QALE changes when disease is present; disease can affect health (and thus HRQL) or life expectancy, or both. It also changes when different medical interventions are administered. Like disease, health interventions have an effect on the quality and quantity of life. The number of QALYs gained when a health intervention is implemented is calculated using the following equation:

$$QALE_{Intervention\ 1} - QALE_{Intervention\ 2}$$

where intervention 1 is the more effective intervention.

How do we go about this? Simple. We just estimate the change in life expectancy and the change in HRQL associated with an intervention, calculate QALE with and without the intervention, and voilà!

Now think back to Figure 8.1. This figure showed that the health pathways between people given an intervention and people not given an intervention differ from year to year. Here, we see that a quality-adjusted life table does precisely that.

Exercises 1 to 4

To complete these exercises, you'll need to download the 2015 QALE calculator from http://www.wiley.com/WileyCDA/WileyTitle/productCd-1119011264.html.

Table 8.5   A Quality-Adjusted Life Table

Age (years) X+N (1)	Probability of Dying Between Ages X and X+N (1)	Number Surviving to Age X (2)	Number Dying Between Ages X and X+N (Col. 1 × Col. 2) (3)	Person-Years Lived Between Ages X and X+N (4)	HRQL Score (Obtained from MEPS) (5)ª	Quality-Adjusted Person-Years Lived Between X and X+N (Col 4 × Col 5) (6)	Total Quality-Adjusted Number of Person-Years Lived Above Age X (Sum of Col. 4 Values) (7)	Quality-Adjusted Expectancy of Life at Age X (Col.7/Col. 2) (8)
0–1	0.006058	100,000	606	99,472	0.95	94,498	6,091,835	60.9
1–5	0.001054	99,394	105	496,709	0.94	466,907	5,997,337	60.3
5–10	0.000603	99,289	60	496,298	0.93	461,557	5,530,430	55.7
10–15	0.000709	99,230	70	495,972	0.92	456,294	5,068,873	51.1
15–20	0.002438	99,159	242	495,192	0.9	445,673	4,612,579	46.5
20–25	0.004296	98,917	425	493,525	0.89	439,237	4,166,906	42.1
25–30	0.004824	98,493	475	491,275	0.89	437,235	3,727,669	37.8
30–35	0.005638	98,017	553	488,705	0.84	410,513	3,290,434	33.6
35–40	0.006985	97,465	681	485,622	0.84	407,922	2,879,921	29.5
40–45	0.010006	96,784	968	481,499	0.84	404,459	2,471,999	25.5
45–50	0.016018	95,816	1,535	475,241	0.84	399,202	2,067,540	21.6
50–55	0.024459	94,281	2,306	465,639	0.79	367,855	1,668,338	17.7
55–60	0.035105	91,975	3,229	451,802	0.79	356,923	1,300,483	14.1
60–65	0.049332	88,746	4,378	432,785	0.79	341,900	943,560	10.6
65–70	0.07331	84,368	6,185	406,377	0.79	321,038	601,660	7.1
70–75	0.110896	78,183	8,670	369,239	0.76	280,622	280,622	3.6

ªValues for those under 18 were not available in the Medical Expenditure Panel Survey (MEPS) and were obtained using predictive linear regression.

1. Desperate for a job out of public health school, you have taken a position with a health foods company. It has produced a new product called Super Holistic Chakra Enhancer, which it claims reduces mortality by 50 percent. It has asked you to translate this miraculous effect into life-years gained. You shrug your shoulders and set to the calculations. What number do you give for the total years gained by an infant given this formula for the rest of his or her life? Tip: Enter the risk ratio into the column labeled "Crude Risk Ratio," and see how the overall life expectancy changes.

2. You quit your job working on Super Holistic Chakra Enhancer and decide to join a group working on the cost-effectiveness of a new drug to lower blood sugar in patients with diabetes. The target audience has a mean age of disease onset of 60 years. You wish to know how the drug compares to the current practice. You find that the average diabetic over age 60 is at 10 percent greater annual risk of mortality than the average person in the United States. The new drug has been shown to have a risk ratio (RR) of 0.95 compared to current practice among diabetics. How many years of life will be gained on average? Hint: Be sure to enter risk ratios starting at age 60 in the table.

3. Your next step is to calculate the gain in QALE. You go to the Medical Expenditure Panel Survey linked to mortality data and find that the mean HRQL for people over age 60 is 0.7. Your team finds that there is a 10 percent improvement in HRQL. How many QALYs are gained when this new treatment is consistently given to diabetics?

4. Just for fun, let's see what your life expectancy is relative to the average person in your country. If you are from the United States, use the life table provided. Otherwise, you can build your own life table by copying age-specific mortality probabilities from a life table from your ministry of health (any search engine should get you there). Assuming you are on your way to some graduate degree, here is a rough indicator of your risk of death at any given age: (1) If you are from a country with very few college-educated people, give yourself a risk ratio of about 0.5 beginning at your current age. (2) If you are from a country with a high number of college-educated people (e.g., the United States, Japan, countries in Europe, Cuba), give yourself a risk ratio of about 0.65. (This is lower because the average person is somewhat more likely to have a college or graduate degree, putting him or her closer to you.) Note that the answer to this exercise is age and country dependent, so there is no answer provided in the key.

Using Markov Models to Calculate QALE

In Chapter 6, you saw that life expectancy is calculated in a Markov model by granting survivors one year of life. To calculate QALE, we simply substitute the one-year gain every year with the age-specific HRQL score.

Recall that every time the tree cycles, we gain one year of life expectancy (Incr Rwd = 1) and that the annual risk of death is obtained from a life table. In Figure 8.2, this is represented as tDead[_stage]. In this diagram, [_stage] indicates how many cycles have been completed. So when the subject is 10 years of age, _stage = 10. A subject who has an HRQL of 0.9 rather than 1.0 would have lived 9 QALYs over these 10 cycles.

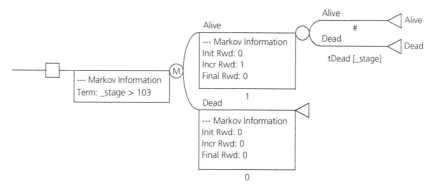

Figure 8.2   Basic Markov Model Used to Calculate Life Expectancy

Let's take this to the next level to see how we might calculate the QALYs gained by a particular intervention using Markov models. Suppose that you are comparing two surgical treatments for a congenital heart valve defect. This defect affects newborns but can be corrected using one of these two procedures at birth.

The first procedure is called the Filmore procedure (after Ignacious Danenhousen Filmore) and does a pretty good job of fixing the problem at no initial risk to the infant to speak of. However, each year, the person will be at a 25 percent increased risk of mortality due to the incomplete nature of this surgical technique.

Recently Ludviga Elmore Reinkenshein modified the Filmore procedure so that it completely fixes the heart defect. However, she patented her surgical technique, so it's expensive, requiring the hospital to pay $10,000 to her every time it's used. Let's first look at these two procedures in terms of effectiveness alone.

We know that babies who receive the Reinkenshein procedure have an approximately normal life expectancy. Those who receive the Filmore procedure will be at 25 percent increased risk of death. Therefore, if tDead[_stage] in Figure 8.2 reflects the mean life expectancy in the United States, the risk of death among those receiving the Filmore procedure is simply 1.25 × the age-specific mortality rate. (In other words, the age-specific mortality rate increased by 25 percent.) This change can

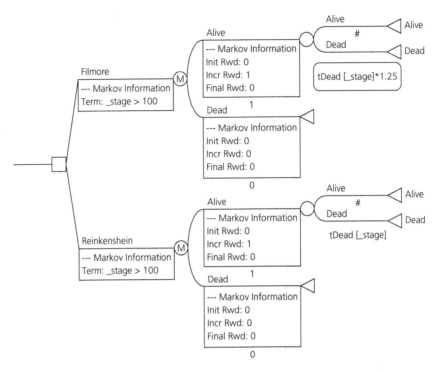

Figure 8.3   Markov Models Designed to Calculate the Life Expectancy of Subjects Receiving the Filmore and Reinkenshein Procedures

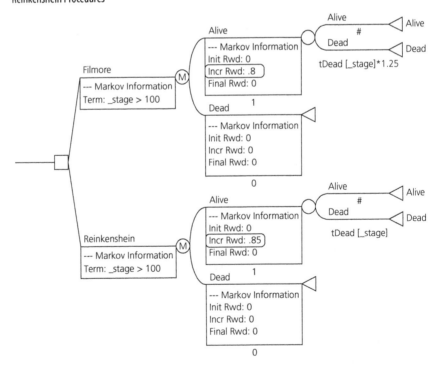

Figure 8.4   Difference in HRQL Among Subjects Who Received the Filmore or the Reinkenshein Procedure

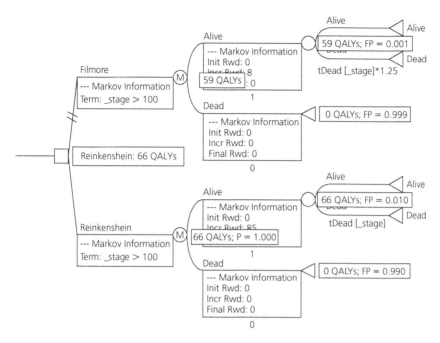

Figure 8.5   Filmore Versus Reinkenshein Model Rolled Back to Reveal Gains in Quality-Adjusted Life Expectancy Associated with Each Strategy

be seen in the top portion of Figure 8.3. Notice that `tDead[_stage]` is multiplied by 1.25 to reflect the higher mortality in this group.

Now let's add a measure of HRQL to each arm. Suppose that we take a group of patients living with the Filmore procedure and a group living with the Reinkenshein procedure and have them fill out the EQ-5D. We find that those with the Filmore procedure have an average HRQL of 0.8, and those who have the Reinkenshein procedure have an average HRQL of 0.85. To calculate the difference in QALE, we give subjects with the Filmore procedure a gain of 0.8 for every year that they lived and those who had the Reinkenshein procedure a gain of 0.85 (Figure 8.4).

Now let's see what happens when we calculate the QALE of each competing alternative (Figure 8.5). Here we see that greedy Ludviga's procedure does result in a significantly longer QALE—about seven years of additional life lived in perfect health. The next logical question is: Is this worth the extra cost?

More On Discounting

In Chapter 4, we discussed how and why we discount costs. But what about health benefits, such as QALYs? Should they also be discounted?

Let's consider a simple thought experiment. Suppose a patient has cancer and needs lifesaving therapy right away. Postponing this therapy will likely result in death. In other words, waiting will result in some amount of health benefit that is discounted over time. If the health benefit is lost due to delays or postponements, then we need to apply discounting (Gold, Siegel, Russell, & Weinstein, 1996; Neumann, Sanders, Russell, Siegel, & Ganiats, 2016).

So what should the discount rate be for health benefits (e.g., QALYs)? For decades, there have been many debates about the appropriate discount rate that should be applied to the health benefit component (e.g., QALYs) of a cost-effectiveness analysis. This debate has sparked numerous suggestions for how to discount health benefits in cost-effectiveness analysis.

The U.S. Panel on Cost-Effectiveness in Health and Medicine recommends using a uniform discount rate of 3 percent for both costs and health benefits per (Gold et al., 1996; Neumann et al., 2016). However, other researchers argue that the discount rate for benefits should be different from (and possibly lower than) the discount rate used for costs (Katz & Welch, 1993; Nord, 2011; Parsonage & Neuburger, 1992).

One argument that has defended the uniform discounting rate being applied to cost and health benefits (e.g., QALYs) is the Keeler-Cretin paradox. Keeler and Cretin (1983) demonstrated that a health benefit that is postponed could artificially decrease the incremental cost-effectiveness ratio (ICER) as time increases if the discount rate for health benefits was less than the discount rate for costs. For example, if a lifesaving surgery was needed now but was costly (due to the ICER being quite large), then a decision maker would postpone the surgery until next year when the ICER would be lower. Imagine that we fast-forward to the future by one year; the decision maker has to face the same issue once again. Predictably, the decision maker will postpone the surgery in order to have a favorable ICER the following year. As a consequence, a decision maker would always postpone having the surgery because the ICER the following year will always be lower than the ICER in the current year. This is called the Keeler-Cretin paradox and has been the main reason that uniform discounting for cost and health benefits should be applied rather than differential discounting (Keeler & Cretin, 1983).

For now, we will go with the recommendations from the U.S. Panel on Cost-Effectiveness in Health and Medicine and use a discount rate of 3 percent for both costs and QALYs. One way to deal with this problem is to perform sensitivity analyses on the discount rates. We will show you how to perform sensitivity analyses in Chapter 9.

Issues with QALYs

QALYs are a great way to capture health benefits in a cost-effectiveness analysis. However, they are not a perfect metric, and there are some concerns with using them. One of the concerns with QALYs is rooted in how the utility score is estimated. In Chapter 7, you were introduced to different methods to capture preference scores (otherwise known as "utility") for a given health state. Now, in the examples in this chapter, you used the preference scores (e.g., HRQL scores) to estimate the QALYs with a variety of methods. But how are these preference scores captured? Were they captured ex ante (before the event) or post ante (after the event)? And are QALYs independent across time? Researchers have struggled with this problem for years and have not come up with a good solution.

Another issue with QALYs has to do with fairness. Does society value someone who is older versus someone who is younger? How about someone who has a disease that is self-inflicted versus someone who develops a disease because of genetics? Even though the QALYs are similar, who should be given priority? This issue has come up with liver transplantation in alcoholics (Ubel, 1997). Society tends to value you differently depending on your preexisting conditions. For example, in a hypothetical example where subjects were asked to value a lifesaving treatment in patients with and without preexisting paraplegia, the value of a treatment that saved the lives of patients with preexisting paraplegia was equivalent to a lifesaving treatment that restored a patient without preexisting paraplegia to perfect health (Ubel, Richardson, & Prades, 1999). In other words, society does not value QALYs equally.

Another criticism of QALYs is the assumption of additive utility independence (Bleichrodt & Filko, 2008; Gandjour & Gafni, 2010; Spencer, 2000). When health status varies across time, we normally add up the QALYs to give us the total QALYs experienced during that time frame. In order to do this, we have to assume that the QALYs at different time points are independent of each other. This makes calculating QALYs across time very simple. However, there is some concern that QALYs are correlated over time, meaning that the sequence of the preferences is important and some adjustment should be made. Fortunately, there is evidence to support the additive utility independence assumption (Spencer, 2000; Spencer & Robinson, 2007; Treadwell, 1998). For the purposes of this text, we will assume that the additive utility independence assumption holds.

Calculating Incremental Cost-Effectiveness

Now we add cost differences to the model and show how a Markov model calculates incremental cost-effectiveness ratios. Let's say that we know that each procedure costs $12,500 to perform. (It would actually be a lot more, but I want to avoid shocking anyone reading this book.) We also know that the Reinkenshein procedure costs an additional $10,000 in patent fees to perform, bringing the cost of this procedure up to $22,500. (Look at the initial cost entries in Figure 8.6.)

PROJECT MAP

1. Think through your research question.

2. Sketch out the analysis.

3. Collect data for your model.

4. Adjust your data.

5. Build your model.

6. *Run and test the model.*

7. Conduct a sensitivity analysis.

8. Write it up.

In Chapter 4, you learned that both costs and effectiveness values must be discounted, and at the same rate. In this case, the cost of the procedure is incurred at birth, so there is no discounting applied. Therefore, we'll want to discount only the HRQL values we enter into these models. (Recall that the Panel of Cost-Effectiveness in Health and Medicine's reference case uses a discount rate of 3 percent.)

Figure 8.7 shows the model with the discounting equation $\left(\frac{\text{HRQL}}{1.03^{\text{time}}}\right)$ added. Remember that the time that passes is represented as _stage, so the formula is $\left(\frac{\text{HRQL}}{1.03^{[\_\text{stage}]}}\right)$.

Finally, Figure 8.8 shows the incremental cost-effectiveness of the Reinkenshein procedure. Notice that the gains in QALE have shrunk considerably after we discounted the values. Nonetheless, the incremental cost charged by greedy Ludviga ($10,000) is more than justified by the gains in QALYs (2 QALYs). The incremental cost-effectiveness is just $5,000 per QALY gained.

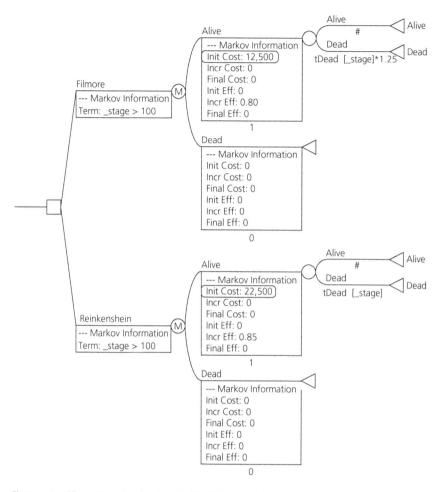

Figure 8.6   Filmore Versus Reinkenshein Model with Costs Added

Exercises 5 to 9

You are running a small needle exchange organization for intravenous drug users in Lagos. You estimate that the program will reduce the seroprevalence of HIV infection by 5 percent among a group of subjects who are being treated for HIV infection. You look through the literature and are able to find the cost of treating HIV for a year ($1,000). You also know the cost of running the program for one year ($100,000) and life expectancy for HIV-negative persons (20 years) and HIV-positive persons (15 years).

5. You are asked to evaluate the cost returns associated with one year of operation. Which costs are counted over the one-year period, and which costs go beyond this one-year period? (Hint: Think about the future cost savings associated with the initial investment.)

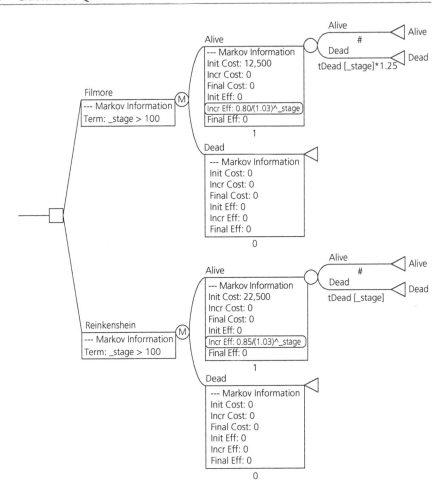

Figure 8.7   Filmore Versus Reinkenshein Model with Discounting Added to the HRQL Values

6. You estimate that the program prevents 100 cases of HIV per year. How much money will preventing these 100 cases save over their lifetimes? Assume that none of the cases prevented by your program will later become infected with HIV.

7. What is the lifetime cost savings of the 100 cases in Exercise 5 at a 3 percent rate of discount? Recall that the formula is: Cost/$(1.03)^t$, where t is time in the future. For simplicity, assign year 1 savings equal to $1,000 and begin discounting in year 2.

8. HIV-positive patients in Lagos have an average HRQL score of 0.6. What is their discounted quality-adjusted life expectancy? (Use a discount rate of 3 percent here, too.)

9. HIV-negative persons in Lagos have an average HRQL of 0.9. What is the incremental gain in QALYs per HIV case prevented? (Again, assume that none of the subjects for whom HIV was prevented in year 1 will later become HIV positive.)

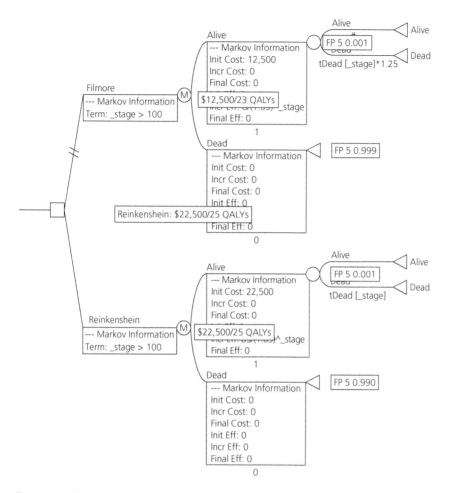

Figure 8.8   Filmore Versus Reinkenshein Model Rolled Back

Disability-Adjusted Life-Year (DALY)

The disability-adjusted life-year (DALY) is sometimes used in international cost-effectiveness analyses. Because it was designed for burden-of-disease analysis, it's meant to estimate years of perfect health lost rather than gained. For this reason, the DALY score is equal to 1 − HRQL. Thus, if the HRQL is 0.9, the disability weight is 1 − 0.9 = 0.1. Likewise, to convert a DALY score to an HRQL score, we can simply subtract it from 1.0. The scores have been published in a huge book by Lopez, Mathers, Ezzati, Jamison, & Murray (2006) and are available for many conditions and diseases.

The general formula for the DALYs lost to disease is:

$$\text{Years of life lost (YLL)} + \text{years lost to disability (YLD)}. \qquad (8.3)$$

In other words, we first add up the future years of life lost for every death and then add up all of the years of perfect health lost while the individual was still alive to get the total DALYs lost. Thus, if a 30-year-old dies who was expected to live to 80, the years of life lost (YLL) are $80 - 30 = 50$ DALYs. If those 30 years of life had a DALY value of 0.1, then the person also lost $30 \times 0.1 = 3$ DALYs. The total DALYs lost is 50 DALYs + 3 DALYs = 53 DALYs.

The DALY is not based on the reference case analysis and for many different reasons does not produce a QALY-compatible HRQL score (Muennig & Gold, 2001; Neumann et al., 2016). For this reason, it generally should not be used in cost-effectiveness analysis. One exception might be in fieldwork in developing countries where no other HRQL measure is available.

Summary

There are several methods to calculate QALY for a cost-effectiveness analysis. You have learned to calculate QALYs using the summation method and the life table method, and with a Markov model. In addition, you learned to apply discounting when estimating QALYs for future years and then estimating the incremental cost-effectiveness ratio. Despite the limitations of the QALY, it is still useful in research on cost-effectiveness. More important, it is a tool that should be used alongside other sources of evidence to help policymakers with their final decisions.

Further Readings

Constructing life tables is easy, but there are some very difficult parts that require additional assumptions and adjustments. For a detailed description of how life tables are constructed, students should read the U.S. Vital Statistics Special Report (Greville & Carlson, 1953). Life tables and other reports on methodology can be found at the National Center for Health Statistics web site (National Center for Health Statistics, 2015).

For more discussion about the fairness and limitations of QALYs, students should read papers by Ubel et al., 1999; Dolan & Kahneman, 2008; and Nord, Daniels, & Kamlet, 2009. They provide some excellent background and history behind the debates and proposed solutions.

Curious students will find that the Keeler-Cretin paradox is nicely explained by Keeler and Cretin in their short but insightful manuscript (Keeler & Cretin, 1983).

References

Anderson, R. N. (2000). A Method for Constructing Complete Annual U.S. Life Tables. *Vital and Health Statistics. Series 2: Data Evaluation and Methods Research* (129): 1–28.

Bleichrodt, H., and M. Filko. (2008). New Tests of QALYs When Health Varies over Time. *Journal of Health Economics* 27(5): 1237–1249. http://doi.org/10.1016/j.jhealeco.2008.05.009.

Dolan, P., and D. Kahneman. (2008). Interpretations of Utility and Their Implications for the Valuation of Health. *Economic Journal* 118(525): 215–234. http://doi.org/10.1111/j.1468-0297.2007.02110.x.

Drummond, M. F., M. J. Sculpher, G. W. Torrance, B. J. O'Brien, and G. L. Stoddart. (2005). *Methods for the Economic Evaluation of Health Care Programmes*, 3rd ed. New York: Oxford University Press.

Erickson, P., R. Wilson, and I. Shannon. (1995). Years of Healthy Life. *Healthy People 2000 Statistical Notes/National Center for Health Statistics* (7): 1–15.

Gandjour, A., and A. Gafni. (2010). The Additive Utility Assumption of the QALY Model Revisited. *Journal of Health Economics* 29(2): 325–328; author reply 329–331. http://doi.org/10.1016/j.jhealeco.2009.11.001.

Gold, M. R., J. E. Siegel, L. B. Russell, and M. C. Weinstein. (1996). *Cost-Effectiveness in Health and Medicine*. New York: Oxford University Press.

Greville, T. N. E., and G. A. Carlson. (1953). Method for Constructing Abridged Life Tables for the United States, 1949. *Vital Statistics: Special Report* 3(15). Washington, DC: U.S. Public Health Service.

Hoyert, D. L., and J. Xu. (2012). Deaths: Preliminary Data for 2011. *National Vital Statistics Reports: From the Centers for Disease Control and Prevention, National Center for Health Statistics, National Vital Statistics System* 61(6): 1–51.

Hsieh, J. J. (1991). Construction of Expanded Continuous Life Tables—A Generalization of Abridged and Complete Life Tables. *Mathematical Biosciences* 103(2): 287–302.

Katz, D. A., and H. G. Welch. (1993). Discounting in Cost-Effectiveness Analysis of Healthcare Programmes. *PharmacoEconomics* 3(4): 276–285.

Keeler, E. B., and S. Cretin. (1983). Discounting of Life-Saving and Other Nonmonetary Effects. *Management Science* 29(3): 300–306.

Lopez, A. D., C. D. Mathers, M. Ezzati, D. T. Jamison, and C. J. Murray. (2006). *Global Burden of Disease and Risk Factors*. New York: Oxford University Press.

Muennig, P., and M. R. Gold. (2001). Using the Years-of-Healthy-Life Measure to Calculate QALYs. *American Journal of Preventive Medicine* 20(1): 35–39.

Murray, C. J. L., and A. D. Lopez. (1997). Global Mortality, Disability, and the Contribution of Risk Factors: Global Burden of Disease Study. *Lancet* 349(9063): 1436–1442. http://doi.org/10.1016/S0140-6736(96)07495-8.

National Center for Health Statistics. (2015). Products—Life Tables—Homepage. Retrieved March 27, 2015, from http://www.cdc.gov/nchs/products/life_tables .htm.

Neumann, P. J., G. D. Sanders, L. B. Russell, J. E. Siegel, and T. G. Ganiats. (2016). *Cost-Effectiveness in Health and Medicine.* New York: Oxford University Press.

Nord, E. (2011). Discounting Future Health Benefits: The Poverty of Consistency Arguments. *Health Economics* 20(1): 16–26. http://doi.org/10.1002/hec.1687.

Nord, E., N. Daniels, and M. Kamlet. (2009). QALYs: Some Challenges. *Value in Health* 12: S10–S15. http://doi.org/10.1111/j.1524-4733.2009.00516.x.

Parsonage, M., and H. Neuburger. (1992). Discounting and Health Benefits. *Health Economics* 1(1): 71–76.

Reed, L. J., and M. Merrell. (1995). A Short Method for Constructing an Abridged Life Table. 1939. *American Journal of Epidemiology* 141(11): 993–1022; discussion 991–992.

Spencer, A. (2000). *Testing the Additive Independence Assumption in the QALY Model* (Working Paper No. 427). Queen Mary University of London, School of Economics and Finance. Retrieved from https://ideas.repec.org/p/qmw/qmwecw/wp427.html.

Spencer, A., and A. Robinson. (2007). Tests of Utility Independence When Health Varies over Time. *Journal of Health Economics* 26(5): 1003–1013. http://doi .org/10.1016/j.jhealeco.2007.04.002.

Treadwell, J. R. (1998). Tests of Preferential Independence in the QALY Model. *Medical Decision Making* 18(4): 418–428.

Ubel, P. A. (1997). Transplantation in Alcoholics: Separating Prognosis and Responsibility from Social Biases. *Liver Transplantation and Surgery* 3(3): 343–346.

Ubel, P. A., J. Richardson, and J. L. Prades. (1999). Life-Saving Treatments and Disabilities. Are All QALYs Created Equal? *International Journal of Technology Assessment in Health Care* 15(4): 738–748.

Weinstein, M. C., G. Torrance, and A. McGuire. (2009). QALYs: The Basics. *Value in Health* 12: S5–S9. http://doi.org/10.1111/j.1524-4733.2009.00515.x.

CHAPTER 9

CONDUCTING A SENSITIVITY ANALYSIS

Overview

At various points in this book, we have seen how the value of model inputs can be difficult to establish with absolute certainty. For instance, HRQL scores can be obtained from various generic preference-weighted instruments, each producing a slightly different number (Gold & Muennig, 2002). Because these differences arise due to differences in the way the studies are designed, they represent a form of nonrandom error. Most model inputs will be derived from a sample and therefore also contain random error. (For a discussion of random and nonrandom error, see Chapter 11.)

Each model input has some level of uncertainty that can influence the results of a cost-effectiveness analysis. But how much do our results change due to uncertainty? In order to find out, sensitivity analyses are performed to test how much the initial (or base-case) results change.

Performing a Sensitivity Analysis

We can usually guess the range of plausible values within which the true value might lie. For instance, looking through the literature, we might see that the HRQL score for the disease we are studying varies by roughly 20 percent when using different instruments. We might also know the standard error in datasets or published values. (Again, if standard error is unfamiliar to you, check out Chapter 11 before going further.) In this chapter, you will learn how to test the effect of this uncertainty on the output of the decision analysis model.

LEARNING OBJECTIVES

- Explain why a sensitivity analysis is performed.

- Distinguish between different types of sensitivity analyses.

- Define what it means to have a model that is robust.

- Define one-way, two-way, and multiway sensitivity analyses.

- List the advantages and disadvantages of using different types of sensitivity analyses.

- Identify proper distributions for model inputs for a probabilistic sensitivity analysis.

- Interpret the results of a cost-effectiveness acceptability curve.

PROJECT MAP

1. Think through your research question.

2. Sketch out the analysis.

3. Collect data for your model.

4. Adjust your data.

5. Build your model.

6. Run and test the model.

7. *Conduct a sensitivity analysis.*

8. Write it up.

After you've built your model and obtained results, it is time to perform a sensitivity analysis. A sensitivity analysis allows you to test how your model output changes over ranges of uncertain inputs. This procedure will let others know that you've thought about potential errors and outcomes that may not have been fully captured with the model or parameters you used. Sensitivity analyses are also important because they will help guide future research in the field you are studying. This is because they help you find important variables for which there is inadequate data.

For the purpose of this chapter we will talk about two types of uncertainties where sensitivity analysis is performed in cost-effectiveness analysis: (1) model uncertainty and (2) parameter uncertainty.

Model uncertainty (otherwise known as **structural uncertainty**) involves testing the way that you built your decision model and helps you decide whether you need to make some changes. For instance, in our flu vaccine example from Chapter 5, we constructed a decision analysis model where an unvaccinated patient becomes ill and sees a doctor for treatment. What if the patient does not see the doctor? Instead, what if the patient became so ill that he called 911 and was admitted through the emergency department (ED)? According to Self and colleagues (2013), the incidence of ED visits due to pneumonia was 7.6 visits per 1,000 person-years in 2008–2009 (Self et al., 2013). If we believe that this is large enough to affect the conclusions of our cost-effectiveness results, we should investigate this scenario by including a branch in the decision tree where the patient does not see the physician. How will that change our results?

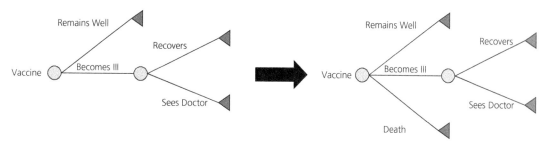

Figure 9.1   Sensitivity Analysis Focusing on Structure for the Vaccine Event Pathway

Sensitivity Analysis

Sensitivity analysis is a "stress test" of the decision model. Sensitivity analysis can focus on the *structure* and *parameters* of the model. The structure of the model involves a design such as that used for pathways and events. For example, in Figure 9.1 there are two events that would occur after a patient receives vaccine treatment (Remains Well and Becomes Ill). However, if there was a strong possibility that a patient could die from the vaccine, then another event could be added, such as Death. Consequently, we would need to rerun the model and evaluate the impact of Death on the overall conclusion. This is an example of sensitivity analysis on model *structure*.

Sensitivity analysis on the *parameters* of the model involves adjusting or testing the values of the inputs in the model. For example, if we were not confident about the probability of the event Remains Well, we would test the effect of this uncertainty by using a range of possible values. In Figure 9.2 the probability of Remains Well was 0.97. We would perform a sensitivity analysis across a range of 0.80 to 1.00 and see if this changes or affects the conclusions of the study. If our conclusions change, then we state that the model is sensitive to the probability that a patient Remains Well. This is an example of sensitivity analysis on a single model parameter.

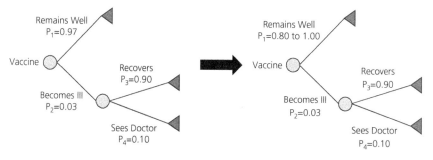

Figure 9.2   Sensitivity Analysis Focusing on the Parameter Change (Remains Well) for the Vaccine Event Pathway

> We can also perform a sensitivity analysis on two or more parameters simultaneously using more complex methods. (We discuss these methods later in this chapter.)

The second type of uncertainty that is normally addressed using sensitivity analysis is parameter uncertainty. The inputs we are least likely to be certain about are the assumptions we have made. For example, we might have made an assumption about the amount of time it takes for a nurse to administer the influenza vaccine. Or we might be unsure of the probability of being protected by an influenza vaccine because the quality of the data we used to make that estimate was low. There are other values that we might be fairly confident about, such as the cost of the influenza vaccine itself. (For instance, the average wholesale price is usually easy to get.)

The parameters we are least certain about should be tested over the widest range of values (because it is plausible that the values are much higher or much lower than our baseline estimate). Parameters that we are somewhat more confident about can be tested over a narrower range of values. When a particular strategy remains dominant over the range of plausible values for the inputs that we are uncertain about, the model is said to be **robust**.

There are many different ways of testing variables in a sensitivity analysis. In a **one-way** (univariate) sensitivity analysis, a single variable is tested over its range of plausible values while all other variables are held at a constant value. In a **two-way** (bivariate) sensitivity analysis, two variables are simultaneously tested over their range of plausible values while all others are held constant. In a **tornado diagram**, each variable is sequentially tested in a one-way sensitivity analysis. The tornado diagram is used to graphically rank the different variables in order of their overall influence on the magnitude of the model outputs. More complex sensitivity analyses include first-order Monte Carlo simulation (stochastic) and second-order Monte Carlo simulation (probabilistic sensitivity analysis).

Sensitivity analyses can also be used to test for errors in the decision analysis model. By showing how a variable affects the output of a model over a range of values, a sensitivity analysis will bring to light inconsistencies in the model's design. This chapter concludes with a discussion of Monte Carlo analysis, which allows the researcher to generate a confidence interval around the cost-effectiveness ratio.

Because the actual value of any given model input is almost always unknown, we usually enter the inputs as variables in the decision analysis

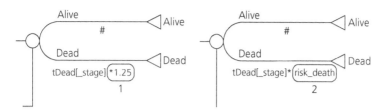

Figure 9.3   Terminal Branch of the Filmore Arm Represented in Figure 8.3

tree rather than a fixed number. A variable is a kind of placeholder for a number. It can assume a range of values rather than one fixed value. In Chapter 8, we saw that those who had the Filmore procedure were at 25 percent greater risk of mortality. To measure this higher risk of mortality, we multiplied the annual mortality rate by 1.25. But we might have obtained this 1.25 risk of death from a study that found that the higher risk of death was 1.25 with a 95 percent confidence interval of 1.1 to 1.4. So there is a small chance that the value could be 1.1 and a small chance that the value could be 1.4, but most likely the real-world value is closer to 1.25.

Rather than enter a value of 1.25 here, we can enter a variable (Figure 9.3), which we will call "risk_death," which represents the risk ratio of mortality. We can now assign risk_death a range of values rather than a fixed number (e.g., 1.1 to 1.4). We can also assign it a **baseline value** so that whenever we roll back the tree, this variable assumes a value of 1.25. The range of values that this variable might assume comes into play only when we conduct a sensitivity analysis on the overall model.

One-Way Sensitivity Analysis

What happens to the incremental effectiveness of the Reinkenshein intervention when we vary the effectiveness between 1.1 and 1.4? If we entered each value by hand and then calculated the effectiveness by scratch each time, we might come up with a plot of effectiveness values that looked something like Figure 9.4. This type of analysis is called a one-way sensitivity analysis because we held all other variables constant while changing only the risk ratio of mortality among the recipients of the Filmore procedure.

Here, we see that the greater the risk of death among recipients of the Filmore procedure, the greater the incremental gain in QALYs for recipients of the Reinkenshein procedure. Of course, if the Filmore procedure turns out not to put recipients at increased risk of death, then both procedures will be equally effective.

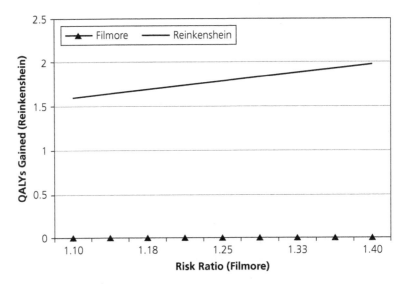

Figure 9.4   Incremental Effectiveness of the Reinkenshein Procedure Relative to the Filmore Procedure over a Range of Risk Ratios

Just as we can assign variables to effectiveness data, we can assign variables to costs. Let us briefly return to the question of vaccine costs in the influenza research question. Suppose that we were comparing three strategies: supportive care, vaccination, and treatment with anti-influenza drugs. We want to know the overall cost of each of these strategies when we vary the cost of the vaccine. Now suppose that we're unsure about the cost of providing the vaccine itself, and we think it might vary between $6.99 and $48.79.

In Figure 9.5, the *y*-axis indicates the expected value (overall cost) of each strategy, and the *x*-axis indicates the different vaccine costs at which the model was tested. For example, if the cost of the vaccine were $6.99, the expected cost of the Vaccinate arm of the decision analysis model would be about $32 per person, and the Support arm would cost around $44. The Treat strategy comes in at $49 per person.

Note that the Vaccinate and Support arms cross at $20.92. This means that if the cost of the vaccine were $20.92, the model predicts that the strategy of vaccinating all subjects would cost about the same amount as providing only supportive care. When a variable is set to a value that changes the dominance of one intervention relative to another (the point at which one intervention becomes more cost-effective than another), the value is called the threshold value of that variable (or the "break-even" point).

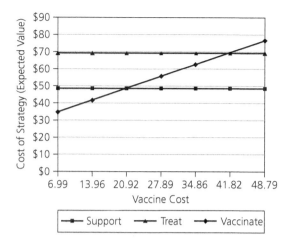

Figure 9.5   One-Way Sensitivity Analysis Examining How the Cost of Providing the Influenza Vaccine Influences Intervention

If the cost of the vaccine were $48.79, our model predicts that the strategy of vaccinating all persons in our cohort would cost around $77—about $28 more than the cost of providing supportive care alone and $7 more than the cost of providing treatment with an anti-influenza drug.

Exercise 1

1. Using Figure 9.5, determine the threshold cost of the influenza vaccine where the expected costs of the vaccination strategy is less than the other strategies. Determine the threshold cost where the vaccination strategy's expected cost is greater than the other strategies.

Using One-Way Sensitivity Analyses to Validate a Model

When examining the results of a one-way sensitivity analysis, always ask yourself whether the expected value of a strategy changes in a predictable way. For example, in Figure 9.5, we would expect that the vaccination strategy would become increasingly less attractive as the cost of the vaccine increases. We would also expect that the amount paid for the influenza vaccine would have no influence on the expected value of any of the other strategies. Thus, they should appear as straight lines (assume the same expected value at all costs of the vaccine).

The easiest way to test that the model has no glaring errors is to consider how you might expect changes in a particular cost or probability to affect a model and then to vary that cost or probability over a wide range of values. Varying a probability from zero to one, or a cost from zero to a very large number, allows you to see the relationship between the strategies under study at predictable end points.

For instance, if your intuition tells you that the direction of the relationship is positive, then any negative relationship in the plot would be a red flag that something might be wrong with the model. It could mean that another element of the model was built incorrectly or there is an error in one of your parameter values. This should be considered a final step in model validation, so it is a good idea to check your model for any errors prior to running these types of tests.

Answering Secondary Questions Using One-Way Sensitivity Analyses

Imagine that you are working for the Ministry of Health in Ghana. Ghana is one of many lower-income countries that has a national health insurance system. You are working to set up a drug formulary, but many of the drugs on your list are "unaffordable" given your current budget. That is, you have a league table with the cost and effectiveness values, but you do not have the funds on hand to buy QALYs above and beyond what you would get with spending money on basic surgical programs. However, your citizens are complaining about the high cost of medications eating into their quality of life. Wouldn't it be great to have information on exactly how much lower the cost of the drug would need to go (given any level of effectiveness) before it was affordable? With that information in hand, you could decide which drugs are worth bargaining for and which are simply out of reach.

Sensitivity analyses can also be used to help you understand where to spend the scarce resources you have. For parasitic diseases, drugs are sometimes given to everyone in high-risk areas (a process called deworming). Wouldn't it be great to know where you should target your efforts? With information on the relationship between disease prevalence and the incremental cost-effectiveness of a drug, you can decide whom you should give presumptive treatment to, and whom you should not. These values can be obtained using one-way sensitivity analyses.

One-way sensitivity analyses are frequently employed to address clinical or policy questions. For example, in a cost-effectiveness analysis comparing one drug with another, they have been used to set drug prices.

When constructing decision analysis models, there are many parameters for which the investigator will have sufficient data. These base-case parameters may not have a lot of uncertainty associated with them, providing the decision makers with confidence that they will not influence their final decisions by much. However, some parameters may have few supporting data or none at all. Researchers may "guess" what the actual parameter value is and assign a wide confidence interval to represent that uncertainty. A range from 0 to 1 for the probability of the effectiveness of a drug is not uncommon. In fact, policymakers may prefer to see that in order to examine whether or not an extreme case would affect their decisions. For instance, an extreme case would be when the treatment strategy (i.e., drug) had a probability of 100 percent effectiveness (or 0 percent effectiveness). The additional costs and payoffs for using a treatment strategy that is 100 percent effective may result in an overall net benefit for the decision maker. However, if the probability of effectiveness was 0 percent, the net benefit may not be enough for the policymaker to support such a strategy.

For instance, we might wish to conduct a broad one-way sensitivity analysis on the cost of oseltamivir, the drug used to treat influenza virus infection. If we demonstrate that there is a price point for this medication that renders it cost-effective relative to the other strategies, the pharmaceutical company that makes the drug may wish to lower its market price.

Two-Way Sensitivity Analysis

Many variables in a cost-effectiveness analysis are interdependent. For instance, the effectiveness of influenza vaccination is dependent on both the incidence rate of influenza (or the more commonly measured influenza-like illness) and the efficacy of the vaccine in preventing influenza. If the vaccine is 100 percent effective but the incidence of influenza is 0 percent, there is little gain associated with vaccination.

Now suppose that we overestimated the mean efficacy of the influenza vaccine in our hypothetical example. Vaccination might still have been cost-saving so long as the overestimation was not large. But if both our estimate of the incidence rate of influenza-like illness and our estimate of vaccine efficacy were too high, the cost savings that we initially found to be associated with vaccination might not be real. In other words, there might be some interaction between vaccine efficacy and incidence rate of influenza-like illness that attenuates the net benefit of vaccination.

In Figure 9.6, any intersection of values on the x-axis and the y-axis will fall into one of two zones: solid or clear. Each zone indicates which arm will be dominant with respect to costs. For example, if the efficacy of the influenza vaccine at preventing influenza-like illness were 0.4 and the incidence rate of influenza-like illness were 40 cases per 100 persons,

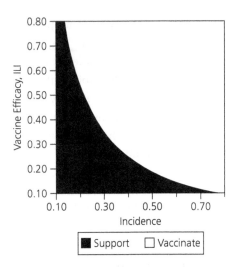

Figure 9.6   Two-Way Sensitivity Analysis Comparing Changes in the Efficacy of the Influenza Vaccine and the Incidence of Influenza-Like Illness

the vaccination strategy would be dominant with respect to cost (because the intersection of these two values falls in the clear zone). However, if the actual efficacy of the influenza vaccine were 0.3 and the actual average annual incidence rate of influenza were 20 cases per 100 persons, then supportive care would be dominant with respect to cost.

Two-way sensitivity analysis figures provide a convenient map of the interaction effects between two parameters in the decision analysis model. Policymakers can easily determine whether the strategy they select would continue to provide a net benefit or would result in reduced cost-effectiveness.

Tornado Diagram

Conducting sensitivity analyses may seem like a lot of fun the first few times you do it, but no researcher would want to spend an entire week conducting one-way sensitivity analyses on all of the variables used in the model. If we knew which variables had the most influence on the relative cost (or effectiveness) of each intervention, we could focus on just those variables.

A **tornado diagram** (also known as influence analysis) is a handy way of determining how much influence each of the variables has on the overall model. These analyses, which produce a graph that assumes the appearance of a tornado, conduct a one-way sensitivity analysis on every variable in the model.

In this type of analysis, each variable is tested independently. Tornado diagrams provide the investigator with a method for quickly deciphering which parameter has the most influence on the cost-effectiveness of treatment strategy. Normally, the most influential parameter is at the top and the least influential parameter is at the bottom. The x-axis can be the net benefit, incremental costs, or incremental cost-effectiveness ratio; it depends on the purpose of the scientific question. In some cases, the interest is focused on the incremental costs of treatment strategy relative to the comparator; therefore, the investigators will create a tornado diagram of the parameters with the most effect on incremental costs.

However, the limitation with a tornado diagram is that it does not evaluate the effects of varying multiple parameters simultaneously. It's easy to see how this can deceive students. The tornado diagram provides all the results of the one-way sensitivity analyses in one convenient diagram, creating the illusion that they are all being varied simultaneously. It's important that researchers indicate in the figure that this is a summary of multiple one-way sensitivity analyses and not a sensitivity analysis that tests all variables at the same time.

TORNADO DIAGRAM

Figure 9.7 is an example of a tornado diagram because of the funnel shape, which is widest at the top and narrowest at the bottom. In the tornado diagram in Figure 9.7, Cost of Treatment has the most influence on the ICER. This figure provides a nice graphical representation of the influence each variable has on the main outcome, the ICER (just to jog your memory, this is the incremental cost-effectiveness ratio). The horizontal bar gives you an idea of how wide the variation in the ICER is due to a change in the plausible range. In Figure 9.7, the Cost of Treatment is varied across a plausible range of $0 to $100. The result in the tornado diagram shows us that the ICER crosses $0. Depending on whether the numerator is positive and the denominator is negative or if the numerator is negative and the denominator is positive, the strategy could be dominated or dominant, respectively. (Oh, stop it with the Craigslist jokes already.)

Similarly, the Probability of Success is varied across a plausible range between 10 percent and 50 percent. The horizontal bar does not cross the ICER threshold of $0; therefore, we can't conclude that the strategy is dominant or dominated. Recall from Chapter 3 how threshold analysis is used in cost-effectiveness analysis. Here, our decision rule for cost-effectiveness is the "willingness-to-pay" threshold. In other words, we have set the amount that we would be willing to pay to save an additional QALY. If the ICER dips below this threshold, the intervention is considered cost-effective relative to the competing alternative. If the ICER is

TORNADO DIAGRAM (*Continued*)

above this threshold, the intervention is considered not cost-effective relative to the competing alternative.

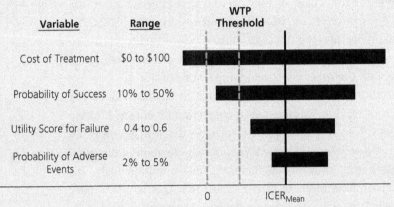

Figure 9.7   Tornado Diagram Example

The least influential variable is the Probability of Adverse Events. There is very little variation on the ICER after varying the plausible range of Probability of Adverse Events (2 percent to 5 percent). Therefore, it is positioned at the very bottom of the tornado diagram.

A limitation with one-way sensitivity analysis and two-way sensitivity analysis is the constraints that they impose on the number of parameters that are evaluated. In one-way sensitivity analysis, policymakers focus on only one parameter (e.g., probability of vaccine efficacy, probability of adverse reactions, cost of vaccine, or frequency of office visits). And in two-way sensitivity analysis, policymakers can see how varying two parameters (cost of vaccine and incidence of influenza-like symptoms) can result in the strategy being cost-effective or not. However, the policymakers will want to see what the potential net benefits would be if they were interested in varying multiple parameters at once. An analysis that tests all variables in the model is known as a multiway sensitivity analysis.

Multiway Sensitivity Analysis

Imagine that your boss has asked you to come up with the sampling error associated with the average cost of hospitalization for influenza infection among a cohort of people infected with influenza in Brazil. The cost was calculated by multiplying the probability of hospitalization by the average cost of hospitalization using a national dataset. You are told that the probability is 0.0002 with a standard deviation of 0.00005 and that the cost is $500 with a standard deviation of $50. You know that the average cost of hospitalization among this group is 0.0002 × $500 = $0.1, or 10 cents. But what is the standard deviation of this 10-cent value? The problem is that when you have two variables, each with its own standard deviation, it's no simple task to figure out what the standard deviation of the product of these two variables might be.

Now imagine that instead of trying to figure out what the error is for two variables, you must estimate the cumulative effect of the error in 20 variables on your cost-effectiveness model output. Theoretically, if all the variables were associated with sampling error alone, you should be able to estimate a 95 percent confidence interval around your incremental cost-effectiveness value. But how?

One solution is **Monte Carlo simulation**. Named after the famous gambling enclave, this type of analysis allows the generation of a single confidence interval around multiple variables. In cost-effectiveness analysis, there are two types of Monte Carlo simulations: (1) first-order Monte Carlo simulations, and (2) second-order Monte Carlo simulations. Each one investigates a different type of uncertainty. These are discussed in the next sections.

First-Order Monte Carlo Simulation

One way of easily understanding a Markov model is to think of it as a framework for watching people grow old. As they grow old, they incur costs, get sick, and die. This is a way of understanding a Markov model. In reality, it just estimates a bunch of weighted values over time.

However, in a first-order Monte Carlo simulation, a Markov model really does work this way. A hypothetical cohort of individual subjects enters into the decision analysis model. As each individual passes through the model, he or she encounters a number of different probabilities, such as the chance of developing influenza-like illness, the chance of seeing a doctor, and the chance of being hospitalized. Each individual experiences a unique path through the decision model, accumulating costs and outcomes as he or she grows older. For example, the first patient might pass through the decision model and develop influenza-like illness, and see the doctor, but not be hospitalized (Figure 9.8). On the other hand, the second patient might not develop influenza-like illness. What you get at the end is an estimate of the average costs and effects for each arm of the decision model.

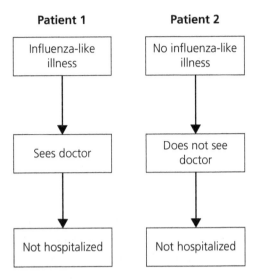

Each patient experience through the decision tree is unique. Not all patients experience the same events.

Figure 9.8   Microsimulation of Individual Patients Through a Decision Path

Since the probabilities are fixed, first-order Monte Carlo simulation does not provide any information regarding the uncertainty around each model input. Rather, what we get is the uncertainty or variation of the population as it passes through the decision model. This simulation is also called a microsimulation. Most software packages are capable of performing this.

However, what we are more concerned with in cost-effectiveness analysis is the uncertainty surrounding the model inputs, otherwise known as parameter uncertainty. To investigate parameter uncertainty, we use a second-order Monte Carlo simulation.

Second-Order Monte Carlo Simulation

In the two-way sensitivity analysis, two model inputs were varied to estimate the effect on the outcome of a cost-effectiveness analysis. But what if we wanted to vary more than two model inputs? How do we do it? And how do we present it?

In a second-order Monte Carlo simulation, also known as **probabilistic sensitivity analysis**, multiple model inputs are allowed to vary

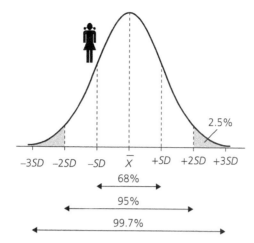

Figure 9.9   Chance of Incurring Any Given Value of a Normally Distributed Variable

Note: The female figure is at −1 standard deviation from the mean. If the mean is $500 and the standard deviation is $50, this subject would be assigned a value of $450.

simultaneously. Each time a subject encounters one of the model inputs, the value of that model input is determined by its probability distribution. (If the word *probability* coupled with the word *distribution* sounds daunting to you, read Chapter 11 for a quick and simple brushup on biostatistics. It's easy to understand and will be well worth the time spent.)

For instance, imagine that the cost of hospitalization for influenza in Brazil is $500 with a standard deviation of $50, and say that the cost is normally distributed (Figure 9.9). We know that there is a 68 percent chance that the actual cost of hospitalization is between +1 and −1 standard deviations from the mean. When the decision analysis software samples this distribution, it will sample between $450 and $550 approximately 68 percent of the time, since those values lie within 1 standard deviation of the mean. Using a normal distribution, the chance that a cost will be sampled around 2 standard deviations above or below the mean is just 5 percent, with a 2.5 percent chance of a high value and a 2.5 percent chance of a low value.

In a second-order Monte Carlo simulation, the process of running subjects through the model and sampling at each variable is repeated thousands of times. Once the simulation is completed, the expected value of each arm of the decision analysis model will be associated with a distribution of incremental cost or effectiveness values (Figure 9.10).

To look at this in more detail, let's examine the tree that was built to capture the expected value of diabetes in Chapter 7 (see Figure 7.3).

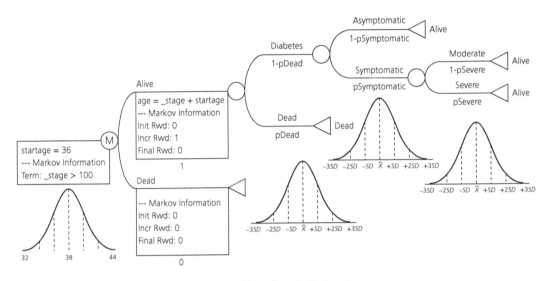

Figure 9.10   Diabetes Model in Which Values of Each Variable Are Normally Distributed

Note: Each time a subject is run through the model, the subject is assigned a value sampled from each distribution. As a result, the expected value of the variable is normally distributed. In this case, the baseline-expected QALE associated with diabetes is 38 QALYs, but there is a 2.5 percent chance that it could be as low as 32 QALYs or as high as 44 QALYs.

We labeled the probability of mortality, having symptoms, and having severe symptoms as pDeath, pSymptomatic, and pSevere, respectively. Pretend for a moment that all of the variables in this model are normally distributed. At the first juncture the model samples pDead, it then samples pSymptomatic, and finally it samples pSevere. If thousands of subjects run through the model, the mean value of each of these variables will determine the expected value of the overall model (38 QALYs). The model now has a distribution of samples as well and can report the approximate 95 percent confidence interval around the mean incremental cost-effectiveness.

Picking Distributions

When the time comes to conduct a second-order Monte Carlo simulation, you may find that few of the variables you wish to include in your model are normally distributed. For example, you may have a series of influenza incidence values you obtained from the medical literature. Even if each study was conducted in a similar way, the mean value in each study will probably not be identical or even close to the mean value in other studies. This occurs because there is often more than random error involved in generating each mean.

For instance, you might be studying the effect of influenza vaccination on the average German, but have data on samples from three different studies in different parts of Germany. Differences in the geographical location of the study and the income, race, and age of the subjects studied can also lead to very different results because the north of Germany is very different from the south. The best way of dealing with this variation is to conduct a

TIPS AND TRICKS

Always be certain to save a backup copy of your decision analysis tree under a different name before you assign distributions to the variables in your model. Once a distribution has been assigned to a variable, you will not be able to conduct further n-way sensitivity analyses using fixed probabilities or costs. Some software may give you an option to have multiple values and distributions for a single parameter.

meta-analysis. That might not only provide you with the best "mean" value for Germany in this example, but also a range of values around this mean. (See For Example: Meta-Analysis.) But when a meta-analysis isn't possible, you can pick the value that you think is most likely and a high and low value that you think are quite unlikely, and then artificially distribute your values. In this example, you might have to get expert input as to whether the mean value would be higher or lower.

FOR EXAMPLE: META-ANALYSIS

In cases in which many similar studies are available, the ideal way to obtain a value for your decision analysis tree is to conduct a meta-analysis and then use the resulting distribution. A meta-analysis provides information about the mean value and a confidence interval from two or more different studies. Meta-analysis is beyond the scope of this book but typically involves selecting many separate studies with a sound research design and then analyzing the data across all studies as if they were a single study. As long as you've been careful in selecting your studies, though, a Monte Carlo simulation comes fairly close to accomplishing what a meta-analysis would without as much effort.

No matter what distribution you use, the final sample will be normally distributed. One way of distributing the values is to use a **triangular distribution**. In this distribution, the lowest and highest values are assigned a probability of zero, and the middle value is assigned the highest probability

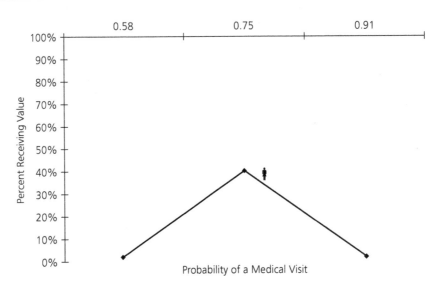

Figure 9.11   The Triangular Distribution

Note: We have distributed the variable representing the probability of a medical visit using a triangular distribution. The values fall into a range from 0.58 to 0.91, with a middle value of 0.75. The chance of sampling the middle value is 50 percent, but the chance of sampling either extreme is 0 percent.

(Figure 9.11). This distribution is unpretentious. It tells the reader that you are unsure what the distribution looks like but that you want low values and high values to be sampled infrequently.

Certain model inputs are associated with specific distributions. A beta distribution is used for probability and utility values because the range is bounded by a lower bound of 0 and an upper bound of 1. Since probability and utility values also are bounded between 0 and 1, a beta distribution makes perfect sense. A gamma distribution is sometimes used for cost variables because the range has a lower bound of 1 and an upper bound of infinity. It's not often that we spend negative dollars, but we accrue a large amount. Therefore, using a distribution that mimics how we

TIPS AND TRICKS

When a tree containing distributions is rolled back, the average cost or average effectiveness values assigned to each arm of the decision analysis model may differ from those generated from a tree that does not contain distributions. This occurs because the mean or midpoint value of the distributions you enter may not be equal to the baseline value you used for each variable. Do not be alarmed. Report what you see and explain that you applied a distribution to your model parameters.

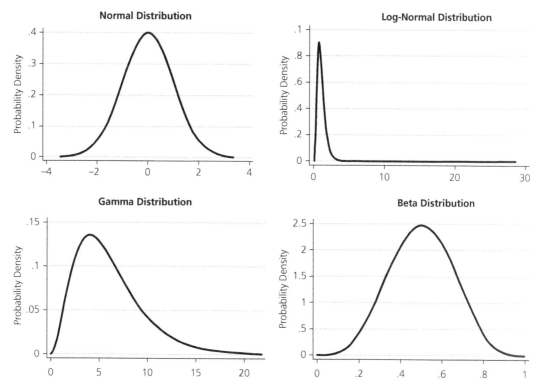

Figure 9.12   Other Distributions Used in Monte Carlo Simulations

spend makes sense. A normal distribution can also be used for cost variables in some instances. However, this presents some problems. One is that you need to be concerned with getting negative costs. Another is that a lot of cost value inputs are not normally distributed because health cost data often have a lot of zeros for participants who were not charged for their care.

Figure 9.12 provides some examples of the different distributions used in Monte Carlo simulations. One great thing about a second-order Monte Carlo simulation is that even if you distribute your values using triangular distributions, the incremental cost-effectiveness value will still be normally distributed!

Determining the Plausible Range of Each Variable

There are a few guiding principles to follow in determining the range of plausible values for a given variable. These principles can be applied to n-way sensitivity analyses and Monte Carlo simulations alike:

• If the parameter is based on an assumption or expert opinion, it should be tested over a very broad range of values in a one-way analysis. Expert opinion should also be used to determine the plausible high and low boundaries for the variable.

- If the parameter was derived from a random sample, you may use 95 percent confidence intervals when most of the error in the value of a parameter will be sampling error. But you should consider ways that nonrandom error may also influence your estimated value.

- If multiple estimates of the value of a parameter are available, consider conducting a meta-analysis or setting the lowest and highest believable values as boundaries in your analysis. You might use these high and low values as end points in a Monte Carlo simulation and opt not to conduct a meta-analysis.

- If two sources of error are interdependent, conduct a two-way sensitivity analysis on each source of error. Do not go overboard with two-way analyses, though! They can be difficult to interpret.

- If the parameter was obtained from electronic sources, check the data documentation for error estimates. Many data sources comment on both random and nonrandom sources of error.

Although we do not discuss it in this book, using a Delphi panel to systematically gather expert opinions in the absence of published data is a reliable method to estimate model parameters. For more information, see the RAND Corporation's web site (RAND Corporation, 2015).

Presenting the Results of the Probabilistic Sensitivity Analysis

How do we present the results of a second-order Monte Carlo simulation (or probabilistic sensitivity analysis)? There are two common methods that are used. The first method involves using a cost-effectiveness plane, and the second method uses a cost-effectiveness acceptability curve.

Figure 9.13 illustrates how a second-order Monte Carlo simulation is presented on a cost-effectiveness plane. (This is a concept that was introduced in Chapter 2.) The outcome is the ICER comparing Strategy A versus Strategy B, which is represented by a circle. The x-axis represents the incremental effectiveness (e.g., QALYs) and the y-axis represents the incremental costs. The cost-effectiveness plane is divided into four quadrants: northeast (NE), northwest (NW), southeast (SE), and southwest (SW).

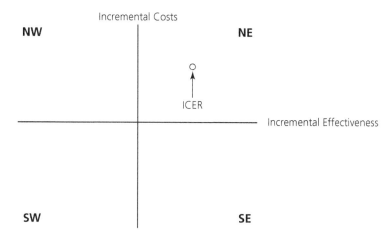

Figure 9.13 Cost-Effectiveness Plane with a Single Simulation

In the northeast quadrant, the ICER reflects a strategy that is more costly and more effective relative to a standard comparator. In the northwest quadrant, the ICER reflects a strategy that is more costly and less effective relative to a standard comparator. If the ICER is in the northwest quadrant, of course, we call this strategy dominated. In the southeast quadrant, the ICER reflects a strategy that is less costly and more effective relative to a standard comparator. If the ICER is in the southeast quadrant, we call this strategy dominant. In the southwest quadrant, the ICER reflects a strategy that is less costly and less effective. (We first introduced the ideas of dominant and dominated in Chapter 2. Here we see them being used again but within a cost-effectiveness plane.)

The single ICER point in the quadrant represents only a single simulation. If there were 10 simulations performed, then there would be 10 ICERs plotted on the cost-effectiveness plane. If there were 100 simulations performed, then there would be 100 ICERs plotted on the cost-effectiveness plane. In the past, performing these simulations was not easy. With powerful personal computers, we can now perform simulations in the tens of thousands. Figure 9.14 provides a hypothetical example of a probabilistic sensitivity analysis plotted on a cost-effectiveness plane with 100 simulations.

Another method for presenting the results of a probabilistic sensitivity analysis is the cost-effectiveness acceptability curve. The cost-effectiveness

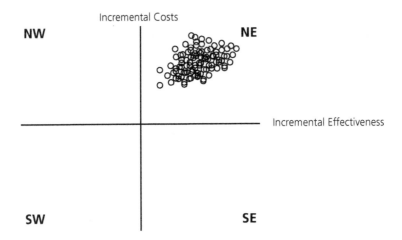

Figure 9.14   Hypothetical Results of 100 Simulations on the Cost-Effectiveness Plane

acceptability curve takes the results of the probabilistic sensitivity analysis and plots the probability of a strategy being cost-effective (relative to whatever the competing alternative is) against the willingness to pay.

The willingness to pay is different for different payers and countries. In order to capture the different willingness-to-pay thresholds, the cost-effectiveness acceptability curve plots the proportion of ICERs that are below the willingness-to-pay threshold. ICERs that are below the line tell us that Strategy A is cost-effective compared to Strategy B.

In Figure 9.15 (top panel), five different willingness-to-pay thresholds are presented (indicated by WTP in the figure). For each willingness-to-pay threshold, the proportion of ICERs that are below the line is given. Imagine pivoting the willingness to pay from WTP_1 to WTP_2. Notice how the number of ICERs underneath the willingness-to-pay line starts to increase from 0 percent to 10 percent. If the WTP line increased to WTP_5, then 100 percent of the ICERs are below this line.

The bottom panel in Figure 9.15 shows the associated cost-effectiveness acceptability curve. Notice how the proportion of ICERs that fall below the willingness-to-pay threshold aligns with the probability of a strategy being cost-effective. This is a pretty cool way of showing the proportion of ICERs that are cost-effective depending on the willingness to pay. In other words, it represents the probability that a treatment strategy is cost-effective (relative to a standard alternative) at different willingness-to-pay thresholds. Therefore, payers or countries with different willingness-to-pay thresholds can estimate the probability that choosing a strategy is cost-effective relative to a competing alternative.

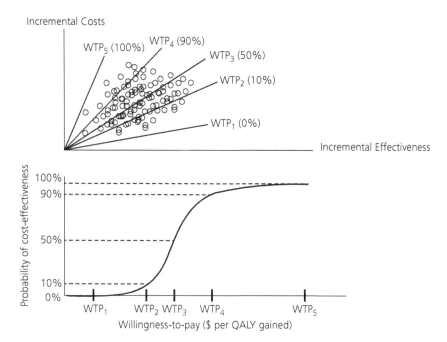

Incremental Costs

WTP$_5$ (100%) WTP$_4$ (90%)
WTP$_3$ (50%)
WTP$_2$ (10%)
WTP$_1$ (0%)

Incremental Effectiveness

Figure 9.15   Cost-Effectiveness Acceptability Curve

Exercises 2 and 3

2. Use Figure 9.16 to answer the next two questions. Suppose that a U.S. pharmacy benefits management organization is reviewing a new therapy called "Expensive." The decision makers want to know whether this is a cost-effective drug compared to the competing alternative "Old." They hired you to perform a cost-effectiveness analysis. You conduct a probabilistic sensitivity analysis on the probability of cure, the utility values, and the cost of the two medications. You then generate a cost-effectiveness acceptability curve using a range of willingness-to-pay thresholds. The pharmacy benefits management organization has a willingness to pay threshold of $100,000 per QALY gained. What is the probability that the drug Expensive is cost-effective compared to the competing alternative, Old?

3. Suppose a developing country was interested in using the results of your cost-effectiveness analysis for their national pharmacy drug coverage decision. They use the cost-effectiveness acceptability curve you generated, but their willingness to pay is $30,000 per QALY gained. What is the probability that the new drug, Expensive, is cost-effective relative to the competing alternative, Old?

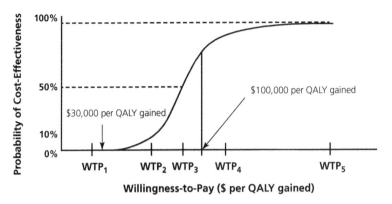

Figure 9.16   Cost-Effectiveness Acceptability Curve for Exercises 2 and 3

Summary

Sensitivity analyses are performed to test how much influence the uncertainty surrounding our model inputs affects our base-case results. One-way, two-way, and multiway sensitivity analyses are some commonly used sensitivity analyses. A tornado diagram is a special case of the one-way sensitivity analysis that ranks individual model inputs in descending order from greatest to least influential.

First-order Monte Carlo simulation is used to evaluate the population average cost and average outcomes by running an individual patient through a decision model repeatedly without variations in the probabilities. Unlike first-order simulation, second-order Monte Carlo simulation tests the uncertainty surrounding multiple model inputs, simultaneously, by randomly drawing from a distribution. This is more important for decision analysis because it provides an estimate for the ICER and its distribution (e.g., 95 percent confidence interval).

Presenting the results of a probabilistic sensitivity analysis on a cost-effectiveness plane can give us a graphical representation of ICER distributions. However, a cost-effectiveness acceptability curve allows decision makers with different willingness-to-pay thresholds to determine whether the new intervention is cost-effective relative to the competing alternative.

Further Readings

Students interested in learning more about sensitivity analysis are encouraged to read *Decision Modeling for Health Economic Evaluation* by Andrew

Briggs, Karl Claxton, and Mark Sculpher from the University of York (2006). Other works of interest include Sonnenberg and Beck (1993), and the ISPOR Report of the ISPOR-SMDM Modeling Good Research Practices Task Force Working Group (A. H. Briggs et al., 2012).

References

Briggs, A., K. Claxton, and M. Sculpher. (2006). *Decision Modelling for Health Economic Evaluation*. New York: Oxford University Press.

Briggs, A. H., M. C. Weinstein, E. A. L. Fenwick, J. Karnon, M. J. Sculpher, and A. D. Paltiel. (2012). Model Parameter Estimation and Uncertainty Analysis: A Report of the ISPOR-SMDM Modeling Good Research Practices Task Force Working Group–6. *Medical Decision Making* 32(5): 722–732. http://doi.org/10.1177/0272989X12458348.

Gold, M. R., and P. Muennig. (2002). Measure-Dependent Variation in Burden of Disease Estimates: Implications for Policy. *Medical Care* 40(3): 260–266.

RAND Corporation. (2015). Delphi Method. Retrieved March 27, 2015, from http://www.rand.org/topics/delphi-method.html.

Self, W. H., C. G. Grijalva, Y. Zhu, C. D. McNaughton, T. W. Barrett, S. P. Collins, . . . M. R. Griffin. (2013). Rates of Emergency Department Visits due to Pneumonia in the United States, July 2006–June 2009. *Academic Emergency Medicine* 20(9): 957–960. http://doi.org/10.1111/acem.12203.

Sonnenberg, F. A., and J. R. Beck. (1993). Markov Models in Medical Decision Making: A Practical Guide. *Medical Decision Making* 13(4): 322–338.

CHAPTER 10

PREPARING YOUR STUDY FOR PUBLICATION

Overview

The publication format of cost-effectiveness analyses differs from that of other types of scientific investigations in subtle ways. In a cost-effectiveness analysis, the basic format is the same as that of other medical studies; however, the methods and results sections are presented in a way that is structurally quite different from most other studies. In addition, cost-effectiveness analysis may include a technical appendix that contains important information for reproducibility and transparency.

Content and Structure of Cost-Effectiveness Articles

One of the most agonizing aspects of research, many students tell us, is writing the manuscript. This is true especially when you have a deadline at the end of the semester. Thankfully, there is a standard that all students and researchers can use that will help guide what should be in the manuscript. Most experimental and observational studies use a format that contains an introduction (or back ground), methods, results, and discussion section (some-times a conclusion section is added). But for cost-effective-ness analysis, these sections may be slightly different.

For example, in an experimental study (or obser-vational study), the first table is usually reserved for the demographics of the sample. Unless the analysis is a **piggy-back study** (following a cohort in a prospective study), the description of the cohort is brief for a cost-effectiveness analysis, and the first table is often used to describe the values assigned to each variable rather than demographic characteristics, as is done in traditional studies.

LEARNING OBJECTIVES

- Describe the main elements in a cost-effectiveness analysis manuscript based on the CHEERS guidelines.

- Know which key elements should be included in the methods section.

- Given the results of an incremental cost-effectiveness analysis, present it in an effective and systematic manner.

- Use tables to summarize your findings, and provide further descriptions in the text.

- Prepare figures and illustrations appropriate for manuscript submission.

There are several checklists available. These checklists include one developed by the Panel on Cost-Effectiveness in Health and Medicine. For example, the Panel recommends that an abstract be included that clearly states the study objective, what the intervention is, who the target population is, whether the analysis is a cohort or a whole population, what the study perspective is, the time horizon, the discount rate, the data source, outcome measures, results, limitations, and conclusions. These points are covered in Chapter 3, since they really need to be thought out before you start your analysis. It's pretty unrealistic to include all of these in the actual abstract of a paper. We instead focus on guidelines that all journal editors will be familiar with: the Consolidated Health Economic Evaluation Reporting Standards (CHEERS), developed by the International Society for Pharmacoeconomics and Outcomes Research (Husereau et al., 2013). According to the CHEERS checklist (Exhibit 10.1), the following elements should be included in a cost-effectiveness analysis manuscript:

- Title and Abstract
- Introduction
- Methods
- Results
- Discussion
- Other

TIPS AND TRICKS

Checklists are guides to help you organize your manuscript in a manner that is efficient and comprehensive to your audience. If you feel that certain elements from the checklist are unnecessary, you should not feel compelled to include them.

The "other" elements that should also be considered as part of the manuscript in this case mostly refer to a technical appendix. The technical appendix is an important element that does not always appear in manuscripts but is posted on the journal's web site or the author's web site (in the case of low-budget journals). In addition, journals have developed standard requirements for the submission of figures and illustrations. We will discuss these additional elements at the end of the chapter.

EXHIBIT 10.1. THE COMPLETE CHEERS CHECKLIST

Section/Item	Item Number	Recommendation
Title and Abstract		
Title	1	Identify the study as an economic evaluation, or use more specific terms such as "cost-effectiveness analysis" and describe the interventions compared.
Abstract	2	Provide a structured summary of objectives, perspective, setting, methods (including study design and inputs), results (including base case and uncertainty analyses), and conclusions.
Introduction		
Background and Objectives	3	Provide an explicit statement of the broader context for the study. Present the study question and its relevance for health policy or practice decisions.
Methods		
Target population and subgroups	4	Describe characteristics of the base-case population and subgroups analyzed including why they were chosen.
Setting and location	5	State relevant aspects of the system(s) in which the decision(s) need(s) to be made.
Study perspective	6	Describe the perspective of the study and relate this to the costs being evaluated.
Comparators	7	Describe the interventions or strategies being compared and state why they were chosen
Time horizon	8	State the time horizon(s) over which costs and consequences are being evaluated and say why appropriate.
Discount rate	9	Report the choice of discount rate(s) used for costs and outcomes and say why appropriate.
Choice of health outcomes	10	Describe what outcomes were used as the measure(s) of benefit in the evaluation and their relevance for the type of analysis performed.
Measurement of effectiveness	11a	Single study–based estimates: Describe fully the design features of the single effectiveness study and why the single study was a sufficient source of clinical effectiveness data.

(Continued)

Section/Item	Item Number	Recommendation
	11b	Synthesis-based estimates: Describe fully the methods used for the identification of included studies and synthesis of clinical effectiveness data.
Measurement of valuation of preference-based outcomes	12	If applicable, describe the population and methods used to elicit preferences for outcomes.
Estimating resources and costs	13a	Single study–based economic evaluation: Describe approaches used to estimate resource use associated with the alternative interventions. Describe primary or secondary research methods for valuing each resource item in terms of its unit cost. Describe any adjustments made to approximate to opportunity costs.
	13b	Model-based economic evaluation: Describe approaches and data sources used to estimate resource use associated with model health states. Describe primary or secondary research methods for valuing each resource item in terms of its unit cost. Describe any adjustments made to approximate to opportunity costs.
Currency, price date, and conversion	14	Report the dates of the estimated resource quantities and unit costs. Describe methods for adjusting estimated unit costs to the year of reported costs if necessary. Describe methods for converting costs into a common currency base and the exchange rate.
Choice of model	15	Describe and give reasons for the specific type of decision-analytic model used. Providing a figure to show model structure is strongly recommended.
Assumptions	16	Describe all structural or other assumptions underpinning the decision-analytic model.
Analytic models	17	Describe all analytic methods supporting the evaluation. This could include methods for dealing with skewed, missing, or censored data; extrapolation methods; methods for pooling data; approaches to validate or make adjustments (e.g., half-cycle corrections) to a model; and methods for handling population heterogeneity and uncertainty.

Section/Item	Item Number	Recommendation
Results		
Study parameters	18	Report the values, ranges, references, and, if used, probability distributions for all parameters. Report reasons or sources for distributions used to represent uncertainty where appropriate. Providing a table to show the input values is strongly recommended.
Incremental costs and outcomes	19	For each intervention, report mean values for the main categories of estimated costs and outcomes of interest, as well as mean differences between the comparator groups. If applicable, report incremental cost-effectiveness ratios.
Characterizing uncertainty	20a	Single study–based economic evaluation: Describe the effects of sampling uncertainty for estimated incremental cost, incremental effectiveness, and incremental cost-effectiveness, together with the impact of methodological assumptions (such as discount rate, study perspective).
	20b	Model-based economic evaluation: Describe the effects on the results of uncertainty for all input parameters, and uncertainty related to the structure of the model and assumptions.
Characterizing heterogeneity	21	If applicable, report differences in costs, outcomes, or cost-effectiveness that can be explained by variations between subgroups of patients with different baseline characteristics or other observed variability in effects that are not reducible by more information.
Discussion		
Study findings, limitation, generaliza-bility, and current knowledge	22	Summarize key study findings and describe how they support the conclusions reached. Discuss limitations and the generalizability of the findings and how the findings fit with current knowledge.

(Continued)

Section/Item	Item Number	Recommendation
Other		
Source of funding	23	Describe how the study was funded and the role of the funder in the identification, design, conduct, and reporting of the analysis. Describe other nonmonetary sources of support.
Conflicts of interest	24	Describe any potential for conflict of interest among study contributors in accordance with journal policy. In the absence of a journal policy, we recommend authors comply with International Committee of Medical Journal Editors' recommendations.

PROJECT MAP

1. Think through your research question.
2. Sketch out the analysis.
3. Collect data for your model.
4. Adjust your data.
5. Build your model.
6. Run and test the model.
7. Conduct a sensitivity analysis.
8. *Write it up.*

Title and Abstract

Although this may not seem super important, having a complete and clear title helps your audience in determining what kind of study you are performing. You should have a title that describes the type of analysis and the comparators being studied. For example, "Cost-Effectiveness Analysis of Linezolid vs. Vancomycin in Treating Methicillin-Resistant *Staphylococcus aureus* Complicated Skin and Soft Tissue Infections" identifies the study as a cost-effectiveness analysis between linezolid and vancomycin (Boun-thavong, Hsu, & Okamoto, 2009). Some journals will have a word limitation on the title, so be sure to always check the author guidelines.

Obviously, cost-effectiveness papers do not usually have catchy titles like "Your Money or Your Life: Strong Medicine for America's Health Care System (Cutler, 2004)." That is good, because it is almost always the case that they are botched. (Here, this famous economist titled a bunch of papers starting with "Your Money or Your Life," but those words almost never bear any relation to what follows the semicolon.)

TIPS AND TRICKS

It's always a good idea to test your title by pasting it into Google Scholar and seeing what comes up. If there is a very similar title, that can lead to confusion, but if there are very few hits, it is a sign that you are on the wrong track.

Another reason why it is important to have a good title is for indexing purposes. Search engines such as PubMed and EMBASE will be able to identify your manuscript more easily if the title has keywords that distinguish it as an economic analysis comparing specific interventions. It will also make it easier for other researchers to identify your work when they perform a search.

An abstract is a structured summary of the research project. Unlike the manuscript, the abstract is much shorter and has just enough information to capture a reader's attention. Do not include information in the abstract that is not in the manuscript. Every journal will have specific requirements for constructing an abstract, but most will usually include objectives, methods, results, and conclusions. Most journals will have a word limit on the abstract. *Value in Health,* an important journal for health technology assessment, has a 250-word limitation for their abstracts (http://www.ispor .org/publications/value/submit.asp).

Introduction

Every good study should begin with a good story. The introduction is your opportunity to explain why your research is important. The introduction should begin by describing the impact of the disease under study and the need for a cost-effectiveness analysis that evaluates the interventions used to treat or prevent this disease. We will refer to the former as the **impact statement** and the latter as the **statement of need**. The impact statement describes the epidemiological and economic impact of a disease on society. The statement of need outlines why there is sufficient uncertainty to warrant the analysis.

TIPS AND TRICKS

Make sure to always check the authors' guidelines for the journal first, before writing your manuscript. You don't want to spend a lot of time writing an amazing manuscript only to find out that the journal you want to submit to requires a different format or word limitation. What if you don't know which journal you want to submit to? Once you have a draft of your abstract down, you can paste it into a "journal selector" search engine such as: http://www.edanzediting.com/journal_advisor or http://journalfinder.elsevier.com.

The impact of the disease on society usually includes facts pertaining to the incidence rate, the disease severity, or mortality associated with the disease. For example, the influenza article might begin "Influenza virus infections account for approximately 30,000 deaths, upward of 200,000 hospitalizations, and over a million ambulatory care visits and days of lost work in the United States each year" (Neuzil, Reed, Mitchel, & Griffin, 1999; Nichol, Margolis, Wuorenma, & Von Sternberg, 1994). If the economic impact of the disease has been published elsewhere, these data and their sources might be cited.

When describing the need for a cost-effectiveness analysis, the researcher should indicate why it is unclear whether the costs, risks, and efficacy of one intervention might outweigh those of another. For example, the cost-effectiveness of vaccination versus supportive care hinges on the fact that vaccination must be administered to every healthy adult (Muennig & Khan, 2001). But it's also quite clear that the elderly or chronically ill should be vaccinated, since they are at high risk of death or complications if they get the flu.

You might try something like this: "Although there is good evidence that the chronically ill and elderly will benefit from vaccination, healthy adults are at lower risk of hospitalization or death from influenza-virus infections. Nevertheless, complications do arise among younger persons, and otherwise healthy persons can spread disease to the elderly and infirm. Therefore, there is uncertainty as to whether vaccination is cost-effective among healthy adults." Here, you are telling the reader that the analysis will help solve a critical policy question.

A large part of the art of writing journal articles is in the prose. Avoid the use of jargon and painstaking detail. The introduction and discussion sections are less formal and technical than the methods and results sections. Therefore, you should take the opportunity to clearly set up the story you intend to tell in the introduction and tie it all together in the conclusion section.

Methods

The methods section contains more detailed technical terms; nonetheless, it should be written for the audience of the journal you are submitting to. If it is a journal of epidemiology, use epidemiological terms; most of your readers will have a master's degree or doctorate in this field. If it is a journal geared toward policymakers, consider moving the technical details to the technical appendix.

The methods section should include the following information:

* The demographic profile of the cohort or hypothetical cohort
* The setting and location (e.g., the U.S. healthcare system)
* The perspective of the study (societal, governmental, patient, or payer)
* Whether the model adhered to the reference case scenario recommended by the Panel on Cost-Effectiveness in Health and Medicine or chose a different comparator
* The time horizon (length of the analysis)
* The discount rate used
* The basic event pathway(s) for your analysis
* The type of outcome used (e.g., QALY, effectiveness)
* The sources used to obtain cost and effectiveness data
* The year to which all costs were adjusted
* All assumptions used in the analysis
* The types of sensitivity analyses performed

If you are using a hypothetical cohort, mention how the subjects from your different data sources matched or deviated from your cohort. If differences existed, explain how the problem was addressed.

Details such as the perspective of the analysis, the discount rate used, the year to which all costs were adjusted, and location (e.g., United States) do not have to take a lot of space. This section should, however, give a complete description of the setting and location of your analysis. For instance, you can write "A cost-effectiveness analysis comparing linezolid to vancomycin was performed using a decision analytic model from the U.S. healthcare payer perspective adjusted for 2013 $U.S. A uniform discount rate of 3 percent was applied to both cost and health benefits." These simple statements provide a lot of information that the reader will appreciate.

It is important to indicate whether your results include a reference case scenario (or whether the entire study is a reference case analysis). You should also indicate ways in which your results may have strayed from the reference case scenario. For instance, you may not have been able to capture an environmental cost that was likely to have been relevant, or you may not have used a QALY-compatible health-related quality-of-life instrument (Gold, Siegel, Russell, & Weinstein, 1996; Neumann, Sanders, Russell, Siegel, & Ganiats, 2016).

The **time horizon** (or analytical horizon), which we introduced in Chapter 3, is the period over which all costs and outcomes are considered (Haddix, Teutsch, Shaffer, & Dunet, 1996). For every cost-effectiveness analysis you perform, the time horizon should be included as part of the methods. For instance, the time horizon for an acute infection may be between 7 and 14 days, but a time horizon for type II diabetes may be three months. If the time horizon is greater than one year, then you should consider performing discounting on both costs and health benefits.

The event pathway should be described in as much detail as possible given the space limitations. Frequently, the decision analysis model will be too large to include in the analysis, and the event pathway will be too detailed to describe. If this is the case, be sure to highlight the key points of the pathway. If you generated the event pathway using clinical practice guidelines, you may wish to cite the guidelines you used. You can also use a table to describe the event pathway. For example, a study on the cost-effectiveness of linezolid compared to vancomycin included a table that described the assumptions and resources of each event pathway in the decision tree (Bounthavong et al., 2009). This provides a clear and transparent portrait of the event pathways.

The bulk of the methods section describes the sources of the cost and effectiveness data you used in your analysis. It should include descriptions of the ways in which you adjusted your data using secondary sources and formulas. In Chapter 4, we described different sources of cost data. These should be listed, and any type of adjustments should be provided. You should also include the year and edition of the references. Including this as part of a table helps organize the methods section (Table 10.1).

You should provide information on how the data were synthesized. Were the data based on a single study or from multiple studies? For instance, a cost-effectiveness analysis comparing different biologics for rheumatoid arthritis performed a network meta-analysis to combine multiple studies to synthesize parameter values for a Markov model (Nguyen, Bounthavong, Mendes, Christopher, Tran, Kazerooni, & Morreale, 2012).

Table 10.1   Simple Summary of Costs Used in a Cost-Effectiveness Model

Cost	Cost per Day	Reference
Linezolid 600 mg twice a day	$14	*RED BOOK* (2009)[a]
Vancomycin 1000 mg twice a day	$250	*RED BOOK* (2009)
Microbiologic culture	$25	HCUP (2009)[b]
Monitoring costs	$10	HCUP (2009)

[a] AWP: average wholesale price (2009)
[b] HCUP: Healthcare Cost and Utilization Project (2009)

The methods section should explicitly mention the type of analysis you chose to perform (a cost-effectiveness analysis or a cost-benefit analysis). This is also where you want to describe the model you are using. Is the analysis going to be based on a decision tree model, state-transition model, or some combination?

Economic analyses in health almost always require a lot of assumptions. It is important that you be as transparent as possible about your assumptions. Readers and other researchers will not know what assumptions you make unless you write them down. For instance, if you assume that patients received other medications besides linezolid for broad-spectrum coverage, then you should state this. (The reader will not be able to read what's in your mind.) These assumptions can be listed in the text or they can be inserted as part of a table. Placing the assumptions in a table is convenient for a number of reasons. First, one of the nagging difficulties with writing a journal article is that the word count has to be kept within the journal's limits. By placing the assumptions in a table, they are not counted as words in the body text. Second, the reader does not have to scan through the text to find them.

The method should contain a section that describes the types of sensitivity analyses you are going to perform. In Chapter 9, you have learned to perform a sensitivity analysis on the structure and/or the parameters of the model. The section should specify if a one-way and/or multivariate sensitivity analysis was performed.

Results

After completing the analyses, the results section should be a report of what you discovered. It should not include explanations or speculations for how the results were derived (leave that for the discussion section). Instead, focus on presenting the results concisely and effectively for your audience.

Table 10.2   Cost-Effectiveness Table

Row Intervention	Total Cost	Total Effectiveness	Incremental Cost	Incremental Effectiveness	Incremental Cost-Effectiveness
	A	B	C	D	E
Usual care	Cost of usual care	Total QALYs in usual care cohort			
Intervention 2	Cost of intervention — savings from intervention	Total QALYs in intervention cohort	A2 – A1 (= C2)	B2 – B1 (= D2)	C2/D2
Intervention 3	Cost of intervention — savings from intervention	Total QALYs in intervention cohort	A3 – A2 (= C3)	B3 – B2 (= D3)	C3/D3

Note: Interventions are first ranked by their effectiveness, with least effective interventions listed first. The incremental cost and incremental effectiveness values are then sequentially calculated. Finally, the incremental cost-effectiveness ratios are presented.

The results section of a cost-effectiveness analysis should include the cost, effectiveness, and incremental cost-effectiveness (if the intervention is not cost saving) of each intervention under study. It should also contain a presentation of the results of the sensitivity analysis. (The results section is where you will present most of your figures such as the one-way sensitivity analysis, two-way sensitivity analysis, or tornado diagram.)

There is a standard format for presenting the results of cost-effectiveness analyses in table form (see Table 10.2). In a cost-effectiveness table, interventions are ranked in order from the least effective at the top of the table to the most effective at the bottom of the table. The incremental cost-effectiveness ratios are then sequentially calculated by subtracting the cost of usual care from the intervention (Gold et al., 1996; Neumann et al., 2016). Some decision analysis packages can generate a publication-quality cost-effectiveness table for you.

In a cost-effectiveness table, interventions that are dominated (are both less effective and more costly than others) should not contain incremental cost-effectiveness ratios (Gold et al., 1996; Neumann et al., 2016). Instead, the word *dominated* should appear where you would have placed the ratio. The table should be divided into two or three sections listing the results of the analysis at a 3 percent discount rate, undiscounted results, and the results of the analysis at a 5 percent discount rate or higher (Gold et al., 1996; Neumann et al., 2016).

Let's look at an example table where the results from a hypothetical cost-effectiveness analysis are presented in Table 10.3. We order the different interventions according to the total effectiveness in ascending order.

Usual care has the lowest number of QALYs so it is listed first. Intervention 2 is listed next since it has the second lowest QALY, followed by Intervention 3. The ICER comparing Intervention 2 to Usual Care is $750 per QALY gained. Intervention 3 is a dominant strategy compared to Intervention 2 because it costs less and has greater effectiveness.

The sensitivity analysis description should outline:

* The variables that exerted the most influence on the model
* How these variables affected the dominance of each strategy
* The results of bivariate analyses (if any are relevant)
* How assumptions affected the model
* The results of a sensitivity analysis on the discount rate
* The results of statistical analyses, such as a Monte Carlo simulation
* Additional analyses of interest to policymakers

Rather than use technical terms such as *tornado diagram*, it is generally better to make descriptive statements. For example, in describing the influence of each variable, you might state, "The incidence of influenza-like illness, the cost of transportation, and the cost of caregiver support exerted the greatest influence over the relative cost and effectiveness of each intervention." You should also describe how each assumption affected the relative dominance of each strategy in one-way sensitivity analyses.

Figures are a great way to graphically present the results of the sensitivity analysis. Tornado diagrams, ICER distributions in a cost-effectiveness plane, and cost-effectiveness acceptability curves can be included as part of the results section. (Details regarding formatting are discussed later in this chapter.)

Table 10.3   Example of a Cost-Effectiveness Table

Row Intervention	Total Cost	Total Effectiveness	Incremental Cost	Incremental Effectiveness	Incremental Cost-Effectiveness
	A	B	C	D	E
Usual care	$100	0.5 QALY			
Intervention 2	$250	0.7 QALY	$250 – $100	0.7 – 0.5	$750 per QALY gained
Intervention 3	$200	0.78 QALY	$200 – $250	0.78 – 0.7	Dominant

Discussion

After presenting your results, the discussion section is where you have an opportunity to revisit your original research question and expand on how the results support your conclusions. For example, were the results a surprise or did they fit with the current knowledge and thinking? What have other studies reported, and do the results support or refute them? How do the conclusions of the study add to the current literature? And what other questions were generated from the study?

You also want to demonstrate that your work is meaningful. In order to do this, the discussion section should include the implications your work will (or can) have on policy and decision making. In the introduction, you provided the impact statement (or statement of need). You want to revisit this in the discussion and tie it all together nicely.

This is also where the limitations of the study should be highlighted and discussed. Dedicating a paragraph or two to the limitations provides an honest discussion of problems that were encountered during the study. This provides transparency and also helps the audience to avoid or prepare for these limitations in future research.

The discussion section also includes a statement or two on how the results of the study should help direct future research. In some journals, this is where you will make a concluding statement (or two) based on the results.

Other

According to the CHEERS checklist, the last section should include disclosure statements and conflicts of interest (Husereau et al., 2013). This is done in order to provide transparency on the motivation and potential

EXHIBIT 10.2. THE IMPACT INVENTORY CHECKLIST

Sector	Type of Impact (list category within each sector with unit of measure if relevant)[a]	Included in This Reference Case Analysis From. . . Perspective?		Notes on Sources of Evidence
		Health Care Sector	Societal	
Formal Health Care Sector				
Health	Health outcomes (effects)			
	Longevity effects	☐	☐	
	Health-related quality-of-life effects	☐	☐	
	Other health effects (eg, adverse events and secondary transmissions of infections	☐	☐	
	Medical costs			
	Paid for by third-party payers	☐	☐	
	Paid for by patients out-of-pocket	☐	☐	
	Future related medical costs (payers and patients)	☐	☐	
	Future unrelated medical costs (payers and patients)	☐	☐	
Informal Health Care Sector				
Health	Patient-time costs	NA	☐	
	Unpaid caregiver-time costs	NA	☐	
	Transportation costs	NA	☐	
Non-Health Care Sectors (with examples of possible items)				
Productivity	Labor market earnings lost	NA	☐	
	Cost of unpaid lost productivity due to illness	NA	☐	
	Cost of uncompensated household production[b]	NA	☐	
Consumption	Future consumption unrelated to health	NA	☐	
Social Services	Cost of social services as part of intervention	NA	☐	
Legal or Criminal Justice	Number of crimes related to intervention	NA	☐	
	Cost of crimes related to intervention	NA	☐	
Education	Impact of intervention on educational achievement of population	NA	☐	
Housing	Cost of intervention on home improvements (eg, removing lead paint)	NA	☐	
Environment	Production of toxic waste pollution by intervention	NA	☐	
Other (specify)	Other impacts	NA	☐	

bias that can occur with cost-effectiveness analysis. Because most of cost-effectiveness analysis is based on model and simulation, there is a risk that the influence of funding agencies and financial incentives can result in data that are favorable to one product over another. Although we cannot be certain whether bias occurs, this section provides some transparency.

The second Panel on Cost-Effectiveness in Health and Medicine (Neumann, 2017) recommends that an "Impact Inventory" be included with each analysis. This is a checklist that they developed that, like the CHEERS guidelines, helps the reader make sure that you have included all of the relevant pieces of information in your cost-effectiveness analysis. (See Exhibit 10.2. This can also be downloaded from our book's website.) The Impact Inventor can be incorporated into supplementary materials that go along with your analysis. This brings us to the Technical Appendix.

Technical Appendix

It is somewhat more difficult to communicate the results of a cost-effectiveness analysis effectively than it is to present the methods and results of other studies in the health literature. Therefore, extra care must be taken to ensure that all of the relevant issues are addressed while the less important aspects of the analysis are left out. Still, most of the nuances of the cost-effectiveness analysis cannot adequately be described within the word count limitations of most journals.

By including a technical appendix, you will be able to present to the reviewer every assumption, each piece of data used, and all of the mundane details of the sensitivity analyses performed. The reference case recommends that the event pathway in the decision analysis model be described (including changes in the HRQL in each pathway). The technical appendix can also contain codes from a software program (e.g., WinBUGS) used to perform simulations such as probabilistic sensitivity analysis (introduced in Chapter 9). It may include a program and files, such as TreeAge Pro, to allow the reader an opportunity to replicate the results.

TIPS AND TRICKS

Most decision analysis programs do not produce publication-quality graphs; however, many programs allow the user to export the information used to build a chart into a spreadsheet program such as Excel (Microsoft), a charting program such as SPSS Graph (SPSS), or an illustration program such as Adobe Illustrator (Adobe Systems). Free software, such as R (http://www.r-project.org), WinBUGS (http://www.mrc-bsu.cam.ac.uk/software/bugs), and OpenBUGS (http://www.openbugs.net) are available with manuals and tutorials for interested users.

Some journals may not accept such supplementary materials. In this case, it is generally acceptable to provide the technical document on the Internet, so that all readers can have access to the details of the analysis if they so desire. Your institution's web master or technical folks should help with the task. However, as more journals take advantage of the online capabilities of the Internet, many journals offer to post supplementary materials along with your manuscript. An example technical appendix detailing the methods for a meta-analysis used to generate parameter values for a decision analysis model is available from the journal's web site under Supplementary Materials (Bounthavong, Zargarzadeh, Hsu, & Vanness, 2011).

Figures and Illustrations

In cost-effectiveness analysis, figures of the decision model (or Markov model) and sensitivity analyses are necessary elements that highlight, summarize, and illustrate the concepts, results, and message that you are telling the audience. When submitting to a journal, always check their requirements for figures and illustrations. Most print journals will require black-and-white images that have a resolution of at least 300 DPI in specific file formats. For example, *Value in Health* requires that the figures be at least 300 DPI (line illustrations should be at least 1,000 DPI) and in the following formats: TIFF, JPEG, EPS, and PDF (http://www.ispor.org/publications/value/submit.asp). Many journals will charge you for color figures or illustrations in print versions, but not for online versions. Be careful deciding whether or not you want to spend extra resources on color figures.

Many journals also have limits on how many figures and tables you can submit. For example, *Value in Health* has a limit of six figures or tables for each manuscript that is considered original research. Therefore, don't go overboard in presenting everything as a figure or a table. You will need to exercise practicality and logic when selecting what you want to present in figure and table formats.

Figures and illustrations that are used from other sources require permission from the copyright holder (usually the publisher). All journals require the author to acknowledge the source and gain written permission from the copyright holder to reproduce the figure and/or illustration.

Each figure and illustration will require a title and a legend, which is usually provided as a separate page from the manuscript. The legend should contain all the notes and details such as an explanation of the symbols and abbreviations used.

Summary

Preparing your manuscript for publication is an exciting but challenging enterprise. There are standards for setting up the format of your manuscript that includes the Introduction, Methods, Results, and Discussion. Each part follows specific formats that are designed to facilitate the presentation of your results. Furthermore, you want to demonstrate that your work has value. A lot of the information in this chapter is generalizable to many journals. However, you should always carefully read the journal's Author Guidelines for additional directions and formatting.

Further Reading

Students are encouraged to read the entire CHEERS guidelines, which can be downloaded from the ISPOR web site (http://www.ispor.org/taskforces/economicpubguidelines.asp). Details for each section, with more examples, are provided.

The International Committee of Medical Journal Editors (ICMJE) has further guidelines on the conduct, reporting, editing, and publication of manuscripts for submission to scientific journals (http://www.icmje.org/recommendations/). Students interested in the roles and responsibilities of authors should download and read their guidelines.

References

Bounthavong, M., D. I. Hsu, and M. P. Okamoto. (2009). Cost-Effectiveness Analysis of Linezolid vs. Vancomycin in Treating Methicillin-Resistant Staphylococcus Aureus Complicated Skin and Soft Tissue Infections Using a Decision Analytic Model. *International Journal of Clinical Practice* 63(3): 376–386. http://doi.org/10.1111/j.1742-1241.2008.01958.x.

Bounthavong, M., A. Zargarzadeh, D. I. Hsu, and D. J. Vanness. (2011). Cost-Effectiveness Analysis of Linezolid, Daptomycin, and Vancomycin in Methicillin-Resistant Staphylococcus Aureus: Complicated Skin and Skin Structure Infection Using Bayesian Methods for Evidence Synthesis. *Value in Health* 14(5): 631–639. http://doi.org/10.1016/j.jval.2010.12.006.

Cutler, D. (2004). *Your Money or Your Life: Strong Medicine for America's Healthcare System*. Oxford, U.K.: Oxford University Press.

Gold, M. R., J. E. Siegel, L. B. Russell, and M. C. Weinstein. (1996). *Cost-Effectiveness in Health and Medicine*. New York: Oxford University Press.

Haddix, A., S. Teutsch, P. Shaffer, and D. Dunet (1996). *Prevention Effectiveness: A Guide to Decision Analysis and Economic Evaluation*. New York: Oxford University Press.

Husereau, D., M. Drummond, S. Petrou, C. Carswell, D. Moher, D. Greenberg, . . . ISPOR Health Economic Evaluation Publication Guidelines–CHEERS Good Reporting Practices Task Force. (2013). Consolidated Health Economic Evaluation Reporting Standards (CHEERS)—Explanation and Elaboration: A Report of the ISPOR Health Economic Evaluation Publication Guidelines Good Reporting Practices Task Force. *Value in Health* 16(2): 231–250. http://doi.org/10.1016/j.jval.2013.02.002.

Muennig, P., and K. Khan. (2001). Cost-Effectiveness of Vaccination Versus Treatment of Influenza in Healthy Adolescents and Adults. *Clinical Infectious Diseases* 33(11): 1879–1885. http://doi.org/10.1086/324491.

Neumann, P. J., G. D. Sanders, L. B. Russell, J. E. Siegel, and T. G. Ganiats. (2016). *Cost-Effectiveness in Health and Medicine*. New York: Oxford University Press.

Neuzil, K. M., G. W. Reed, E. F. Mitchel, and M. R. Griffin. (1999). Influenza-Associated Morbidity and Mortality in Young and Middle-Aged Women. *Journal of the American Medical Association* 281(10): 901–907.

Nguyen, C. M., M. Bounthavong, M. A. S. Mendes, M. L. D. Christopher, J. N. Tran, R. Kazerooni, and A. P. Morreale. (2012). Cost Utility of Tumour Necrosis Factor-A Inhibitors for Rheumatoid Arthritis: An Application of Bayesian Methods for Evidence Synthesis in a Markov Model. *PharmacoEconomics* 30(7): 575–593. http://doi.org/10.2165/11594990-000000000-00000.

Nichol, K. L., K. L. Margolis, J. Wuorenma, and T. Von Sternberg. (1994). The Efficacy and Cost Effectiveness of Vaccination Against Influenza Among Elderly Persons Living in the Community. *New England Journal of Medicine* 331(12): 778–784. http://doi.org/10.1056/NEJM199409223311206.

BASIC CONCEPTS IN EPIDEMIOLOGY AND APPLICATION TO COST-EFFECTIVENESS ANALYSIS

Overview

One of the reasons that cost-effectiveness analysis is fun is that you get to criticize everyone else's hard work. One of the most often used sources of information in cost-effectiveness analysis is the medical literature, and you must be good at tearing it apart to be certain that you are obtaining the highest-quality data possible. Data for cost-effectiveness analyses are also obtained from electronic data sources, expert opinion, the authors of published studies, and, in some cases, ongoing randomized controlled trials. Although it is not as much fun to criticize electronic data as it is to criticize the medical literature, the same basic sources of error are present in both.

To understand data commonly used in cost-effectiveness analysis, you need to know how to work with risks and rates. You also need to know how to work with distributions, and how to weight means. This chapter provides a basic overview of the epidemiology skills needed for cost-effectiveness analysis in health. The point of this chapter is not to cover any of these topics in detail. Rather, it's here for readers who don't have a degree in biostatistics or epidemiology and need a review of some of the pieces of those disciplines that are most relevant to cost-effectiveness analysis.

LEARNING OBJECTIVES

- Calculate the cumulative incidence and incidence rate and when to use one versus the other.

- Explain why adjustments are needed in determining risks and rates.

- Distinguish between prevalence and incidence and how each are used in epidemiology.

- Understand when to use the mean and standard deviation in a cost-effectiveness analysis.

- Distinguish between cross-sectional, retrospective, and prospective studies and when each should be used.

- Analyze the difference between risks and rates and when each should be used.

- Explain the importance of generalizability in cost-effectiveness analysis.

Review of Incidence

To understand the medical literature and use data in electronic datasets, you should have a basic understanding of the different measures of incidence and know how to calculate them. "Incidence" falls into two broad categories: cumulative incidence and incidence rate.

Cumulative incidence provides a proportion of the number of new events divided by the number of persons initially at risk for the event (Weiss & Koepsell, 2014). The cumulative incidence is based on a fixed time period. But the basic calculation is the same:

$$\frac{\text{Number of new events occurring in a given year}}{\text{Population at risk of event}} \times 10^n \qquad (11.1)$$

"Number of new events" in the numerator of Equation 11.1 refers to the number of diseases, hospitalizations, deaths, and so on, that occur in a population of people in the time period you are interested in. The "Population at risk" in the denominator is the population in which an event might conceivably have occurred. For example, if we knew the number of cases of uterine cancer in the United States during 2007, the population at risk would be all females in the United States at the midpoint of 2007.

The multiplier, 10^n, is usually tacked on to the end of a rate to make the cumulative incidence easier to understand. While it is not easy to grasp the meaning of the cumulative incidence for uterine cancer in the United States, 0.00013, it is easy to grasp the cumulative incidence for uterine cancer per 100,000 persons: 13 per 100,000 persons. Very common events are usually described per 100 persons (10^2), and very uncommon events, such as death, are usually described per 100,000 persons (10^5). One very common mistake that students make is to forget to remove the 10^n when using an incidence rate in their models. You won't make this mistake if you get why this is important.

For example, suppose there were 700 passengers on a cruise from Long Beach, California, U.S.A., to Ensenada, Baja California, Mexico. Everyone at the start of the cruise was healthy. However at the end of the five-day cruise, there were 155 cases of diarrhea. The cumulative incidence of diarrhea is calculated as:

$$\frac{155}{700} \times 10^2 = 22.1 \text{ cases per 100 population}$$

In other words, in a five-day cruise population of 100 people, there were 22 to 23 cases of diarrhea. Chalk it up to Cortez, whose conquest of Montezuma rained smallpox on the native population. Montezuma has been waging, and winning, revenge ever since.

The **incidence rate** is the number of new events divided by the amount of time contributed by the person at risk in a given observation period. Unlike cumulative incidence, the amount of time at risk affects the calculation of the incidence rate. Time is an important factor that is part of the calculation. The incidence rate is calculated as:

$$\frac{\text{Number of new events}}{\text{Person-time at risk}} \times 10^n$$

The "Person-time at risk" is sometimes counted as the amount of time that a *single person* contributes to the denominator. For example, a group may be at risk for developing cancer due to exposure to radiation. The exposure period for one member of the group may be 10 days. Imagine that another person who is also at risk for developing cancer had an exposure period for 300 days. The incidence rate captures the contributions of each person in the group based on the amount of time they are at risk for developing the disease. Table 11.1 provides an example for calculating incidence risk.

The incidence rate of cancer due to radiation exposure is calculated as:

$$\frac{3 \text{ cases}}{2491 \text{ days}} \times 10^5 = 120 \text{ cases per } 100,000 \text{ person-days.}$$

Table 11.1 Calculating the Incidence Rate of Developing Cancer due to Exposure to Radiation in a Two-Year Observation Period, 2011–2012

Patient Number	Developed Cancer (Y/N)?	Person-Time Exposed to Radiation (Days)
1	Yes	500
2	Yes	658
3	No	33
4	No	200
5	No	59
6	No	94
7	Yes	469
8	No	244
9	No	156
10	No	78
Total	3 cases of cancer	2491 days

In other words, for every 100,000 person-days of radiation exposure, there are 120 cases of cancer. The incidence rate provides us with a frequency for how many cases we can expect based on the amount of time at risk.

Distinguishing between cumulative incidence and incidence rate is not easy. Very often, you will encounter examples in the literature where these terms are interchangeable. For now, try to focus on how the two are interpreted and curse the statisticians for trying to make an already confusing world even less clear than it might otherwise be.

Note that another measure of disease frequency is mortality rate, which can be calculated as:

$$\frac{\text{Number of deaths}}{\text{Person-time at risk}} \times 10^n$$

We take some liberty with this calculation because we make an assumption that each person contributes 1 person-year to the denominator. Therefore, if the population was 1,000 people at risk of developing cancer, then the denominator can be assumed to be 1,000 person-years at risk.

Crude, Category-Specific, and Adjusted Rates

So far, the incidence measures (cumulative incidence and incidence rate) that we just calculated are based on the assumption that the population is homogeneous and uniform. In reality, the population is heterogeneous and diverse. What we have learned, thus far, is how to calculate a crude rate.

A **crude rate** is the rate measure that is unadjusted for differences in the population such as age, gender, and sociodemographic characteristics. Crude rates apply to everyone in the population who could have experienced an event and therefore do not account for differences in the characteristics of different groups of people, such as the elderly or the poor. Older people are generally at much greater risk of disease and death than young people, and poor people are generally at much greater risk of disease and death than wealthy people (Muennig, Franks, Jia, Lubetkin, & Gold, 2005). Recall from Chapter 7 how a patient's characteristics can affect his or her HRQL score. Therefore, we want to use QALYs that take into account these differences in patient characteristics. It is critically important that the rates you use are specific to the age, race, gender, and socioeconomic status of your hypothetical cohort.

Category-specific rates correspond to a subpopulation with different characteristics you might be interested in. Age is a common category-specific rate that is applied in most epidemiological studies. Age-specific rates refer to the number of events occurring in a particular age group. For instance, the rate of influenza among 20- to 25-year-olds is defined as:

$$\frac{\text{Total cases of influenza among persons 20 to 25 years old}}{\text{Midpoint U.S. population among persons 20 to 25 years old}} \times 10^n$$

(11.2)

One of the sad facts of life is that as people get older, the risk of illness and death increases. If we do not carefully account for differences in the rate of disease for each age group, our estimate of the rate of disease may lead to errors in our analysis.

Suppose we have a situation where the number of deaths due to influenza was categorized into different age groups (Table 11.2). We can calculate the crude mortality rate by dividing the number of deaths (column 1) by the number of people in each age group (column 2). We can get the total crude mortality rate for the entire cohort by dividing the total number of deaths (row 9 column 1) by the total number of people (row 9 column 2). The crude mortality rate for the cohort is 287.2 deaths per 100,000 persons. This is very similar to the life table example you were given earlier. Recall that the distribution of deaths is higher in the older population, which the crude mortality rate does not properly capture. In order to

Table 11.2 Calculating the Age-Adjusted Mortality Rate Using a Hypothetical U.S. Population

		(1)	(2)	(3)	(4)	(5)	(6)
Row	Age Group	Number of Deaths	Number of Subjects	Mortality Rate[a]	U.S. 2011 Standard Population	Age Distribution of Standard Population	Adjusted Mortality Rate[b]
1	0–10	1	10,000	10.0	42,135	0.13765	1.4
2	10–20	2	15,000	13.3	40,906	0.13363	1.8
3	20–30	5	20,000	25.0	42,907	0.14017	3.5
4	30–40	18	40,000	45.0	39,457	0.12890	5.8
5	40–50	23	25,000	92.0	42,576	0.13909	12.8
6	50–60	81	30,000	270.0	41,519	0.13564	36.6
7	60–70	122	15,000	813.3	29,590	0.09667	7.7
8	70+	219	9,000	2,433.3	27,018	0.08826	214.8
9	**Total**	**471**	**164,000**	**287.2**	**306,108**	**1.00000**	**355.3**

[a] Per 100,000 persons
[b] Per 1,000 persons

properly address the higher mortality in the older age groups, we need to perform some kind of adjustment.

In order to adjust for age, we need to use a technique called the direct standardization method for age-adjusted death rates (Curtin & Klein, 1995). The standardization method uses the U.S. population as the reference population for estimating weights for the standard population. In Table 11.2, weights are calculated by determining the proportion of people in each age group divided by the total U.S. population in 2011. (Note that most standardized populations are based on the U.S. population in 1940 or in 2000, but we use 2011 as a hypothetical illustration.) For instance, in order to determine the weight for the 0–10 age group, divide 42,135 by 306,108, which is 0.13765. Once you've determined the weights for each age group, you can calculate the mortality rates. The age-adjusted mortality rate for the 0–10 age group is the mortality rate (column 3) multiplied by the standardized weight for the 0–10 age group (column 5), which is 1.4 deaths per 100,000 persons. Summarizing all the age-adjusted mortality rates for each age group will give you the mortality rate for the entire cohort, which is 355.3 deaths per 100,000 persons. This is higher than the crude mortality rate of 287.2 deaths per 100,000 persons.

There are two lessons from this section. First, adjusted rates obtained from a study will have been adjusted to some standard population and will therefore usually be useless for your study. The second lesson is that crude rates also almost always are useless. Whenever you conduct a cost-effectiveness analysis, it is necessary to apply age-specific mortality rates to your hypothetical cohort. You will also need to match other demographic characteristics to the characteristics of your hypothetical cohort.

Exercises 1 to 5

1. Two hospitals collected data on the number of deaths due to postoperative surgical infections. Hospital A reported 54 deaths among 1,500 surgeries. Hospital B reported 156 deaths among 1,000 surgeries. What is the cumulative incidence of deaths in each hospital per 1000 surgical patients?

2. Suppose that there were more surgical patients in the intensive care unit (ICU) at Hospital A compared to Hospital B. Hospital A had 1,000 surgical patients in the ICU and Hospital B had 500 patients in the ICU. Calculate the ICU-specific mortality rates for each hospital by completing the following table.

	Hospital A			Hospital B		
Location	Deaths	Number of Surgeries	Deaths per 1,000	Deaths	Number of Surgeries	Deaths per 1,000
ICU	50	1,000		100	500	
Non-ICU	4	500		56	500	

3. Using the number of surgeries from both hospitals, determine the standard population for the number of surgeries in the ICU. (Hint: Use the following table to assist you.)

Location	Hospital A Number of Surgeries (1)	Hospital B Number of Surgeries (2)	Standard Population Size (1) + (2)
ICU			
Non-ICU			

4. Use the ICU-specific mortality rates and the standard population for each hospital to calculate the expected number of deaths for the ICU and non-ICU locations. (Hint: Use the table below to assist you.)

	Hospital A			Hospital B		
	ICU	Non-ICU	Total	ICU	Non-ICU	Total
Mortality rate per 1,000						
Standard population size						
Expected number of deaths						

5. Using the expected number of deaths for the ICU and non-ICU locations for both hospitals, estimate the ICU-adjusted mortality rate.

Prevalence Versus Incidence

Prevalence refers to the total number of cases of a disease in society (it is also referred to as **prevalent cases**). The **prevalence ratio** is the total number of prevalent cases divided by the number of people at risk for the disease. The ratio is often erroneously described as prevalence rate. Because it refers to the proportion or percentage of people with a disease rather than the number of cases that develop over a period of time, it is a ratio rather than a rate.

Recall from Chapter 1 that the incidence refers to the number of new cases over a period of time, usually one year, and that the incidence rate refers to the number of new cases divided by the population at risk of the disease over a defined period of time. In other words, the incidence rate of diabetes in the year 2007 would include only persons who were newly diagnosed with the condition in the year 2007.

Relationship Between Risks and Rates

Rates, such as incidence rates and mortality rates, are usually good estimators of the risk of disease. The risk of disease is defined as:

$$\text{Number of events over period/Population at the beginning of period} \tag{11.3}$$

As you can see, the formula for rates, Equation 11.1, is very similar to the formula for risk, Equation 11.3. Notice that the denominator of Equation 11.1 incorporates the midpoint population for the year in which the events occurred as an estimator of the population in which the events can occur, while Equation 11.3 includes all subjects over the same period (Jeckel, Elmore, & Katz, 1996).

Suppose that we followed a group of 1,000 people over a year to see how many would develop an influenza-like illness. If 410 subjects develop an influenza-like illness, the risk of developing the flu is $410 \div 1,000 = 0.41$. Rates are typically calculated using information from the general population. In the general population, people are constantly moving, dying, and being born. We use the denominator value with the midpoint of the period over which the events were tabulated (the rate) only when we do not have data on a specific cohort of people who have been followed over time (the risk).

So how might the risk and the rate differ in the real world? Imagine that there was a horrible influenza epidemic in February that wiped out 15 percent of the population. If we were to use the midpoint population of that year, we would be underestimating the population in which the events (cases of influenza) actually occurred. Why? Because those who died of influenza would not be counted by the census workers who come around in June. This would result in an overestimation of the risk of influenza, because the denominator would be smaller than it would have been if the true population of persons at risk for influenza had been known.

Technically speaking, any calculation of the risk of influenza, or any other disease that occurs early or late in the year, should be adjusted to better reflect the risk of disease before it is used in a cost-effectiveness analysis. However, for most diseases, the difference between a risk and a rate will not be large. Therefore, a rate can usually be used in a decision analysis model as a substitute for a measure of risk. (The more doubt we have about it, the larger we make the upper and lower bounds of our sensitivity analysis.)

There are four things to consider when deciding whether a rate is a good estimator of risk. First, the period over which the events occur in the rate should be short (one year or less). If the period is long, the chances are greater that the events in the numerator will fail to mesh with the population in the denominator. Second, if the event is a death, the proportion of the population affected by the event in the rate should be small (less than 3 to 5 percent). If many people die from the event, the population that is susceptible to the event (the denominator) will shrink, resulting in a rate that is larger than the risk. Third, we must consider whether the event occurs once or many times over the period of measurements. Finally, we must be certain that the susceptible population in the denominator of the rate is truly the population at risk of the event. For example, if we knew the total number of influenza cases and were to apply Equation 11.1, it would be tempting to divide the total number of cases in each age group by the total population in each age group. However, some people in the general population will have received the influenza vaccine and will not be as susceptible to infection as those who did not.

If we were epidemiologists rather than cost-effectiveness researchers, we might be more interested in the rate of influenza

TIPS AND TRICKS

Always be careful to remove the constant (10^n) multiplier when using rates in cost-effectiveness analyses. This may seem obvious, but some published rates appear in decimal form despite the 10^n multiplier. For example, the crude mortality rate per 100,000 persons for tuberculosis was 0.1 in 2006 (National Center for Health Statistics, 2005). To obtain the actual mortality rate, this number must be divided by 100,000, yielding a rate of 0.000001 or 10^{-6}.

in the general population than the rate of influenza among unvaccinated people, because we would be more concerned with the severity of the epidemic than some abstract notion of risk. However, in cost-effectiveness analysis, we are more interested in knowing the chances of contracting influenza virus infections among unvaccinated and vaccinated people, and we should be careful to include only unvaccinated subjects in the denominator.

Understanding Error

For every measurement, rate, probability, and cost value used in a cost-effectiveness analysis, there exists a true mean value that is applicable to the hypothetical cohort. For example, there is an average risk of developing influenza-like illness in any given year. Unfortunately, only an omniscient being would know what this value is. Being fallible, humans must rely on imperfect scientific methods to estimate the true value of each input into a cost-effectiveness model. The extent to which the measured value of an input is representative of its real value is referred to as the **accuracy** of that measurement. If the value of the input is similar each time that it is measured, it is said to be **reproducible** or **reliable**.

Once you have obtained the articles from the medical literature that you need to conduct your cost-effectiveness analysis, you must determine whether the information you extract from these articles is likely to be accurate. To evaluate the data for accuracy, you will need to have a basic understanding of the common types of error and statistical distributions (such as the normal distribution), and you will need to understand the different ways in which studies are conducted.

The more you read and systematically analyze the methods sections of original research articles, the more comfortable you will become with judging the quality of these articles. Although the basic elements of bio-statistics and epidemiology presented in this section will be sufficient as a brief review of error estimation, students who have never had exposure to epidemiology and biostatistics or have never had to critically read the medical literature may require further study.

The most common types of error found in the medical literature are **random error** and **bias**. The extent to which a value is subject to random error is dependent on the size of the sample from which it was derived. Random error is sometimes referred to as sampling error and can be reduced by increasing the size of a statistical sample. We will see examples of how this works in the section "Frequency Distributions and Random Error" later in this chapter.

Bias, or **nonrandom error**, occurs when error affects the data in a systematic way. Consider surveillance data. These data are obtained by asking physicians who see a patient with a communicable disease of public health importance to fill out a card and send it to a local health department. Because only some physicians take the time to fill out the reporting card, reportable diseases are almost always undercounted. This type of error is called "nonrandom" because it has nothing to do with the sample size. The error in the number of cases reported always occurs in one direction. Because nonrandom error is systematic, it is sometimes referred to as **systematic bias** or differential error.

To understand the difference between random error and nonrandom error, consider the case of two different people shooting arrows at a target. A highly trained but cross-eyed sharpshooter's target might look like Figure 11.1, while a clear-sighted amateur's target might look like Figure 11.2.

In the first case, the sharpshooter's problem was systematic error or bias. In the second case, the amateur's arrows did not miss the target in a systematic way. Rather, the arrows were randomly distributed around the target. If the amateur kept shooting arrows, the arrows would be distributed around the target in such a fashion that the average distance between arrows was at the center, even if the arrows were scattered all over the wall. Note that this implies that a dataset can be populated with accurate data but contains a good deal of random error. Nonrandom error is, by definition, inaccurate.

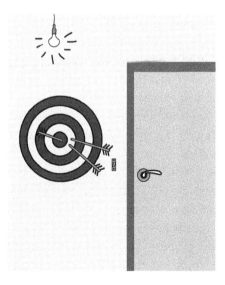

Figure 11.1 Nonrandom Error

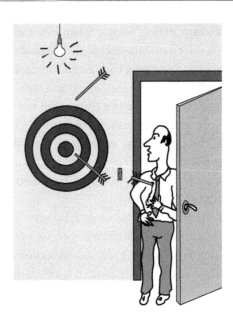

Figure 11.2   Random Error

Most medical data contain either random or nonrandom error simply because it is very expensive to eliminate both types of error. For example, the National Health Interview Survey (NHIS) is a health survey of about 100,000 people living in the United States (National Center for Health Statistics, 2014b). Because it is administered to a large number of people, it is relatively free of random error when it is used to tabulate the incidence or prevalence of common diseases. However, the NHIS asks subjects to recall whether they were ill over the preceding year and to record which diseases they had. Since people have trouble remembering whether they were sick, they are likely to forget the number of illnesses they had. (If this seems difficult to grasp, try to remember how many times you had a cold over the past year.) Thus, for some diseases, the NHIS will hit below the bull's-eye (produce an undercount of the number of diseases respondents had), and it will do so consistently. For unforgettable diseases such as cancer there will be little or no bias.

The NHIS has a sister survey, the National Health and Nutrition Examination Survey (NHANES), that is free of recall bias for most variables; however, the sample size is small (National Center for Health Statistics, 2014a). In this survey, the government parks a huge white van outside the door of unsuspecting citizens and invites them into the van to have their health checked. Once inside, they are poked, prodded, and tested for a number of diseases. By actually testing subjects, the study greatly reduces bias (nonrandom error), but the testing is very expensive, so only a small sample of subjects can be tested. Therefore, random error presents a bigger problem. (To overcome this, the survey is adding subjects each year. This way, researchers can add many years of data together to increase the sample size.)

Managing Error in Cost-Effectiveness Analysis

Virtually every source of data you will use in cost-effectiveness research will be subject to random or nonrandom error. Cost-effectiveness researchers must therefore learn how to manage error and demonstrate how error affected the accuracy and reliability of the cost-effectiveness ratios they present to the people who read the analysis.

Random error is usually easy to measure, but nonrandom error cannot always be perfectly quantified. Sometimes, though, it is possible to estimate the extent to which an input is subject to nonrandom error and adjust the input accordingly. This process is akin to nudging the sharpshooter depicted in Figure 11.1 a little to the left. For example, as we learned in Chapter 4, the amount a hospital charges its clients is known to consistently be an overestimate of the actual cost of providing medical services (Centers for Medicare & Medicaid Services, 2014). The cost-to-charge ratio is one example of how to reduce systematic bias in your parameter estimate. In other cases, there may be published data on the direction and magnitude of the error. For instance, in self-report surveys, men are likely to overestimate their height, and women are likely to underestimate their weight. Using data from surveys in which a third party measures height and weight, it is possible to obtain a correction (Strauss, 1999).

In many cases, you will not have a good adjuster like a cost-to-charge ratio or a correction from a published study. In such instances, your best hope is to examine the impact this error might have on your incremental cost-effectiveness ratios using a sensitivity analysis. Recall from Chapter 9 that a sensitivity analysis is a way of testing the effect of error inherent to each input on the overall cost and effectiveness of each of the interventions under study.

Frequency Distributions and Random Error

Suppose we obtain cholesterol test values from 100 people that vary between 115 and 290 mg/dl; the range is 115 to 290 mg/dl. Most of the subjects will

Table 11.3 Frequency Distribution of Hypothetical Cholesterol Values Obtained from 100 Subjects

Cholesterol Level (mg/dl)	Number of Subjects
115 to 135	3
135 to 155	15
155 to 175	30
175 to 195	25
195 to 215	12
215 to 235	7
235 to 255	5
255 to 275	2
275+	1
Total	100

have a cholesterol value somewhere close to the mean of these values, but a few will have values around 130, and a few others will have values around 270. If we were to list the number of people who had a cholesterol level between 115 and 135 mg/dl, 135 and 155 mg/dl, and so on, we would have a frequency distribution of these cholesterol levels (see Table 11.3).

If we were to show Table 11.3 graphically, it would take the form presented in Figure 11.3.

The frequency of events can also be described as a probability. For example, the 30 values between 155 mg/dl and 175 mg/dl, out of the 100 subjects in the sample, can be expressed as $30 \div 100 = 0.3$. When frequency distributions are expressed as probabilities, they are known as **probability distributions**. Figure 11.4 shows the data in Table 11.3 as a probability distribution rather than a frequency distribution.

In Chapter 9, we saw that the Monte Carlo simulation relies heavily on probability distributions. If we are evaluating a cost-effectiveness analysis of anticholesterol drugs, we will need to incorporate a sensitivity analysis on cholesterol values among untreated subjects. We could simply look at what happens when the mean cholesterol value is 115 mg/dl and when it is 275 mg/dl. But we see from Figure 11.4 that the probability of observing either one of these values is less than 0.05. In our Monte Carlo simulation, we'll want to make sure that values between 155 mg/dl and 175 mg/dl are sampled more frequently than on either extreme. In fact, we'll ideally want these values to come up about 30 percent of the time because that is how often they were observed in our sample. By using probability distributions in our sensitivity analysis, we can ensure that we are commonly observing common values and rarely observing rare values.

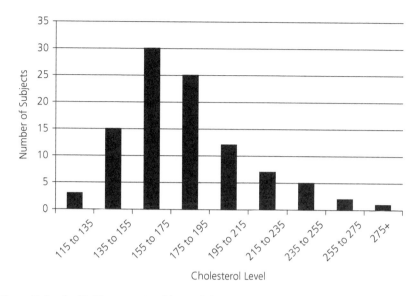

Figure 11.3   Graphical Representation of the 100 Cholesterol Values

Many frequency distributions or probability distributions form a roughly bell-shaped curve known as a **normal distribution** (also known as a *Gaussian distribution*). When perfectly bell-shaped, the peak of the bell (the part that you would hang by a string if it were actually a bell) represents the mean of the sample.

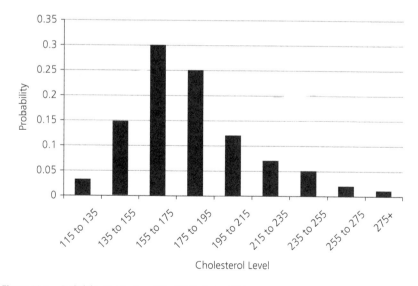

Figure 11.4   Probability Distribution of the 100 Cholesterol Values

When the sample size is small, curves tend to look more like abstract representations of a bell rather than a perfectly drawn bell. (*Skewness* refers to a shift in the peak of a curve to the left or right.) Skewness can occur due to factors other than random error as well, but for now let's just worry about random error.

If we were to increase the sample size, chances are that more people with high cholesterol levels would be randomly selected, thereby rounding out the curve; as the sample size taken from a normally distributed population increases, the distribution of values looks more and more like an actual bell. If we had a sample size of 1,000 subjects rather than 100 subjects, the probability distribution in Figure 11.4 would probably appear more like Figure 11.5. Thus, as the sample size increases in an unbiased sample of values, the accuracy of the mean value is generally improved.

This brings us to the next point. For any set of numbers, it is, of course, possible to calculate a mean. For instance 1, 2, and 3 have a mean of (1 + 2 + 3) ÷ 3 = 2. The sum of deviations of these values from the mean is 0. For instance, 1 is −1 units from 2, 2 is 0 units from 2, and 3 is +1 units from 2. The sum of the deviations is − 1 + 0 + 1 = 0.

If we were to calculate the average deviation of these numbers from the mean, however, we would take a different approach. The average deviation, more commonly known as the **standard deviation**, is calculated by first squaring the deviation of each data point from the mean. This gets rid of the negative sign. We then calculate the average across all deviations, and then

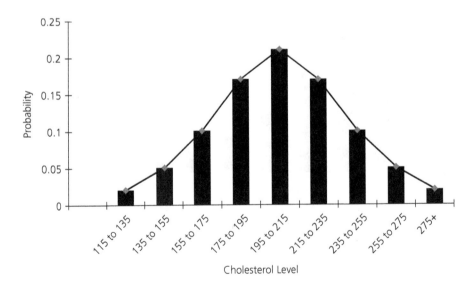

Figure 11.5   Hypothetical Probability Distribution of 1,000 Cholesterol Values

obtain the square root (to undo the square). This average, or "standard," deviation assumes the form:

$$sd = \sqrt{\frac{(x - \bar{x})^2}{n - 1}} \qquad (11.4)$$

where x is the sample value, $\bar{x}$ is the sample mean, and n is the sample size. (We subtract 1 from n just to make sure that we are as conservative as possible or "unbiased" in our estimate.) It turns out that if we obtain the standard deviation of any sample, we can know that chance of observing any range of values.

For instance, look at Figure 11.5. The mean of this sample falls at the peak of the curve, or at 205 mg/dl. If the standard deviation of the sample is 30 mg/dl, then cholesterol values between 175 mg/dl and 205 mg/dl fall within 1 standard deviation of the mean. Knowing the standard deviation, we know that values between 175 mg/dl and 205 mg/dl will be observed 34 percent of the time. We also know that anything above or below 30 mg/dl of the mean will be observed 68 percent of the time (see Figure 11.6). The magic of a standard deviation is that it provides us with a uniform probability distribution from which we can infer the chances of observing any one event.

Basics of Statistical Inference

The normal distribution is very helpful for Monte Carlo simulations because it tells us the chance that we will observe any one value. But it has a much more common use in scientific studies.

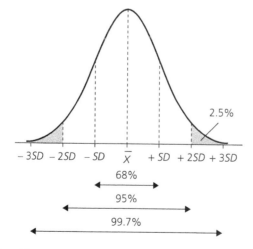

Figure 11.6   The Normal Curve

Note: SD = standard deviation.

Studies in the medical literature often compare two or more sample means. For example, a sample of people who are treated with a cholesterol-lowering drug might be compared with a sample of people who are not so treated. If the drug works, the mean cholesterol level in the treated population should be lower than the mean cholesterol level in the untreated population. However, if the sample size is small, differences between the two population means must be fairly large for a statistically significant difference to be detected. In other words, if the sample size is too small, it is less likely that a real difference between two population means will be detected. Why? If the sample size is small, the standard deviation will be very large. We will therefore not have a good sense of whether the observed difference is due to random error or a real difference between the mean values. The ability of a statistical test to detect a difference between two population means is referred to as **statistical power**.

In cost-effectiveness analysis, we are interested in knowing the **effect size** of a health intervention. The effect size is the magnitude of the expected improvement realized by an intervention or, more technically, the strength of the measured relationship between two variables. If the observed difference between two means in two small groups is large but the error is also large, we might be overestimating the benefits associated with our intervention.

When a real difference between two populations exists but no difference is detected by statistical testing, it is referred to as a *type II error*. When a difference between two populations is detected by statistical testing but no difference between the means actually exists, it is referred to as a *type I error*.

The possible values of true population means are often presented in the medical literature as measured sample means with 95 percent confidence intervals. The 95 percent confidence intervals refer to the range of possible values of the mean over which we can be 95 percent certain the true value of the parent population mean is represented. In other words, we are saying that any two means that differ by two or more standard deviations were probably not observed at random.

Usually, researchers are willing to accept a 5 percent probability that the difference between two samples is due to chance alone. When this threshold is set lower, the chance of making a type II error increases and the chance of a type I error decreases. Conversely, when this threshold is set higher, the chance of a type II error decreases and the chance of a type I error increases.

For each variable used in a cost-effectiveness analysis, there is a value that most likely represents the actual cost, probability, or effectiveness measure that we would expect to see in the real world. Recall that this number is sometimes called the baseline value because it will be used to determine the principal cost-effectiveness ratio you will publish in your study. There will also be high and low values for this variable that are plausible (for example, the highest and lowest observed price of a drug on the market).

In cost-effectiveness analysis, researchers will often know that the baseline value is pretty likely and that the high and low values are pretty unlikely, but they will not have any information on the distribution of these values. In these instances, the triangular distribution might be considered (see Figure 11.7).

Let us return to the example of drug costs. Suppose you call 10 pharmacies across the country to obtain the cost of oseltamivir. The 10 values you obtain might average $53 for a full course of the medication. While the discount drug chains you called were able to sell this medication for less than the mean value, the expensive drug boutique on Rodeo Drive sold it for more. The chance that the actual mean value of this medication is as high as the one you found on Rodeo Drive is very small, and the chance that the mean value is as low as the cheapest drugstore blowout in Joplin, Missouri, is very small. Although you do not have a true statistical sample and do not know the distribution of the values, you want to have a way of telling your decision analysis model that these extreme high and low values are very unlikely. Because you are not certain exactly how unlikely they are, you can simply distribute the probabilities in a triangular shape around the baseline value of $53.

When a triangular distribution is used, values that are more likely representative of the true mean (the baseline values) are assigned a heavier weight than values that represent less likely estimates of the true mean value. In Figure 11.7, the mean cost (about $53 on the left y axis) is assigned a high probability of occurring (about 0.7 on the right y-axis), based on a subjective assessment of the chance that this is the most likely value for the cost of oseltamivir. Likewise, the extreme low value and extreme high value are subjectively assigned a low probability of occurring.

Calculating Weighted Means

Weighted means are commonly encountered in cost-effectiveness analysis. Imagine that you had three groups of people randomly selected from the U.S. population to have their blood cholesterol levels measured. Suppose further that you wanted to know the mean cholesterol level of all of the subjects together. If you knew the number of people in each group and the mean cholesterol value of each of these groups, you could estimate the

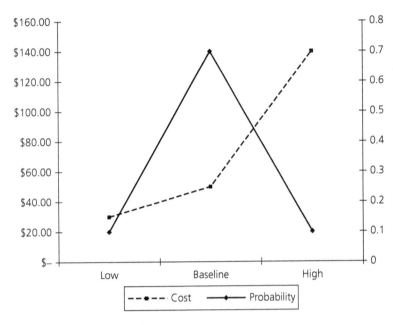

Figure 11.7   Example of a Triangular Distribution

Note: The solid line represents the probabilistic weight assigned to each cost value represented by the dashed line. Thus, a cost of $140 is assigned a very low probability of occurrence

overall mean cholesterol level of all of the subjects combined by calculating a weighted mean. A weighted mean is the average value of a set of numbers that are each weighted by some factor, such as the number of subjects in a group.

In cost-effectiveness analysis, it is often necessary to calculate weighted means for the data that you will ultimately use in your cost-effectiveness analysis. If data from many small **cross-sectional studies** are available, a weighted mean can improve the accuracy of a parameter estimate. Means are also useful for adjusting data retrieved from data extraction tools or from printed tabulations of data. A weighted mean is calculated using the following formula:

$$\text{Weighted Mean} = \frac{\sum (w_i \times x_i)}{\sum w_i}, \tag{11.5}$$

where x_i is the mean of the i-th group and w_i is the weight applied to that group. For example, a study that was conducted reported 15 deaths in sample population 1, but 2 deaths in sample population 2. We would calculate the average number of deaths for the two populations as 8.5 deaths $\left(\frac{15+2}{2} \right)$. However, the number of persons in sample 1 was 50 and the number of persons in sample 2 was 10. Because the sample sizes are different, we need to apply different weights for each population. Therefore, the weighted-average mean number of deaths for the two populations is actually 12.8 deaths $\left(\frac{(50 \times 15) + (10 \times 2)}{50 + 10} \right)$. Another way to think about this is to use Equation 11.6:

(Events in population 1 × number of persons in population 1)

+ (Events in population 2 × number of persons in population 2)

÷ (Number of persons in population 1

+ number of persons in population 2)   (11.6)

Exercise 6

6. Imagine that you are doing a cost-effectiveness analysis that evaluated linezolid, an antibiotic used to treat infections. You are trying to figure out what the average probability of cure is. You collected three randomized clinical trials that reported the number of patients who were successfully cured of their infection with linezolid. In Trial 1, the number of patients cured was 15 out of 20. In Trial 2, the number of patients cured was 2 out of 10. In Trial 3, the number of patients cured was 5 out of 6. What is the weighted mean probability of cure?

Evaluating Study Limitations

This section explains how to identify limitations of studies and also presents some tips for avoiding research efforts that contain mistakes. However, identifying mistakes on the part of researchers is tricky (and sometimes impossible) given the limited amount of information published in the methods section of a research paper.

Review of Medical Study Designs

Medical studies are usually conducted to evaluate risks or rates. For example, they might indicate the risks associated with smoking or the risk of morbidity or mortality among people treated with a new medication relative to untreated people. Alternatively, they might indicate the probability that a screening test will correctly identify people who have a disease. Because cost-effectiveness analyses are constructed using the probabilities of different events, virtually all cost-effectiveness analyses will require information from medical studies.

Medical studies are usually described according to how they follow subjects over time. While cross-sectional studies give a slice of information at one point in time, retrospective studies examine factors that occurred in the past, and prospective studies are designed to examine events that will occur in the future. Each of these different study designs has different limitations, and it is important to understand them.

Cross-Sectional Studies

In a cross-sectional study, data are obtained at one point in time. Cross-sectional studies are useful for obtaining the prevalence of disease or enumerating the number of people at risk for a particular disease (for example, identifying the number of smokers in different age groups). Simple cross-sectional studies can be conducted rapidly using national datasets. For instance, in the United States, the Behavior Risk Factor Surveillance System can be used to determine the percentage of adults who are vaccinated against the influenza virus, the number of smokers, or the number of people with other risk factors for disease.

FOR EXAMPLE: PLACEBO-CONTROLLED STUDIES

The placebo effect is a powerful biopsychological phenomenon. People who are given dummy pills or sham surgery often experience improved health outcomes relative to those who do not. For example, when coronary artery bypass surgery was first evaluated, subjects with angina (chest pain) who were randomized to the placebo group were given nothing more than a superficial cut on the skin of their chest. (Today, this practice would probably be deemed unethical.) Subjects in the experimental group underwent open-heart surgery. While 70 percent of the patients who received the surgery reported improvement in chest pain, all of the patients in the placebo group reported improvement (Fisher, 2000).

Retrospective Studies

Retrospective studies are generally designed to identify risk factors for disease in the past that is associated with an outcome of interest in the present. It is important to note that the outcome of interest has already occurred and that the goal of the investigation is to look back into the past to identify the risk factors associated with the outcome. In a specific type of retrospective study called a **case-control study**, people with a disease are paired with a control group of people who are similar in most ways but

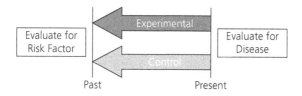

Figure 11.8   Retrospective Study Designs: Case-Control and Cohort Designs

do not have the disease. Each group is then examined for a past exposure to some risk factor for the disease (see Figure 11.8). For example, a group of new mothers whose children had cleft palates might be asked about a potential contributing cause, such as having taken a medication while pregnant. A group of mothers whose children were free of birth defects and gave birth in the same hospital might then be interviewed to determine whether they too had taken that particular medication during pregnancy.

A **retrospective cohort study** is another retrospective study design that identifies risk factors in the past and then follows the patient forward in time to the present (or sometime after exposure to the risk factor) to determine associations. Unlike a case-control design, where the sample selection is determined by the outcome of interest, a retrospective cohort design identifies the sample by their exposure status in the past. For example, suppose you were interested in whether a new group of mothers who were taking a medication while pregnant was at higher risk of having a child with a cleft palate. The study would include mothers who took a medication while pregnant and compare them to mothers who did not take any medication while pregnant. The outcome (cleft palate in newborns) will be determined after the pregnancy, which is after the exposure or risk factor (taking medication during pregnancy).

Retrospective studies are especially susceptible to bias. For instance, recall that bias occurs when the group without the disease fails to remember whether they were exposed to the risk factor. In the case of the new mothers, those whose children had a birth defect may be much more motivated to try to remember whether they had taken medications during pregnancy than mothers whose children did not have the birth defect. If the subjects in the control did not remember having taken the medication (and thus underreported its use), the medication may be falsely implicated as a cause of the birth defect.

Another common type of bias specific to retrospective studies is confounding. This occurs when the control group does not match the experimental group with respect to another risk factor for the disease. For example, one study examining the relationship between coffee drinking and heart disease found a strong association. However, because coffee drinkers are also significantly more likely to smoke than people who do not drink coffee, the control group contained fewer smokers than the experimental group (Thelle, Arnesen, & Førde, 1983; Urgert, Meyboom, Kuilman, Rexwinkel, Vissers, Klerk, & Katan, 1996). (Coffee subsequently was found to be relatively safe.) Because of the great potential for confounding, data from retrospective studies are rarely used in cost-effectiveness analysis.

Prospective Studies

Like retrospective trials, **prospective studies** are generally designed to identify risk factors for disease. Prospective trials offer a number of advantages over retrospective trials. First, they reduce bias by examining people with a putative risk factor relative to those without the potential risk factor before they develop disease. Subjects are then followed over time to see whether the people with the risk factor are more likely to develop the disease (Figure 11.9). Second, they allow the calculation of incidence rates and **risk ratios**. A risk ratio indicates how much more likely people with the risk factor are to develop disease than those who do not have the risk factor.

The risk ratio is calculated as the **incidence rate** of disease among people with the risk factor over the incidence rate of disease in people without the risk factor, or:

$$\text{Risk Ratio} = \frac{\text{Incidence}_{\text{Risk Factor}}}{\text{Incidence}_{\text{No Risk Factor}}} \qquad (11.7)$$

which is often written as:

$$\text{Risk Ratio} = \frac{\text{Risk}_{\text{Risk Factor}}}{\text{Risk}_{\text{No Risk Factor}}} \qquad (11.8)$$

The risk ratio is also referred to as **relative risk**. (Both are conveniently abbreviated RR.)

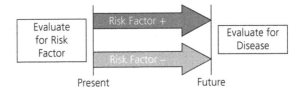

Figure 11.9   Prospective Study Design

The risk ratio produces a number that is easy for most people to understand. For example, the relative risk of developing lung cancer among smokers is about 9.0, indicating that smokers are at nine times the risk of developing lung cancer as nonsmokers (Doll & Hill, 1956). Retrospective trials allow for the

TIPS AND TRICKS

Technically, Equation 11.6 refers to a rate ratio rather than a risk ratio. *Risk ratio* is sometimes used when it is important to distinguish between a ratio of rates and a ratio of risks. In practice, these terms are often used interchangeably.

calculation of **odds ratios** rather than risk ratios, a measure that reflects risk only when applied to relatively rare conditions.

Prospective studies are expensive to conduct and are therefore often generally applied only to major research questions relating to common diseases. Older prospective trials were often targeted toward white male cohorts, and the results may not always be generalizable to other populations.

Another problem with prospective studies is that subjects who are willing to participate in a study may differ from those unwilling to participate. People who are willing to take part in a randomized controlled trial without reimbursement may be healthier, more ideological, or more affluent than people who do not, which can distort the overall severity or impact of a disease. For instance, imagine a study that examines the overall impact of smoking on health outcomes. If mostly healthy subjects enroll in the study, people with diabetes might be excluded from both the experimental and the control groups. Because a diabetic who smokes is at much greater risk of heart disease than the cumulative risk of both of these conditions separately, smoking may appear to be less harmful than it really is.

The tendency for volunteer study subjects to be healthier than the general population is called the **healthy volunteer effect**. If we were to evaluate a nonsmoking intervention in a cost-effectiveness analysis using data obtained from a cohort of mostly healthy smokers, the benefits of smoking cessation would be artificially reduced.

People who drop out of studies differ from those who stick with a study to the end. For example, in a famous prospective study of risk factors for heart disease conducted in Framingham, Massachusetts, subjects who dropped out of the investigation were later found to have a much greater risk of heart attack and death than the subjects who stayed in the study (Dawber, Meadors, & Moore, 1951). Prospective studies are commonly referred to as **longitudinal studies**, because patients are followed over time into the future and the outcome of interest hasn't occurred yet.

Like retrospective studies, prospective studies can be confounded. For instance, people who drink coffee are more likely to smoke. Even if you follow coffee drinkers who are free of heart disease over time, they will still be thought to develop heart disease at a higher rate than noncoffee drinkers simply because they smoke. Therefore, it is important to think long and hard about how the relationship between the risk factor and the disease might be confounded and then ask yourself whether the authors took this into account by controlling for the relevant confounders.

Why so much attention to the problems associated with prospective studies when retrospective studies are so much more problematic? Because they are commonly used as inputs to cost-effectiveness analyses. Therefore, it's very important to understand their limitations.

Randomized Controlled Trials

The **randomized controlled trial** is probably the most often used source of information in the field of cost-effectiveness analysis. A randomized controlled trial is a type of prospective study designed to determine whether those who receive a particular intervention have better health outcomes than those who do not. In this design, subjects are randomly assigned to either an intervention group or a placebo group (Figure 11.10). They are then followed over time to see if there are differences in the rate or severity of disease between the two groups. The difference between a randomized controlled trial and other prospective studies is that some subjects in other prospective studies have something (such as a smoking problem) that may increase their risk of disease, and some subjects in a randomized controlled trial are given something (such as smoking cessation advice) that may reduce their risk of disease.

In a randomized controlled trial, it is common to control for the placebo effect (see the previous "For Example" box on this topic). Unfortunately, in the field of cost-effectiveness analysis, we are interested in how

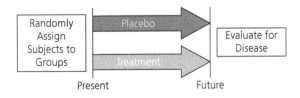

Figure 11.10   Randomized Controlled Trial Study Design

interventions work in the real world. In the real world, people who take a medication benefit from both the treatment effect and the placebo effect.

When a medical intervention is compared with a placebo and the placebo has an impact on the illness under study, the cost-effectiveness of an intervention will be underestimated. Consider the case of clinical evaluations for minoxidil solution, a topical treatment for male pattern baldness. Balding men do not usually spontaneously grow hair. However, this is exactly what happened with men in the placebo group of some of the randomized controlled trials evaluating the clinical efficacy of this drug (Clissold & Heel, 1987). If we were to measure the effectiveness of the drug relative to the placebo, the drug would appear to be less effective than if it were measured relative to each subject's hair pattern when the study was started.

Other subconscious cues, such as the body language of a researcher, can also have an impact on treatment outcomes in a randomized controlled trial. For this reason, the researchers who actually interact with patients are often made unaware of whether the patient has received the intervention. When neither the patients nor the researchers who interact with the patients know who received the placebo and who received the treatment, the study is said to be **double-blinded**.

To keep both the patients and the researchers unaware of who is in the experimental group and who is in the placebo group, patients must be randomly assigned to either group. The status of each patient is hidden until the end of the study, at which point the study is "uncovered," and the effects of the intervention are examined. It is therefore important to examine the characteristics of the patients who were randomly allocated to the placebo group or to the control group (these characteristics are almost always presented in the first table in the article describing the study).

Sometimes chance works against researchers, and subjects receiving the placebo have a lower average income or smoke more often than subjects in the intervention group. When the subjects in the placebo group happen to have more risk factors for disease than the subjects in the experimental group, or imperfections in the randomization process occur, the intervention may appear to be more or less effective than it would have been under perfect conditions. For these reasons, it is important to make sure that the experimental and control groups used in the study are demographically similar. If they differ slightly, the effect size may be more precisely estimated by adjusting for demographic differences between groups.

Meta-Analysis

A **meta-analysis** is a systematic analysis of many studies published in the medical literature. In this design, data are obtained from different prospective or randomized controlled trials and then combined into a single study. For example, if one study evaluated a treatment for heart disease in Chicago and another study evaluated the same treatment using a similar study design in San Francisco, the subjects in the experimental group from each study would be combined into a single group. Similarly, the subjects from the control groups would be combined into a single group. The effect of the treatment on the combined experimental group relative to the combined control group would then be analyzed.

The Cochrane Collaboration is a nonprofit organization dedicated to the promotion of evidence-based decision making through the development and access of systematic reviews and synthesized research. Their web site provides a search engine for systematic reviews and meta-analyses (Cochrane Collaboration, 2014).

As with any other study, the quality of meta-analysis studies is variable. One meta-analysis in a major peer-reviewed journal found that mammography was not effective at reducing mortality rates for breast cancer (Gøtzsche & Olsen, 2000). However, the authors chose to exclude all of the studies demonstrating the clinical effectiveness of this technique because they felt that these studies had problems with the random allocation of subjects. Most experts agree, however, that mammography is effective because the mortality rate for breast cancer has declined more rapidly than improvements in treatments would suggest.

When many studies exist pertaining to a particular parameter of interest in a cost-effectiveness analysis, cost-effectiveness researchers sometimes conduct their own meta-analysis on these studies. For example, if it were necessary to generate an estimate of the incidence rate of influenza infection for the United States

TIPS AND TRICKS

Indirect treatment comparisons can be performed by compiling studies into a network. For example, if you were interested in the treatment effect of Drug A versus Drug C but there were no head-to-head studies available, you could use other studies where Drug A and Drug C are compared to a common comparator, Drug B. Figure 11.11 illustrates how networks of studies can yield indirect comparisons where direct comparisons are unavailable. This figure uses dotted lines to represent indirect treatment comparison, and solid lines are direct comparisons. Advanced users might want to check out the literature on how meta-analysis can also measure treatment effect indirectly using Bayesian methods (Jansen et al., 2011; Lumley, 2002; Nixon, Bansback, & Brennan, 2007).

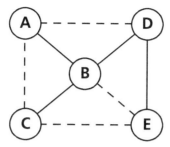

Figure 11.11   Network of Studies Comparing Drugs Directly and Indirectly

but only regional estimates were available, a meta-analysis of all of these studies might provide a better estimate of the rate of influenza nationwide.

Meta-analytical techniques are too advanced for an introductory textbook, and we encourage you to study the topic in more depth.

Primary Cost-Effectiveness Studies

In some instances, a longitudinal study will be primarily directed at collecting cost and effectiveness data. In this study design, a group of subjects is administered a standard of care intervention and one or more health interventions with the primary goal of determining the cost-effectiveness of a particular strategy. In other words, subjects are allowed to behave as they might in a real-world setting and costs are measured as they are incurred. For instance, if the study were evaluating a new antibiotic, patients might see the physician as they normally would. The time spent during the medical encounter is measured, the cost of the antibiotics is recorded, and no unusual measures are taken to ensure that the patients have taken all of their medications. If patients have side effects to the medication, the researchers determine whether the side effects lead to additional medical visits or other costs. Finally, the time patients spend receiving care, driving, and other costs is recorded.

The advantage of a primary cost-effectiveness analysis is that most sources of error can be carefully controlled, costs can be obtained directly from the study, and cost-effectiveness analyses can simulate real-world conditions better than standard longitudinal analyses, providing effectiveness data as well as efficacy data. Unfortunately, try as the researchers may, this approach still yields results obtained under experimental rather than real-world conditions. For instance, patients might be followed in university hospitals, where medical care differs from that in other clinical settings. In a traditional cost-effectiveness analysis (an analysis that uses secondary sources of data), it is often possible to examine longitudinal studies from many different parts of the country and in different clinical settings, improving the validity of the analysis.

Generalizability

When evaluating the medical literature, two questions should immediately come to the cost-effectiveness researcher's mind. The first is "Was this study carefully designed and executed?" The second is "Are the results of this study generalizable to my study population?" If these two questions are consistently asked, cost-effectiveness researchers should be able to get a better idea of whether the data that they wish to extract from the study will be useful. Although there are a number of good books available for evaluating study quality, most pay less attention to issues of generalizability, which is an issue that is paramount in cost-effectiveness analysis.

Are the results generalizable to your study population? A study with external validity will produce results that are generalizable to groups other than those under study. One criticism of medical research conducted in the twentieth century is that the majority of studies examined only the health effects of white men, raising questions as to whether the study results were valid for other groups in the United States. It may be the case that one type of antihypertensive medication is better for African American males and another is better for white women, but these differences in treatment response are usually not known because those cohorts were not represented in the studies. Sometimes the results of studies are undergeneralized as well. Until recently, women with crushing chest pain were sometimes sent home from the emergency room because heart disease was thought of as a "male problem."

Studies applied to specific subgroups of a population can be especially problematic for cost-effectiveness researchers. For example, a cost-effectiveness analysis examining screening mammography versus no screening among African American females would require tricky assumptions on the part of researchers; most studies of the effectiveness of screening and the effectiveness of various treatments were conducted on cohorts of mostly white women.

The following subsets of questions should help you determine whether the results of a published study are generalizable to your study population:

- *Was the study population localized to a particular geographical region?* Results of studies conducted in a specific geographical region of the country may not apply to all persons nationwide. For example, the rate of influenza-like illness in a study conducted in New York City (where winters are cold and people are packed into subways) may not apply to persons living in Los Angeles (where the weather is warm and people spend most of their time alone in cars). It would be best to obtain a national estimate of influenza-like illness or estimates from other parts of the country for comparison.

- *Are the characteristics of the subjects in the study similar to the characteristics of the population you are studying?* Often, researchers conduct studies in specific settings such as a Veterans Affairs hospital or in a health maintenance organization. In the former case, the patients may be likely to be older and have many coexisting illnesses. In the latter case, the subjects may be more likely to be employed and middle or upper-middle class than the general population.

- *What were the inclusion and exclusion criteria?* Sometimes studies examining a treatment for a disease will exclude people with preexisting medical conditions. For example, studies on the efficacy of the influenza vaccine almost always exclude subjects who have diseases that put them at high risk of hospitalization or death from influenza virus infections. Subjects with chronic diseases are excluded from vaccine efficacy studies because subjects in the placebo group have a moderate risk of death if they actually contract influenza. Since we are interested only in the efficacy of the vaccine in healthy adults, this research will be useful to us. However, if we were interested in the efficacy of the vaccine in all adults, the results of these studies would be of little use, because an important subset of our hypothetical cohort would have been excluded (Harper, Fukuda, Uyeki, Cox, Bridges, & CDC, 2004).

- *Does the definition of illness differ in any meaningful way from the definition you are using, or does it differ from the definition used in other studies you are including in your analysis?* Differences in the way that illness is defined can lead to differences across model inputs. For instance, influenza-like illness can be defined as with or without a fever. Cases containing a fever are much more likely to actually be influenza and are more likely to be severe (Hirve et al., 2012). If you use a study that doesn't include fever among the complex of symptoms defining the illness to obtain the likelihood of a medical visit, you are likely to underestimate this probability.

- *Did the subjects who failed to complete the study differ from subjects who successfully completed the study?* Often, subjects who drop out of a study or subjects who fail to complete surveys are sicker than the general population or at higher risk of disease. If a large number of subjects failed to complete a prospective study, the risk ratio for the factor under study is likely to be larger in the real world than in the study. As a very general rule of thumb, at least 80 percent of the subjects should complete the study. However, if 100 percent of the subjects in the group without the risk factor under study completed a prospective study and 80 percent of the subjects with the risk factor completed the study, we can expect the results to be skewed. Often, researchers look back at noncompleters to make sure that they aren't that different from completers.

- *How did the treatment and placebo groups differ in demographic composition and risk factors for disease?* In an economic analysis of influenza vaccination (Bridges et al., 2000), a significantly higher number of subjects exposed to secondhand smoke at home were randomly assigned to receive the influenza vaccine than subjects who were randomly assigned to receive the placebo injection in one part of the study. In that season, the influenza vaccine was poorly matched to the circulating strains of influenza virus, and the subjects who received the vaccine had higher rates of influenza-like illness and more medical visits than subjects in the placebo group.

Other Ways of Identifying Error in the Medical Literature

It is standard practice for authors to discuss the limitations of their studies in the discussion section of their research articles. Here, you often find a good deal of qualified language surrounding the major problems with the analysis. In some cases, authors provide in-depth discussions of the problems they encountered with their research. If an editorial accompanies the article, it may identify additional problems with the research. A final forum for identifying problems with a study is to read the letters to the editor in the months following the study. Medline searches help identify the volume and issue in which the letters were published.

Summary

This chapter was meant to provide a short and very cursory review of basic epidemiology methods. Not all cost-effectiveness analysis will use every tool presented in this chapter, but you should be able to understand the differences between cumulative incidence and incidence rate; crude, category-specific, and adjusted rates; prevalence and incidence; risks and rates; and random and nonrandom error. Knowing these differences and when they are used will go a long way toward improving your research skills.

So far, you've learned how to combine data from multiple studies using meta-analysis and weighted means. Meta-analysis can be complicated and requires you to perform a careful review of the literature. The weighted-means approach presented in this chapter is a simple, alternative way to combine the results from different studies. You should always be clear about which method you used to generate the values for your model inputs.

As you perform your cost-effectiveness analysis, you will need to evaluate the quality of the medical literature. This is a skill that you will develop over time. No one ever becomes an expert at evaluating medical literature overnight. So keep practicing!

Further Readings

Students who are interested in the nuances related to calculating prevalence and incidence should read *Epidemiologic Methods: Studying the Occurrence of Illness,* 2nd edition (Weiss & Koepsell, 2014).

Students interested in further examples for calculating the weighted averages should read Martin Bland and Sally Kerry's wonderful and easy-to-follow tutorial published in the *British Medical Journal* in 1998 (Bland & Kerry, 1998).

Several guidelines are available that provide recommendations on how to properly report the results of different study designs. Students are encouraged to retrieve these guidelines (which are free!) and familiarize themselves with them.

The Consolidated Standards of Reporting Trials (CONSORT) statement provides a 25-item checklist for the proper reporting of randomized clinical trials (Moher et al., 2010). The CONSORT statement can be found at the following web site: http://www.consort-statement.org.

The Strengthening the Reporting of Observational Studies in Epidemiology (STROBE) statement is a series of recommendations for the various observational study designs, such as case-control studies, retrospective cohort studies, and prospective cohort studies (von Elm, Altman, Egger, Pocock, Gøtzsche, Vandenbroucke, & for the STROBE Initiative, 2014). The different checklists for each of these observational study designs can be found at the following web site: http://www.strobe-statement.org.

The Preferred Reporting Items for Systematic Reviews and Meta-Analyses (PRISMA) statement is a set of items for the proper reporting of systematic reviews and meta-analyses (Liberati et al., 2009). The PRISMA statement can be found at the following web site: http://www.prisma-statement.org.

Students interested in learning more about software for performing meta-analysis should consult the Cochrane Collaboration and the use of Review Manager (RevMan) version 5.3 (http://tech.cochrane.org/revman). RevMan is a free tool developed by the Cochrane Collaboration that guides researchers in performing a meta-analysis using the PRISMA statement. Other meta-analysis software include MIX 2.0 (http://www.meta-analysis-made-easy.com) and Comprehensive Meta-analysis Software (http://www.meta-analysis.com).

References

Bland, J. M., and S. M. Kerry. (1998). Statistics Notes: Weighted Comparison of Means. *BMJ (Clinical Research Ed.)* 316(7125): 129.

Bridges, C. B., W. W. Thompson, M. I. Meltzer, G. R. Reeve, W. J. Talamonti, N. J. Cox, . . . K. Fukuda. (2000). Effectiveness and Cost-Benefit of Influenza Vaccination of Healthy Working Adults: A Randomized Controlled Trial. *Journal of the American Medical Association* 284(13): 1655–1663.

Centers for Medicare and Medicaid Services. (2014, October 30). Medicare Fee for Service for Parts A & B. Retrieved March 23, 2015, from http://www.cms.gov/Research-Statistics-Data-and-Systems/Statistics-Trends-and-Reports/MedicareFeeforSvcPartsAB/.

Clissold, S. P., and R. C. Heel. (1987). Topical Minoxidil: A Preliminary Review of Its Pharmacodynamic Properties and Therapeutic Efficacy in Alopecia Areata and Alopecia Androgenetica. *Drugs* 33(2): 107–122.

Cochrane Collaboration. (2014, May 26). Cochrane Community (beta). Trusted Evidence. Informed Decisions. Better Health. Retrieved from http://community.cochrane.org/cochrane-reviews.

Curtin, L. R., and R. J. Klein. (1995). *Centers for Disease Control and Prevention/National Center for Health Statistics: Direct Standardization (Age-Adjusted Death Rates)* (No. 6). U.S. Department of Health and Human Services, Centers for Disease Control and Prevention.

Dawber, T. R., G. F. Meadors, and F. E. Moore. (1951). Epidemiological Approaches to Heart Disease: The Framingham Study. *American Journal of Public Health and the Nation's Health* 41(3): 279–281.

Doll, R., and A. B. Hill. (1956). Lung Cancer and Other Causes of Death in Relation to Smoking: A Second Report on the Mortality of British Doctors. *British Medical Journal* 2(5001): 1071–1081.

Fisher, J. F. (2000). Better Living Through the Placebo Effect. *Atlantic Monthly* 286(4): 16–18.

Gøtzsche, P. C., and O. Olsen. (2000). Is Screening for Breast Cancer with Mammography Justifiable? *Lancet* 355(9198): 129–134. http://doi.org/10.1016/S0140-6736(99)06065-1.

Harper, S. A., K. Fukuda, T. M. Uyeki, N. J. Cox, C. B. Bridges, and Centers for Disease Control and Prevention (CDC) Advisory Committee on Immunization Practices (ACIP). (2004). Prevention and Control of Influenza: Recommendations of the Advisory Committee on Immunization Practices (ACIP). *Recommendations and Reports: Morbidity and Mortality Weekly Report (MMWR). Recommendations and Reports/Centers for Disease Control* 53(RR-6): 1–40.

Hirve, S., M. Chadha, P. Lele, K. E. Lafond, A. Deoshatwar, S. Sambhudas, . . . A. Mishra. (2012). Performance of Case Definitions Used for Influenza Surveillance Among Hospitalized Patients in a Rural Area of India. *Bulletin of the World Health Organization* 90(11): 804–812. http://doi.org/10.2471/BLT.12.108837.

Jansen, J. P., R. Fleurence, B. Devine, R. Itzler, A. Barrett, N. Hawkins, . . . J. C. Cappelleri. (2011). Interpreting Indirect Treatment Comparisons and Network Meta-Analysis for Health-Care Decision Making: Report of the ISPOR Task Force on Indirect Treatment Comparisons Good Research Practices: Part 1. *Value in Health: The Journal of the International Society for Pharmacoeconomics and Outcomes Research* 14(4): 417–428. http://doi.org/10.1016/j.jval.2011.04.002.

Jeckel, J. F., J. G. Elmore, and D. L. Katz. (1996). *Epidemiology, Biostatistics, and Preventive Medicine*. Philadelphia: Saunders.

Liberati, A., D. G. Altman, J. Tetzlaff, C. Mulrow, P. C. Gøtzsche, J. P. A. Ioannidis, . . . D. Moher. (2009). The PRISMA Statement for Reporting Systematic Reviews and Meta-Analyses of Studies That Evaluate Health Care Interventions: Explanation and Elaboration. *Journal of Clinical Epidemiology* 62(10): e1–34. http://doi.org/10.1016/j.jclinepi.2009.06.006.

Lumley, T. (2002). Network Meta-Analysis for Indirect Treatment Comparisons. *Statistics in Medicine* 21(16): 2313–2324. http://doi.org/10.1002/sim.1201.

Moher, D., S. Hopewell, K. F. Schulz, V. Montori, P. C. Gøtzsche, P. J. Devereaux, . . . Consolidated Standards of Reporting Trials Group. (2010). CONSORT 2010 Explanation and Elaboration: Updated Guidelines for Reporting Parallel Group Randomised Trials. *Journal of Clinical Epidemiology* 63(8): e1–37. http://doi.org/10.1016/j.jclinepi.2010.03.004.

Muennig, P., P. Franks, H. Jia, E. Lubetkin, and M. R. Gold. (2005). The Income-Associated Burden of Disease in the United States. *Social Science & Medicine* 61(9): 2018–2026. http://doi.org/10.1016/j.socscimed.2005.04.005.

National Center for Health Statistics. (2005). *Health, United States, 2005: With Chartbook on Trends in the Health of Americans*. Library of Congress Catalog Number 76–641496. Hyattsville, MD: National Center for Health Statistics.

National Center for Health Statistics. (2014a). National Health and Nutrition Examination Survey (NHANES) Homepage. Retrieved August 30, 2014, from http://www.cdc.gov.offcampus.lib.washington.edu/nchs/nhanes.htm.

National Center for Health Statistics. (2014b). National Health Interview Survey (NHANES) Homepage. Retrieved August 30, 2014, from http://www.cdc.gov.offcampus.lib.washington.edu/nchs/nhis.htm.

Nixon, R. M., N. Bansback, and A. Brennan (2007). Using Mixed Treatment Comparisons and Meta-Regression to Perform Indirect Comparisons to Estimate the Efficacy of Biologic Treatments in Rheumatoid Arthritis. *Statistics in Medicine* 26(6): 1237–1254. http://doi.org/10.1002/sim.2624.

Strauss, R. S. (1999). Comparison of Measured and Self-Reported Weight and Height in a Cross-Sectional Sample of Young Adolescents. *International Journal of Obesity and Related Metabolic Disorders: Journal of the International Association for the Study of Obesity* 23(8): 904–908.

Thelle, D. S., E. Arnesen, and O. H. Førde. (1983). The Tromsø Heart Study: Does Coffee Raise Serum Cholesterol? *New England Journal of Medicine* 308(24): 1454–1457. http://doi.org/10.1056/NEJM198306163082405.

Urgert, R., S. Meyboom, M. Kuilman, H. Rexwinkel, M. N. Vissers, M. Klerk, and M. B. Katan. (1996). Comparison of Effect of Cafetière and Filtered Coffee on Serum Concentrations of Liver Aminotransferases and Lipids: Six Month Randomised Controlled Trial. *BMJ (Clinical Research Ed.)* 313(7069): 1362–1366.

Von Elm, E., D. G. Altman, M. Egger, S. J. Pocock, P. C. Gøtzsche, J. P. Vandenbroucke, and for the STROBE Initiative. (2014). Strengthening the Reporting of Observational Studies in Epidemiology (STROBE) Statement: Guidelines for Reporting Observational Studies. *International Journal of Surgery* (London, England). http://doi.org/10.1016/j.ijsu.2014.07.013.

Weiss, N. S., and T. D. Koepsell. (2014). *Epidemiologic Methods: Studying the Occurrence of Illness,* 2nd ed. New York: Oxford University Press.

CHAPTER 12

FINDING THE DATA YOU NEED

Overview

Cost-effectiveness studies often synthesize information from a number of different sources. Usually, researchers require information on the incidence or prevalence of a disease, risk ratios, and costs, among many other inputs. These inputs can be obtained from the medical literature, electronic datasets, unpublished sources (such as ongoing longitudinal studies), or experts on the disease you are studying. In this chapter, we examine different sources of publicly available electronic data, briefly discuss the ways in which alternative data sources can be used, and forward a system for organizing the data you collect.

One question that might immediately come to you is "Why is this chapter near the end of the book?" As you went through sample cost-effectiveness analyses, you learned about many of the data sources mentioned in this chapter. For example, you obtained hospital costs from the Healthcare Cost and Utilization Project (HCUP) in Chapter 4. This chapter isn't really meant for students in a cost-effectiveness class. It's meant for those who are hunkering down to conduct their own analysis and need to know where to look for specific types of data.

Finding Data in the Medical Literature

It is generally easy to find the medical literature that you will need for your cost-effectiveness analysis. You will need three basic tools: a search engine, a way to download the article, and reference managing software. Several search engines are available such as Google Scholar, PubMed,

LEARNING OBJECTIVES

- Describe the different levels of evidence criteria for medical research.

- Identify and locate different sources of publically available datasets.

- Compare and contrast when to use the medical literature and electronic datasets for your cost-effectiveness analysis.

- Find parameter values using data extraction tools for a given dataset.

- Identify the advantages and disadvantages of piggyback studies.

and EMBASE. Among the many sources of freely available research are open source journals, Google Scholar, and repositories such as Research Gate or the National Library of Medicine.

Most researchers these days are completely reliant on Google Scholar for their searches. Google Scholar has a leg up on all of the other search engines in that it gives you the most relevant articles rather than the most recent ones. It ranks results not only according to the number of citations, but also by other measures of their quality. Google Scholar has various other advantages. One is that you can set it (under Preferences on the homepage) to give you citations that you can use in your favorite reference manager software. Just click the package you own and voilà! When you do a search, a link will appear below it that allows you to download the reference. Make sure to check the formatting, because it does make mistakes. Another great feature of Google Scholar is that, if you are part of a wealthy educational institution, you can also get the original PDF. To do this, go to "Library" under settings, and type the name of your institution. Sometimes it will give you a PDF that the author has illegally posted on the Web. (Go ahead, arrest us!)

PubMed is a popular and comprehensive search engine for scientific research that is run by the government and can be accessed on the Internet at http://www.ncbi.nlm.nih.gov/entrez/query.fcgi, which has a helpful tutorial.

Another search engine for medical literature is EMBASE, which contains many more journals outside of North America as well as conferences and meeting presentations and abstracts. Unlike PubMed, which is freely available from the U.S. National Library of Medicine (NLM), EMBASE requires a paid subscription. Check with your library to see if you have access to EMBASE. Cumulative Index to Nursing and Allied Health Literature (CINAHL) is another search engine dedicated to nursing, allied health, and health care.

Recall from Chapter 11 that the Cochrane Collaboration has a repository of systematic reviews and meta-analyses that you can use to identify studies that have already been reviewed and analyzed by other authors. The U.S. Preventive Services Task Force is another outstanding source of synthesized information. Again, the best of all worlds is Google Scholar, which will not only rank "seminal articles (gross)" first (do not touch them without gloves), but also often links to the article free of charge. But just because the article is important doesn't mean that it is high quality. You will need to be the judge of quality yourself.

Grading Published Data

In Chapter 11, we reviewed some of the basic biostatistics and epidemiology concepts pertinent to cost-effectiveness analysis. That section was intended for those who don't have a degree in one of those two disciplines. If you've read that chapter or are familiar with these concepts, you should have some idea about how research studies are designed and some of the common limitations. But how do you decide which ones to use and which to reject? One approach to evaluating the quality of the published data you have gathered for your cost-effectiveness research project is to apply the **levels of evidence** criteria. Levels of evidence is a grading method for organizing published data based on their trustworthiness (Burns, Rohrich, & Chung, 2011).

One useful way of thinking about the levels of evidence is to visualize them as a pyramid, with the most trustworthy study designs at the top and the least trustworthy at the bottom. Multicenter randomized controlled trials and meta-analysis of these studies cap the pyramid. Single-site randomized controlled trials and cohort studies make up the next level, evidence from nonrandomized trials (case-control studies) the next, and on down to expert opinion. Figure 12.1 illustrates the levels of evidence.

Once you've identified the studies you want to collect, it's a good idea to grade the quality of each of them. There are several grading criteria in the

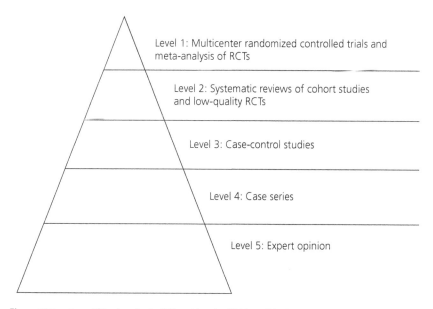

Level 1: Multicenter randomized controlled trials and meta-analysis of RCTs

Level 2: Systematic reviews of cohort studies and low-quality RCTs

Level 3: Case-control studies

Level 4: Case series

Level 5: Expert opinion

Figure 12.1   Pyramid Analogy for the Different Levels of Evidence Criteria

Was the study described as randomized (this includes words such as randomly, random, and
 randomization)? [1=yes; 0=no]

Was the method used to generate the sequence of randomization described and appropriate
 (table of random numbers, computer-generated, etc)? [1=yes; 0=no]

Was the study described as double-blind? [1=yes; 0=no]

Was the method of double-blinding described and appropriate (identical placebo, active
 placebo, dummy, etc)? [1=yes; 0=no]

Was there a description of withdrawals and dropouts? [1=yes: 0=no]

Deduct one point if the method used to generate the sequence of randomization was
 described and it was inappropriate (patients were allocated alternately, or according to
 date of birth, hospital number, etc). [−1=yes; 0=no]

Deduct one point if the study was described as double-blind but the method of blinding was
 inappropriate (e.g., comparison of tablet vs. injection with no double dummy). [−1=yes;
 0=no]

Figure 12.2   An Example of a Jadad Score Grading Form

literature, but the oldest and most familiar grading criterion was developed
by Jadad and colleagues (Jadad, Moore, Carroll, Jenkinson, Reynolds,
Gavaghan, & McQuay, 1996). The Jadad score focuses on the reporting
of randomization, blindness, and withdrawals/dropouts, and ranges from
0 (very poor) to 5 (rigorous) (Figure 12.2). Another grading criterion for
clinical studies was developed by the Cochrane Collaborative (Higgins
et al., 2011). The Cochrane risk of bias tool identifies weakness in the study
design, but it doesn't yield a single score. Instead, it uses a grid to provide
different levels of bias (low, high, and uncertain). While grading scientific
studies is beyond the scope of an introductory textbook, there are some
excellent sources of information available to curious students. An up-to-
date discussion of levels of evidence can be found at the Oxford Center for
Evidence-Based Medicine (Center for Evidence-Based Medicine, 2014).

Unlike studies in the medical literature, it is relatively easy to identify
error in an electronic dataset; most datasets are accompanied by detailed
descriptions of the limitations of the data they contain.

Using Electronic Datasets

Health datasets provide a wealth of information for conducting cost-
effectiveness analyses. Using these datasets, you can obtain much of the
information on medical costs, disease prevalence rates, hospital discharge

rates, or just about any type of cross-sectional health-related data in which you are interested. Some prospective data are also available. Nonhealth datasets contain information related to transportation, crime, and education, all of which are useful for estimating the nonmedical costs of medical interventions or diseases.

Although the words *electronic* and *dataset* instill a sense of fear in many people, obtaining data from electronic databases is not difficult. In fact, a number of tools are designed specifically to make the information that electronic datasets contain more accessible to nontechnical types. These tools take the form of computer programs or web pages that guide would-be researchers through the step-by-step process of obtaining the information they need. These programs or web pages are sometimes referred to as **data extraction tools**. (In Chapter 4, you used one of these tools to get hospitalization costs from the Healthcare Cost and Utilization Project.)

It is also possible to obtain cost-effectiveness data inputs using printed tabulations of data from these datasets. These are large documents containing lists of useful data, such as hospitalization rates or mortality rates, as well as the most commonly used cross-tabulations. A cross-tabulation lists the outcome of interest (such as diseased or healthy) by some other characteristic (such as exposure to a risk factor). Exhibit 12.1 illustrates an example of a table created by cross-tabulation (also called a contingency table).

Virtually all major health datasets in the United States are either associated with a data extraction tool or are available as a printed tabulation. The majority of international data sources require familiarity with statistical packages (see Exhibit 12.2). However, the World Health Organization has organized many data sources from developing countries in various user-friendly ways. We assume that those who can use statistical software

EXHIBIT 12.1. EXAMPLE OF A TABLE CREATED BY CROSS-TABULATION (CONTINGENCY TABLE)

	Diseased	Healthy
Exposed to a risk factor		
Not exposed to a risk factor		

packages are already familiar with how to find and download the health data they need. If you fall into this category but need guidance, Exhibit 12.3 should get you where you need to go.

EXHIBIT 12.2.   MAJOR U.S. HEALTH DATASETS AVAILABLE TO THE PUBLIC

Dataset	Description
Healthcare Cost and Utilization Project (HCUP) www.ahrq.gov	HCUP is a collection of healthcare databases. Datasets include the National Inpatient Sample (NIS), the Kids' Inpatient Database (KID), the Nationwide Emergency Department Sample (NEDS), the State Inpatient Databases (SIDS), the State Ambulatory Surgery and Services Databases (SASD), and the State Emergency Department Databases (SEDD). These datasets contain information on hospital discharges, emergency department visits, outpatient services, and emergency department visits that do not result in admissions. HCUP also contains information on charges.
National Hospital Discharge Survey (NHDS) www.cdc.gov/ nchs	NHDS was conducted annually from 1965 to 2010. It contains a smaller sample of hospitals than the HCUP. This dataset is available in electronic and published form. NHDS has been replaced by the National Hospital Care Survey (NHCS).
National Hospital Care Survey (NHCS) http:// www.cdc.gov/nchs	NHCS integrates the inpatient information from the NHDS along with outpatient information from the National Hospital Ambulatory Medicare Care Survey (NHAMCS). The NHCS is conducted annually.
Medical Expenditure Panel Survey (MEPS) www.meps.ahrq.gov	MEPS contains survey data from clinicians, nursing homes, and the general population regarding healthcare use, expenditures, insurance status, and many other useful variables. Useful for generating ambulatory care costs, MEPS has two main components: Household and Insurance. MEPS is performed annually in a sampling frame of approximately 15,000 people.

Dataset	Description
National Ambulatory Medical Care Survey (NAMCS) www.cdc.gov/nchs	This is a national survey of physicians that includes over 36,000 patient records for ambulatory care services. Does not include hospital outpatient or emergency room data. NAMCS is conducted annually.
National Hospital Ambulatory Medical Care Survey (NHAMCS) www.cdc.gov/nchs	This dataset supplements the NAMCS with hospital and emergency room data. The last one was performed in 2004, with 1,174 participating facilities.
National Nursing Home Survey (NNHS) www.cdc.gov/nchs	This dataset provides information about 8,000 randomly selected nursing home patients.
National Home and Hospice Care Survey (NHHCS) www.cdc.gov/nchs	This is a national sample of 1,500 home and hospice care agencies. The last one was performed in 2007 with 9,416 home health patients and discharges.
Surveillance, Epidemiology, and End Results System (SEER) http://seer.cancer.gov/	This dataset contains information on most major cancers. Variables specific to race, gender, and country of birth are linked to census data.
National Health and Nutrition Examination Survey (NHANES). www.cdc.gov/nchs	This nationally representative dataset contains data from physical examinations and clinical and laboratory tests. Prevalence data are available for specific diseases and health conditions. The NHANES is performed annually, with a sampling frame of 5,000 people.
National Health Interview Survey (NHIS) www.cdc.gov/nchs	A nationally representative survey of the health status, mobility limitations, and disease for noninstitutionalized persons. Also contains the total number of medical visits for each subject. The NHIS is performed annually, with a sampling frame of approximately 87,500 people.

EXHIBIT 12.2.   MAJOR U.S. HEALTH DATASETS AVAILABLE TO THE PUBLIC (Continued)

Dataset	Description
Mortality Statistics www.cdc.gov/nchs	Death certificates contain information on all deaths by ICD-9 code and include the decedent's place of birth, education level, location of the death, as well as the underlying cause of death and other conditions the decedent had. These data are contained in a wide array of data formats.
Combined Health Information Database http://chid .nih.gov	Contains a number of datasets related to chronic disease.
Bureau of Labor Statistics www.bls .gov	Government agency that tracks wages for many professions. This is useful in estimating time costs for patients who undergo an intervention.

EXHIBIT 12.3. MAJOR SOURCES OF INTERNATIONAL HEALTH DATA

WHO Statistical Information System, http://www.who.int/whosis/en/

CHOosing Interventions That Are Cost Effective (WHO-CHOICE), http://www.who.int/choice/en

Unit Costs for Health Services by Country (WHO), http://www.who.int/choice/country/country_specific/en

Harvard International Health Systems Program, http://www.hsph.harvard.edu/ihsg/ihsg.html

Centers for Disease Control and Prevention, International Health Data Reference Guide, http://www.cdc.gov/nchs/data/misc/ihdrg2003.pdf

OECD Health Data 2014: Statistics and Indicators (provides limited public access data), http://www.oecd.org

United Nations Statistics Division, http://unstats.un.org/unsd/default.htm

U.S. Department of Health and Human Services: Global Health, http://www.globalhealth.gov

The advantage of working with an entire dataset is that you have more control over the ways in which different pieces of information are combined, making it possible to conduct more-sophisticated analyses. Because this is an introductory textbook, we will focus on obtaining data from sources that do not require the use of a statistical software package.

Analyses conducted in developing countries previously had to rely on the medical literature or ongoing prospective trials. However, the World Health Organization (WHO) now maintains a useful data repository with information spe-

> **TIPS AND TRICKS**
>
> Active links to major sources of data useful for cost-effectiveness analysis are maintained at http://www.wiley.com/WileyCDA/WileyTitle/productCd-1119011264.html.

cific to cost-effectiveness analysis (http://www.who.int/choice/en). The following sections discuss how to obtain printed data tabulations and data from ongoing studies and how to estimate an input using expert opinion.

Finding the Right Electronic Data

Though electronic datasets are rich sources of information, you will have to familiarize yourself with the contents and limitations of each of the datasets commonly used in cost-effectiveness analysis in your country. Once you are pointed in the right direction, though, it is relatively easy to find the information that you are looking for. For instance, Statistics Canada contains most of the important national health and demographic statistics for Canada (http://www.statcan.ca/start.html). By contacting Statistics Canada officials, it is often possible to find other sources of data, such as provincial health plan datasets that they do not maintain. The same goes for many other countries. (See, for instance, https://www.destatis.de/DE/Startseite.html, which contains statistics for most German agencies.) In fact, researchers examining other contexts can often find statistics for European nations in English. (See, for instance, https://www.destatis.de/EN/Homepage.html.) For the United States, the National Center for Health Statistics (NCHS) has information for all national datasets on a single web site (http://www.cdc.gov.offcampus.lib.washington.edu/nchs). A tutorial is also available from the NCHS to assist researchers in navigating and using the datasets (http://www.cdc.gov/nchs/tutorials).

Most health datasets are designed to meet a particular research need. Therefore, datasets tend to have themes, much the same way that a novel has a central protagonist and plot. Like novels, some datasets essentially replicate the themes of other datasets with varying degrees of success. They differ from novels, though, in that researchers must often examine data from similar datasets to get the full story about the information they are looking for.

For example, the National Hospital Discharge Survey (NHDS) is a dataset containing information on hospital discharges for approximately 300,000 patients from about 500 hospitals. These data were obtained from both electronic hospital tapes and transcripts of actual hospital records (Owings & Lawrence, 1999). The NHDS was replaced by the National Hospital Care Survey (NHCS) in 2010, which integrates the inpatient data from NHDS with the emergency department, outpatient, and ambulatory care data from the National Hospital Ambulatory Medical Care Survey (NHAMCS). The Healthcare Cost and Utilization Project (HCUP) contains several datasets obtained from hospital billing systems, private data organizations, and the federal government, but it is composed of a weighted sample of about eight million hospital stays (Agency for Healthcare Research and Quality, 2014). These datasets contain information on the total number of discharges by diagnosis. Because the NHDS/NHCS was in part built using actual hospital transcripts, it contains less nonrandom error than the HCUP datasets. The HCUP is derived from a very large sample; it has less sampling error and contains a larger number of variables that are useful for cost-effectiveness analysis.

For those of you who are interested in the local county or state, access to these national databases should also give you access to the state-level data. But for state-specific databases not collected by the NHCS, you may need to contact the state department of health directly. Other departments you may want to search for include the epidemiology and public health departments. For example, Los Angeles County has the LA HealthDataNow! portal that runs vital statistics queries specific to areas within the county (Office of Health Assessment & Epidemiology, 2015).

When you are looking for one particular variable contained in many datasets, you probably will want to use various values in a sensitivity analysis. Knowing where to find the datasets containing these variables is another issue altogether. Table 12.1 lists the sources of information that researchers typically turn to when in need of commonly used inputs in cost-effectiveness analyses.

Which Source of Data Do You Turn to?

Students often wonder whether it is best to begin a search for a piece of information in the medical literature or start with electronic data. The answer is simple: Always obtain as much information as possible about any parameter you are looking for and look to both sources. Before the advent

Table 12.1   Datasets Useful for Finding Frequently Needed Cost-Effectiveness Parameters

Variable	Possible Sources
Prevalence rate	NHIS, medical literature, NHANES
Incidence rate	Medical literature, NHIS (acute diseases only), NHANES, SEER
Mortality rate	Medical literature, Multiple Cause of Death Dataset, Mortality Followback Survey, SEER, WONDER
Risk ratio	Medical literature
Population data	U.S. Bureau of the Census, WONDER
Disease severity/distribution	NHIS, NHANES, SEER
Medical utilization (number of hospitalizations, outpatient visits, etc.)	HCFA, HCUP, Medicaid, MEPS, SEER-Medicare, NAMCS, Department of Veterans Affairs Corporate Data Warehouse
Cost of medical care	HCFA, medical literature, HCUP, Medicaid, NMES, SEER-Medicare, BLS, Department of Veterans Affairs Corporate Data Warehouse
Labor costs (salary information)	U.S. Bureau of Labor Statistics
Cost of transportation, labor, environmental impact	U.S. Bureau of the Census, BLS, medical literature, Internet search engines, University of Michigan

Note: NHIS = National Health Interview Survey; NHANES = National Health and Nutrition Examination Survey; SEER = Surveillance Epidemiology and End Results; HCFA = Health Care Finance Administration; HCUP = Healthcare Cost and Utilization Project; MEPS = Medical Expenditure Panel Survey; NAMCS = National Ambulatory Medical Care Survey; BLS = Bureau of Labor Statistics.

of data extraction tools, student researchers sometimes chose to forgo the task of digging through complicated datasets to find information they were able to easily obtain from the medical literature. Today it is so easy to obtain electronic information that there is no excuse for failing to take a peek at parameters that can quickly be obtained from datasets.

Students also wonder whether data from the medical literature are superior to data from electronic sources, or vice versa. When information is available from both published studies and electronic datasets, it is important to weigh the limitations of each source. The medical literature is often the best source of information for data that are difficult to capture in a dataset, such as the incidence rate of a disease or risk ratios. And electronic datasets are often populated with nationally representative information, greatly improving their external validity.

Generally, electronic datasets are most useful for obtaining nationally representative costs, medical care utilization rates, and the prevalence of a disease. Published data are often most useful for finding risk ratios and other forms of data that have been analyzed and processed in experimental trials. Datasets have largely been designed to address research needs that are not often met by scientists publishing in the medical literature. For example, while it would be highly unlikely that you would find a nationally representative sample of cholesterol test results for African American women in the medical literature, you would be able to find such information from the National Health and Nutrition Examination Survey (NHANES). Many national agencies have gone one step further in improving the ease of access to these data by developing data extraction tools.

Data Extraction Tools

Most data extraction tools retrieve information about a particular disease using International Classification for Disease (ICD) codes, Clinical Classification Software (CCS) codes, or Diagnosis Related Groups (DRGs). Table 4.3 in Chapter 4 describes these codes.

Software that takes you step by step through a problem is often referred to as a "wizard." As you proceed through each extraction tool's wizard, you will be asked information about the demographics of the group you are studying, such as age, race, and income; the diagnosis codes you are interested in; and the output that you want. If you did the exercises in the cost chapter, you are familiar with this process. Unfortunately, the categories offered generally cannot be modified, so you are stuck with the age groups and outputs predefined by the tool. Once you have finished, the tool will present you with tables containing the information you need.

The most comprehensive data extraction tool is maintained by the Bureau of the Census. This tool, called the Federal Electronic Research and Review Extraction Tool (also known as DataFerrett), contains both census and health-related datasets (http://dataferrett.census.gov). One of the nice features of the DataFerret is that it allows you to either download any part of a dataset you are interested in or generate cross-tabulations of data. Exhibit 12.4 is a partial listing of available data compilations using extraction tools.

EXHIBIT 12.4. SOME DATA SOURCES FOR WHICH DATA EXTRACTION TOOLS ARE AVAILABLE

National Center for Health Statistics, http://www.cdc.gov/nchs/sets.htm

Centers for Disease Control's WONDER System, http://wonder.cdc.gov/

Healthy People 2020, http://www.healthypeople.gov/2020/data/default.aspx

DataFerret (Includes free software for PC/Mac), http://dataferrett.census.gov/

Perhaps the most comprehensive data extraction tool, WONDER, is maintained by the Centers for Disease Control and Prevention (http://wonder.cdc.gov/). This site contains everything from deaths to population data.

Every data extraction tool has quirks and limitations, but they are generally very easy to use. Students who have never turned on a computer before have produced publication-quality analyses using these tools. Unfortunately, there are few such systems for international data. This is especially tragic in the case of developing countries because fewer researchers have access to statistical software packages. It is perhaps telling that the U.S. government offers many completely redundant software tools for U.S. data (few of which work well) and almost no tools for data sources outside the country.

TIPS AND TRICKS

The WONDER data system is a good source of information but was poorly organized at the time of publication. Many of the hidden data gems are buried in the DATA2010 system (http://wonder.cdc.gov/data2010). If you don't find what you are looking for in the main WONDER system, check the DATA2010 section.

Exercises 1 to 3

1. Suppose you were interested in getting data on the number of breast cancer deaths in the United States for 2011. Which dataset would contain this information?

2. Based on the search results from Exercise 1, how many men died of breast cancer in the United States in 2011?

3. You are going to include a parameter in a decision model that accounts for the cost of a dermatologist's time from the payer's perspective. In your model, the dermatologist spends an average of 30 minutes with a patient. What is the average cost of a dermatologist for 30 minutes? (Hint: Use data from the US Bureau of Labor and Statistics: www.bls.gov/bls/blswage.htm)

Using Printed Tabulations of Electronic Data

A simple way to obtain information is with printed tabulations of data. Like most other data extraction tools, data printouts force the researcher to work with the age, race, and gender groupings the publishers see fit to use. If you use a printed data tabulation, the information must be retyped into your spreadsheet program, but when the data needs are minimal, they are much easier to use than unformatted electronic data. The National Center for Health Statistics (NCHS) offers printed information from the National Health Interview Survey (NHIS) and mortality data, as well as other types of data, for free on its web site (http://www.cdc.gov/nchs). A search engine is also available.

Using Datasets Themselves

Students who know how to load datasets into a statistical software package probably won't be reading this section. For the rest of you, it's probably prudent to seek help before attempting to download a dataset and then open it using a statistical software package. However, readers who have extensively used preloaded datasets and are familiar with a particular statistical package will probably be able to use an electronic dataset without help.

Most datasets are now presented in a format called SAS Transport that can be read by major statistical packages, such as SAS, STATA, and SPSS. There is also a commercial application called Stat/Transfer that will not only convert a dataset into a format readable by your software package, but will even let the user select the variables (https://www.stattransfer.com). Another file format is called the comma-separated values (CSV), which is easily generated by most datasets and is readable by most statistical software packages. The codebook linked to the dataset will help you select the relevant variables.

One caveat to working with datasets is that you must read the documentation in its entirety before working with the data. Many health datasets use complex sampling designs that require familiarity with multiple weighting factors and also require special software. Statistical packages such as STATA, SAS, and SPSS are capable of handling complex sample designs.

For readers from developing nations or without institutional support, a statistical package simply called R works on all major operating systems and is free (http://cran.r-project.org). Unfortunately, free statistical packages are a bit trickier to use than commercial applications. The learning curve for R is steep but rewarding. Students on a budget can purchase the student versions of STATA, SAS, and SPSS.

Datasets need to be loaded (or imported) into the statistical software package before statistical analysis can begin. Students who load datasets for the first time will realize that each software package is a little different. For example, SPSS provides a wizard that assists you in loading data. After loading the dataset, you should inspect it to make sure that it was loaded properly. Oftentimes, there are problems with loading datasets that can frustrate your analyses. It's common to see string text unintentionally shift columns after being loaded. Visual inspection as well as a descriptive inspection is necessary to ensure that the dataset was loaded properly.

Understanding Error in Electronic Data

Electronic health datasets produced by the U.S. government are usually accompanied by a printed discussion of the limitations of electronic data sources that often includes formulas for evaluating the error that they contain. Occasionally researchers need to use smaller datasets that lack a detailed description of the data limitations. In these instances, it is necessary to contact one of the authors to discuss the various limitations of the data, including potential sources of nonrandom error.

While the primary limitation of studies in the medical literature is random error, electronic data are more frequently limited by nonrandom error. For example, hospitalization data and mortality data are primarily affected by **misclassification bias**. Misclassification bias arises when the physician who fills out the death certificate writes down the wrong cause of death.

Imagine that a patient developed heart disease as a result of diabetes mellitus. Sometimes the doctor filling out the death certificate is unsure whether to list the diabetes or the heart disease as the cause of death. Therefore, the enumeration of the number of deaths attributed to these medical conditions may be incorrect.

Using Unpublished Data

For some cost-effectiveness studies, it is possible to obtain unpublished data directly from the authors of studies published in the medical literature. Often, a research project publishes only selected results of studies, leaving out precisely the information you are looking for. Tracking down the authors of a study is usually simple. Authors may be contacted through the medical journal, the institution with which they are affiliated, or, most easily, using a search engine. Contact information for authors, including institutional affiliations, is published in most medical journals. If you don't get a response, try a coauthor. Sometimes unsolicited e-mails get filtered, so don't give up.

A good source for unpublished data is scientific meeting abstracts. Many abstracts do not get published but offer important data that are relevant to cost-effectiveness analysis research. You can browse through the web sites of scientific societies and obtain their meeting abstracts brochure. Alternatively, EMBASE is a good search engine for identifying abstracts presented at scientific meetings.

Using Data from Piggybacked Studies

Piggybacking is the process of adding an economic evaluation to an existing prospective study (Haddix, Teutsch, Shaffer, & Dunet, 1996; Neumann, Sanders, Russell, Siegel, & Ganiats, 2016). When the primary objective of the study is to collect cost and effectiveness data, the study is sometimes called a **primary cost-effectiveness analysis**. In these study designs, data on the cost and efficacy of the health intervention under study are collected over the course of the analysis.

Because no single study can capture all of the costs or changes in mortality rates that result from a health intervention, it is usually necessary to supplement the data that the researchers are collecting with information from other studies or from electronic datasets. For example, Bridges and others (2000) examined the efficacy of the influenza vaccine in preventing influenza-like illness while simultaneously collecting information on the number of medical visits, hospitalizations, and medications consumed in the vaccine and placebo arms of their study (Bridges et al., 2000). They then used the MEDSTAT MarketScan Databases to estimate the cost of each medical visit and each hospitalization that occurred. With this information, they conducted a cost-benefit analysis of influenza vaccination. Unfortunately, they did not capture costs associated with transmission of the flu virus to high-risk populations.

In addition to problems associated with collecting comprehensive data, the piggyback study design usually cannot directly compare the intervention under study with other potentially useful health interventions for preventing or treating a disease. For example, if a pharmaceutical company wishes to compare the product it is evaluating with other products currently on the market, it would have to add more study arms to the randomized controlled trial, which can be very expensive.

Using Expert Opinion

Sometimes information on a parameter is not available through published, electronic, or unpublished sources. When this occurs, the value of the parameter of interest can be estimated using the opinion of experts. Although it would be unusual for a group of experts to correctly guess the true value of a cost-effectiveness input (e.g., the number of people a single syphilis patient will infect on average), they will likely be able to guess the highest and lowest possible values for that parameter. When cost-effectiveness data are collected using the opinion of experts, the reference case analysis requires that a formal process, called the Delphi method, be used. (Discussion of the Delphi method is beyond the scope of this book.)

Organizing Your Data

The bane of any researcher's existence is organizing data. Nevertheless, it is nearly impossible to conduct a research project without a good organizational system. Of course, a good filing system will be necessary to keep track of all of the different medical articles. But it is just as important to keep track of the parameters you will use when it comes time to put all of the information you have collected into a decision analysis model.

There are two major goals to organizing data. The first is to create a summary of each dataset and each study from the medical literature that you will be using. This allows you to quickly review the benefits or the pitfalls of each data element before using it. The second is to have a source of key data elements you will be using to construct your decision analysis model.

No matter how carefully you read a study or a summary of a dataset, you will forget many of its key elements. Having each dataset and study summarized concisely allows you to refer to it quickly. When the Centers for Disease Control and Prevention set out to summarize the medical literature on community preventive services, it hired a small army of public health students and junior researchers. These students summarized the data from each of the thousands of studies they reviewed so that they could quickly put all of the information together in a way that made sense and so that the authors could easily refer to the materials if they had questions. (Both Peter and Mark suffered as student lackeys in their youth.) You would do well to heed their example, albeit on a much smaller scale.

Summary

Finding the data you need is a major challenge. Knowing where to go to find the right data is important to performing a valid cost-effectiveness analysis. Not only do you need to find the data, you also need to judge whether it is of high or poor quality. Levels of evidence provide some guidance on the strength or influence of the study (or studies), which helps to reduce bias.

Data can come from the existing literature or from secondary sources, such as the CDC WONDER. Most national databases are publicly available but may require you to submit a form to gain access. Others have a portal where you can query the information that you need. If the data that you are looking for are unavailable, then communicating directly with experts can yield some important information.

It's always important to keep your data organized. Recording the location, references, dates, and sources of your data will go a long way in helping you write up your manuscript or report. The last thing you want to do is look for some obscure reference to a database you are using. (We're speaking from experience.)

Further Readings

The National Health and Nutrition Examination Survey (NHANES) has a great tutorial that walks you through the survey along with statistical tools for analysis. Students who are interested should go through the tutorial located at http://www.cdc.gov/NCHS/Tutorials/Nhanes/index.htm.

University of California, Los Angeles (UCLA) has a web site with lots of information on loading data into SAS along with other useful resources for R, SPSS, and STATA, located at: http://www.ats.ucla.edu/stat/stat. This is a great resource for any student who will be using statistical software packages to load and analyze data.

Students interested in learning more about the Delphi method should visit the RAND web site at http://www.rand.org/topics/delphi-method .html.

The International Society for Pharmacoeconomics and Outcomes Research provides an interactive questionnaire to determine whether the study you selected is appropriate for your analysis, and it also provides you with an online database to store and retrieve all assessments: http://www.ispor.org/healthstudyassessment_index.asp (International Society for Pharmacoeconomics and Outcomes Research, 2015).

References

Agency for Healthcare Research and Quality. (2014, June). Healthcare Cost and Utilization Project (HCUP) [Text]. Retrieved August 31, 2014, from http://www .ahrq.gov/research/data/hcup/index.html.

Bridges, C. B., W. W. Thompson, M. I. Meltzer, G. R. Reeve, W. J. Talamonti, N. J. Cox, . . . K. Fukuda. (2000). Effectiveness and Cost-Benefit of Influenza Vaccination of Healthy Working Adults: A Randomized Controlled Trial. *Journal of the American Medical Association* 284(13): 1655–1663.

Burns, P. B., R. J. Rohrich, and K. C. Chung. (2011). The Levels of Evidence and Their Role in Evidence-Based Medicine. *Plastic and Reconstructive Surgery* 128(1): 305–310. http://doi.org/10.1097/PRS.0b013e318219c171.

Center for Evidence-Based Medicine. (2014). Oxford Center for Evidence-Based Medicine Levels of Evidence. Retrieved from http://www.cebm.net/ocebm-levels-of-evidence/.

Haddix, A., S. Teutsch, P. Shaffer, and D. Dunet. (1996). *Prevention Effectiveness: A Guide to Decision Analysis and Economic Evaluation.* New York: Oxford University Press.

Higgins, J. P. T., D. G. Altman, P. C. Gøtzsche, P. Jüni, D. Moher, A. D. Oxman, . . . J. A. C. Sterne. (2011). The Cochrane Collaboration's Tool for Assessing Risk of Bias in Randomised Trials. *British Medical Journal* 343: d5928. http://doi.org/10.1136/bmj.d5928.

International Society for Pharmacoeconomics and Outcomes Research. (2015). Assessing the Evidence for Health Care Decision Makers. Retrieved March 30, 2015, from http://www.ispor.org/healthstudyassessment_index.asp.

Jadad, A. R., R. A. Moore, D. Carroll, C. Jenkinson, D. J. M. Reynolds, D. J. Gavaghan, & H. J. McQuay. (1996). Assessing the Quality of Reports of Randomized Clinical Trials: Is Blinding Necessary? *Controlled Clinical Trials* 17(1): 1–12. http://doi.org/10.1016/0197-2456(95)00134-4.

Neumann, P. J., G. D. Sanders, L. B. Russell, J. E. Siegel, and T. G. Ganiats. (2016). *Cost-Effectiveness in Health and Medicine.* New York: Oxford University Press.

Office of Health Assessment & Epidemiology. (2015). LA HealthDataNow! Retrieved March 30, 2015, from http://publichealth.lacounty.gov/epi/.

Owings, M. F., & L. Lawrence. (1999). Detailed Diagnoses and Procedures, National Hospital Discharge Survey, 1997. *Vital and Health Statistics. Series 13, Data from the National Health Survey* (145): 1–157.

CHAPTER 13

A WORKED EXAMPLE

Overview

Up until now, you've been given most of the tools to begin your own investigations into cost-effectiveness analysis. For most complex models, specialized software is used to perform the mathematical calculations and to provide effective data visualization tools. In this chapter, we will introduce you to a decision analysis software package, TreeAge Pro, which is available as a free trial from http://www.treeage.com/. (For the examples in this text, we will be using the 2015 version of TreeAge Pro on the Windows Operating System.) You will be provided with a series of exercises to familiarize yourself with TreeAge Pro and to incorporate the lessons learned from previous chapters. At the end of this chapter, you should feel more confident in conducting your own cost-effectiveness analysis.

Helping Students Learn

The purpose of this chapter is to help students learn by doing. Theory and practice generally need to be combined for effective learning. Students will find that ideas become clearer and are retained for longer periods if their studies have a practical component to them. Thus, we have put together a series of four laboratory exercises that show how Markov models can be put to use in cost-effectiveness analysis.

This chapter is organized into four integrated laboratory exercises. Each exercise will build upon the previous ones in order to take a cost-effectiveness idea from the developmental stages to its final analysis. In Laboratory Exercise One, you will learn how to build a Markov model

LEARNING OBJECTIVES

- Learn to use computer software (e.g., TreeAge Pro) to build a Markov model.

- Compare two competing treatment arms.

- Use the tools from Chapter 9 to perform sensitivity analyses on your model.

- Develop confidence in constructing your own decision analysis model.

that calculates life expectancy. In Laboratory Exercise Two, you will expand the model to compare two medical interventions. In Laboratory Exercise Three, you will learn how to calculate the cost-effectiveness of health insurance in the United States. Finally, you will learn how to conduct sensitivity analyses on the insurance model in Laboratory Exercise Four.

There are a number of software options available for conducting cost-effectiveness analysis. As mentioned, the exercises in this book utilize TreeAge Pro software. However, these exercises can also be conducted using other packages as well. A semi-complete list of alternative packages can be found at: http://www.wiley.com/WileyCDA/WileyTitle/productCd-1119011264.html.

Instructors may wish to install laboratory/institutional packages and teach within computer labs. However, since these exercises provide detailed, step-by-step instructions, these labs can be used as homework assignments or self-study quite effectively. We have found that by performing these exercises, students can learn the art and science of cost-effectiveness analysis quickly and effectively.

This chapter was originally developed as a collaborative effort between Peter Muennig and Andy Sheldon at TreeAge Software, Inc. Any mistakes should be reported via the contact link at http://www.wiley.com/WileyCDA/WileyTitle/productCd-1119011264.html.

Laboratory Exercise One: Building a Markov Tree

It may help to review the section on Markov models in Chapter 6 before starting this exercise.

Step 1. New Tree. When you start TreeAge Pro, you will need to start a new model document. Go to the File tab and select "New Decision Tree" (Figure 13.1).

A window will pop up asking if you want to configure the calculation method of the model (Figure 13.2). Since we are going to perform a cost-effectiveness analysis, select "Yes."

The TreeAge Preference window will appear. Under the Calculation Method option, make sure that the "Cost-effectiveness" option is selected (Figure 13.3).

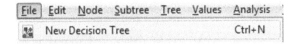

Figure 13.1   Starting a New Project in TreeAge Pro

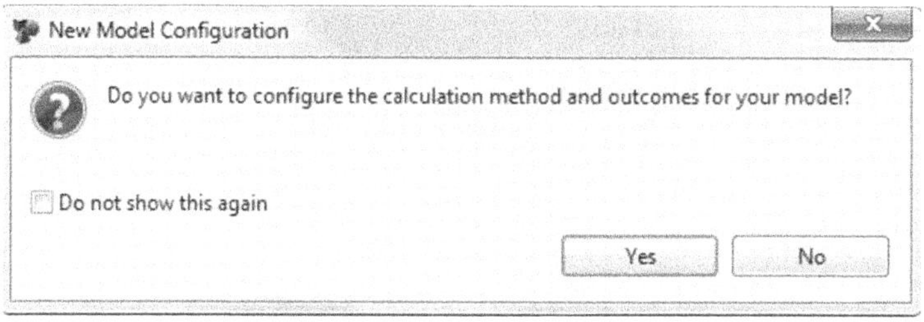

Figure 13.2 Configuring the Model

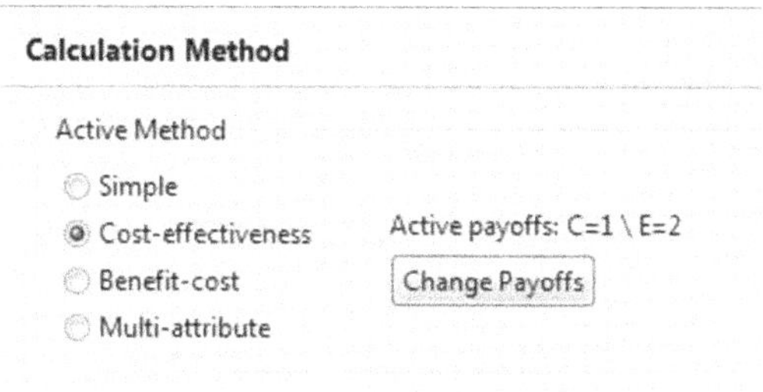

Figure 13.3 Changing the Calculation Method to Cost-Effectiveness

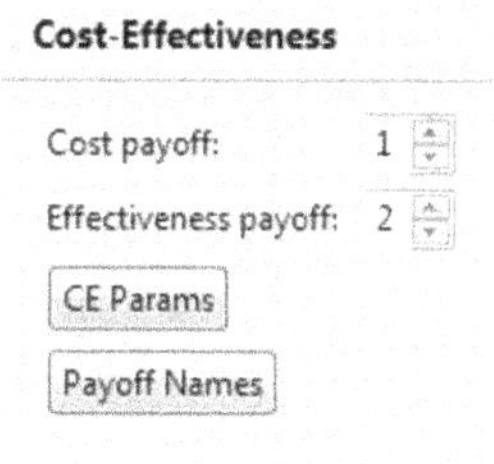

Figure 13.4 Selecting the Payoffs for a Cost-Effectiveness Analysis

After you do this, click "Next." This will bring you to the next option, where you can select the payoffs (cost and effectiveness). You should use the default values of "1" for the Cost payoff and "2" for the Effectiveness payoff (Figure 13.4).

After selecting your payoffs, click "Next." This will bring you to the Cost-Eff Params (WTP) option. For now, we will not change any of these options. (However, if you know what your willingness to pay is, you can change it here.)

Click "Next" to get to the Payoffs option. You can use the default "Number of enabled payoffs" of "2" (Figure 13.5).

Click "Next." This will bring you to the Discounting option. For now, we will do nothing with this. So go ahead and click "Next" again to go to the Custom Names option.

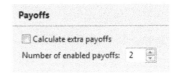

Figure 13.5   Selecting the Number of Payoffs

Custom Names

☑ Use custom payoffs names

Payoff	Custom name
1	Cost
2	Effectiveness

Figure 13.6   Changing Payoffs Names Under the "Custom Names" Option

You can change the name of the Payoffs under Custom Names. Go ahead and check the box "Use custom payoffs names" and type in "Cost" for 1 and "Effectiveness" for 2 (Figure 13.6).

Clicking "Next" will bring you to the top of the Numeric Formatting option. For these exercises, we will use the default formatting, which should have two decimal places for the Cost, Effectiveness, and Cost-Effectiveness values (Figure 13.7).

Click "Finish." This will open up an untitled model document. Start by saving the new document. Open the "Save as" option from the File menu. Use the default file extension "TreeAge Tree Diagram (*.trex)"—this will be the format for all of your work done in TreeAge Pro (Figure 13.8).

Step 2. Add Branches. The new model will start with a single decision node by default. Double-click on the blue square node marker to "sprout" two branches (Figure 13.9).

The new nodes represent *competing alternatives* because they are direct branches of a decision node. If you were comparing three options, you would click on the blue box one more time, and a third branch would be added.

Step 3. Markov Node. In this first lab, however, we aren't ready to compare multiple strategies. In fact, we'll clean things up a little and get rid of one of the strategies. Select either one of the green chance nodes (single-click), open the Node menu from the menu bar, and choose "Delete" (Figure 13.10).

Now use the mouse (or right arrow key) to move to the remaining green chance node. Select this node. We want to turn this into a Markov node, so go to the Node tab, select "Change Type," and select "Markov"

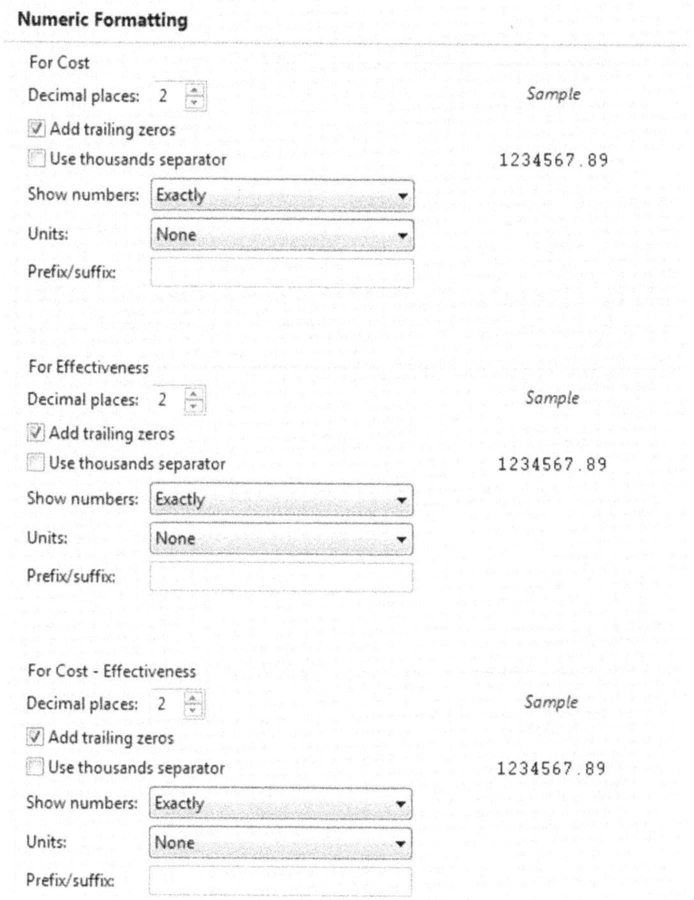

Numeric Formatting

For Cost

Decimal places: 2 ⬍   *Sample*

☑ Add trailing zeros
☐ Use thousands separator   1234567.89

Show numbers: Exactly   ▾

Units: None   ▾

Prefix/suffix:

For Effectiveness

Decimal places: 2 ⬍   *Sample*

☑ Add trailing zeros
☐ Use thousands separator   1234567.89

Show numbers: Exactly   ▾

Units: None   ▾

Prefix/suffix:

For Cost - Effectiveness

Decimal places: 2 ⬍   *Sample*

☑ Add trailing zeros
☐ Use thousands separator   1234567.89

Show numbers: Exactly   ▾

Units: None   ▾

Prefix/suffix:

Figure 13.7   Numerical Formatting for the Cost-Effectiveness Analysis

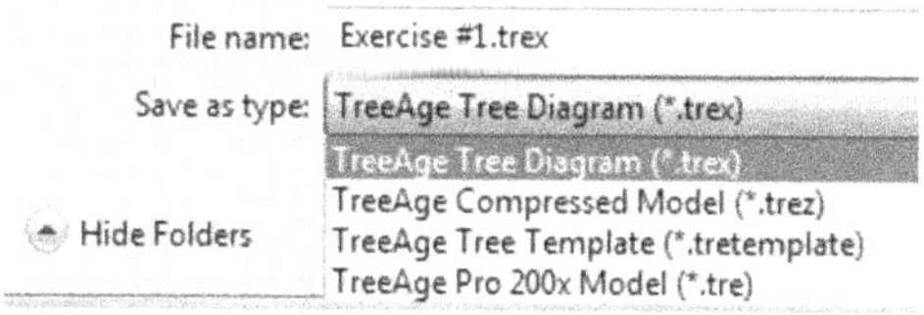

File name: Exercise #1.trex

Save as type: | TreeAge Tree Diagram (*.trex) |
    TreeAge Tree Diagram (*.trex)
    TreeAge Compressed Model (*.trez)
⊙ Hide Folders   TreeAge Tree Template (*.tretemplate)
    TreeAge Pro 200x Model (*.tre)

Figure 13.8   Saving a New Document in TreeAge Pro as a Package Using the *.trex Extension

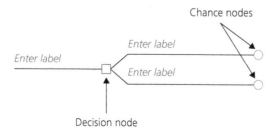

Chance nodes

Enter label

Enter label

Enter label

Enter label

Decision node

Figure 13.9   Adding Two Chance Nodes to the Existing Decision Node

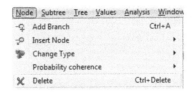

Figure 13.10   Deleting a Branch Using the Table Icons

(Figure 13.11). Alternatively, you can also change the node type by clicking on the icon with various geometric shapes on the button toolbar or right-click on the node and choose the option to Change Type from the context menu.

Once you have selected the Markov node, it should look like Figure 13.12.

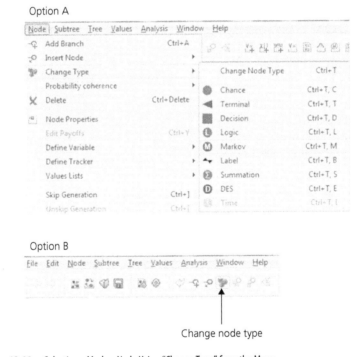

Figure 13.11   Selecting a Markov Node Using "Change Type" from the Menu

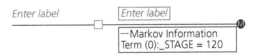

Figure 13.12   Markov Node for a Decision Analysis Model

Step 4. Markov States. Markov health states are the branches directly off the Markov node. To create the Markov health states, add two branches to the new Markov node by double-clicking on the Markov node. Branches will appear curved to indicate that you are in a Markov subtree. Name the states "Alive" and "Dead," as shown in Figure 13.13.

Step 5. Events/Transition Subtrees. Each nondead state will have a subtree to its right representing the events that can occur within a cycle. We have only two events to model at this point—all cause mortality and survival. To represent these outcomes, double-click on the top chance node (Alive) to add two branches. Give the new branches the labels "Survive" and "Die" (Figure 13.14).

If you make any mistakes, you can often use Edit > Undo to fix them.

Step 6. Initial Probabilities. A Markov tree is best thought of as repeatedly transitioning a cohort of subjects between health states over time. Subjects have to start somewhere. In this case, the model starts all subjects as newborns, in Alive at time 0.

The starting state is specified using "initial" probabilities, entered below the Markov states. Clicking just below the square box attached below the Alive state will display the initial probability box. Enter an initial probability of 1 (or 100 percent). Figure 13.15 illustrates where to assign the probability.

Below the Dead state, enter a number sign ("#") to indicate an automatic calculation of the remainder probability for this branch. (The remainder is 0, of course, but it's handy to enter the "#" just in case we were to make the initial probability of Alive a variable later. Being able to have the model calculate your parameters will help ensure that the sum of the probabilities will remain 1. Recall from Chapter 5 that the total probability of the event

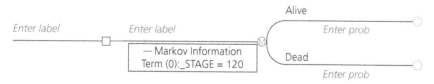

Figure 13.13   Creating Branches on a Markov Tree

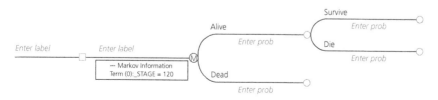

Figure 13.14   Labeling Branches in a Markov Tree

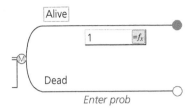

Figure 13.15   Assigning an Initial Probability of 100 Percent to the Alive State in the Markov Model

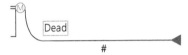

Figure 13.16   Changing the Node from Chance Node to a Terminal Node

must sum to 1. If it doesn't, there could be a problem with the way you entered your variables or the way you designed the tree.

Step 7. Termination Nodes/Jump States. Our next task is to change all rightmost nodes to terminal nodes.

The easiest is the Dead state. Select the Dead state (i.e., the second branch of the Markov node) by clicking on the green circle. Repeat the Change Node Type command, from Step 3, this time selecting Terminal. This will change the green circle to a red triangle (Figure 13.16).

A Markov state with no branches is called an *absorbing state*, because subjects who enter will remain there until the analysis is complete. In this case, as in most Markov models, we need an absorbing Dead state. No one starts out Dead, but the list of states has to represent all possible future health states, including states (like Dead) that can only be reached after time has passed, disease has progressed, and so forth. It's important that you understand this requirement.

Repeat the Change Node Type command for the two other rightmost nodes. These branches represent the different outcomes after one year of life (i.e., whether someone who starts in the Alive state at the beginning of a cycle will continue in Alive or move to Dead at the end of the cycle). Changing each branch to a terminal node indicates that there are no more events occurring during a Markov cycle. When terminating a path in a Markov state, the Edit Jump State dialog box should appear (Figure 13.17).

Each terminal "jump" node must point back to one of the Markov states, so that the cohort can continue processing the next cycle. For the Survive event, select Alive as the jump state. For the Die event, select Dead as the jump state. If you did this correctly, the Markov tree should look like Figure 13.18.

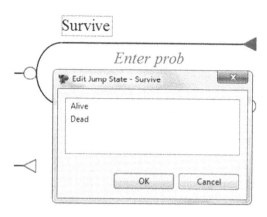

Figure 13.17   Edit Jump State Dialog Box Appears When the Chance Node Is Changed to a Terminal Node

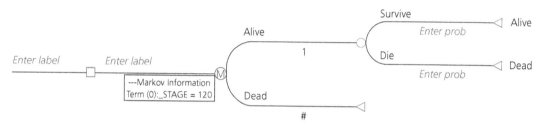

Figure 13.18   Markov Tree After Changing the Remaining Chance Nodes into Terminal Nodes

In this very simple example, these steps may seem redundant, but Markov models are typically more complex. Most health states include a series of different events (treatment complications, failures, etc.) that can occur in each Markov cycle, and the end point in each path must point cohort members to the correct state to start the next cycle.

We'll come back to these branches in a later step, when it's time to assign the per-cycle rates or probabilities of mortality/survival.

Step 8. State Rewards. The basic structure of the Markov subtree has been completed, and now it's time to enter some values required for calculations. Select the Alive state branch by clicking once on the node (Figure 13.19). Now go to the Nodes menu and choose "Values Lists" and then click on "Open Markov Info." (The Markov Info View dialog box can also be opened by clicking on the Open Markov Info View icon on the button toolbar illustrated in Figure 13.20.)

After selecting the Markov Info View, the dialog box will appear at the bottom of your workspace (Figure 13.21). Note that the contents of the Markov Info View are tied to the selected node—the health state Alive.

The Rewards (Active Sets) currently have default values of "0." There are three entries for the state rewards: Initial, Incremental, and Final. The

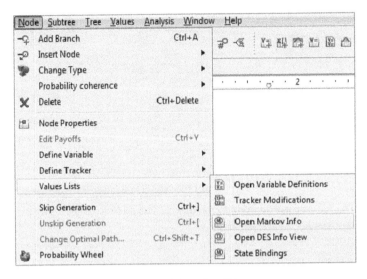

Figure 13.19   Selecting the Markov Info View in Order to Enter Values

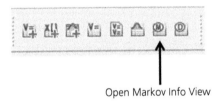

Open Markov Info View

Figure 13.20   Selecting the Markov Info View Using the Icon on the Button Toolbar

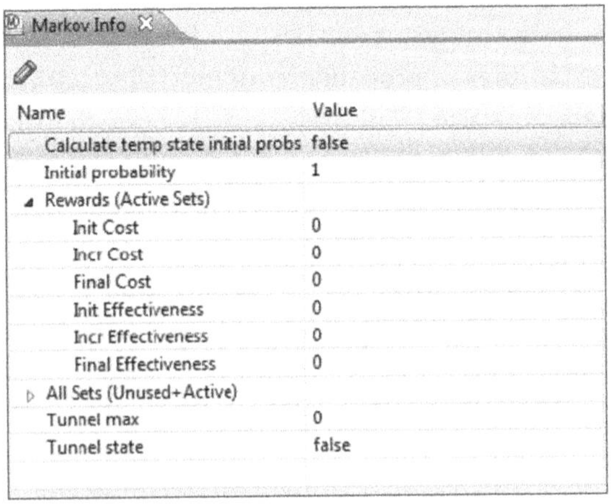

Figure 13.21   Markov Info View Dialog Box

Initial reward for a state defines how much value—that is, life-years or cost—is assigned to subjects spending the first overall Markov cycle in the state. Another way to look at the Initial stage is to equate it to the baseline value (or life-year expectancy). IMPORTANT! The initial state reward will only be given to cohort subjects starting in the state, not those entering it in a later pass/cycle—that is where the Incremental reward value comes in.

An incremental reward value (the second entry box in Figure 13.21 labeled as "Incr Cost" and "Incr Effectiveness") should also be assigned for all subsequent stages (e.g., 1 through n) spent in the state.

Enter a 5 in both the Initial and the Incremental fields, as shown in Figure 13.22. This tells TreeAge Pro to add 5 to the running total life expectancy for each cycle an individual spends in the Alive state. Why are we using 5 as the unit reward? We are assuming the length of one cycle is five years, because we want to use (without transformation) a life table that has five-year age intervals. Cycle length is different for different models; both transition probabilities and state rewards must take into account cycle length.

Disclaimer: Normally, using a five-year cycle is not recommended. Most Markov models settle on a cycle length that is generally less than one year, with a time horizon that spans the lifetime of the cohort. In this example, we chose to focus our lesson on building a Markov mode and have taken liberties with the cycle length.

The Final state reward box tells TreeAge Pro what to do *after* the process stops. (Step 11 will explain how the process is terminated.) For the moment, we won't worry about possible applications of the Final state reward, and leave it as 0.

Name	Value
Calculate temp state initial probs	false
Initial probability	1
⊿ Rewards (Active Sets)	
Init Cost	0
Incr Cost	0
Final Cost	0
Init Effectiveness	5
Incr Effectiveness	5
Final Effectiveness	0
▷ All Sets (Unused+Active)	
Tunnel max	0
Tunnel state	false

Figure 13.22   Setting the Initial and Incremental Rewards

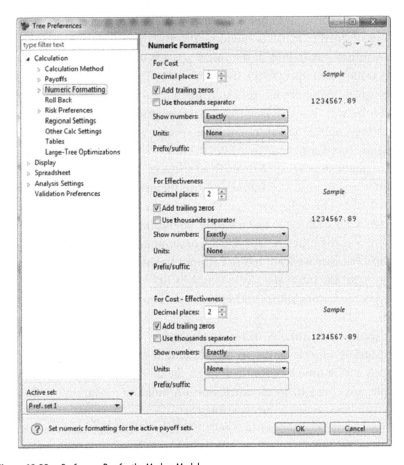

Figure 13.23   Preference Box for the Markov Model

Click OK to save the Alive state rewards. We don't need to make changes to the Dead state—all rewards are 0, of course.

Step 9. Display Preferences. Before we continue, let's tell TreeAge Pro to show us a bit more of the model. Go to the Edit menu and select "Tree Preferences." You get the dialog box shown in Figure 13.23.

Expand the Display option and select the "Variables/Markov Info" option (Figure 13.24). Make sure that "Show definitions" is selected and "Show Markov information" has a check by the box next to it.

Step 10. Termination Condition. Notice the Markov Information box below the Markov node (Figure 13.18), with the word "Term" inside it (short for Termination). The termination condition is required—it tells TreeAge Pro when to stop running the Markov process. Double-click on the Term box to enter a condition (or select the Node tab and go to Values Lists > Open Markov Info).

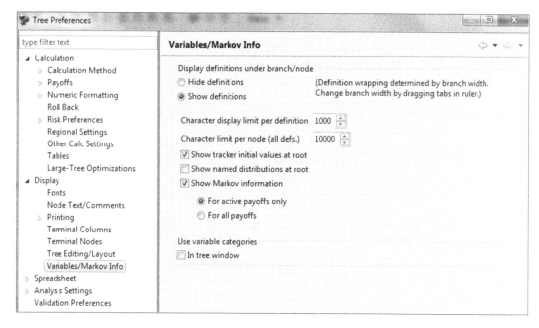

Figure 13.24 Selecting the "Variables/Markov Info" Option from the Tree Preferences Dialog Box

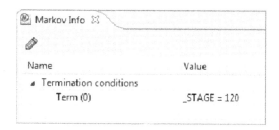

Figure 13.25 Termination Conditions for the Markov Node

Under Termination conditions, TreeAge Pro fills in a default, multipart conditional stopping rule (Figure 13.25). For this laboratory you will not need anything this complex. However, before deleting the default termination condition note the use of the _STAGE keyword. This keyword counts the number of cycles the cohort subjects have completed.

Delete the default termination condition, and in its place type the simpler rule age >= 90 as shown in Figure 13.26. Step 11 will explain what "age" is.

Step 11. Creating a Variable. Once you set your terminal condition, hit the return key. TreeAge Pro will ask if you want to create a new user-defined variable called "age" (it is not a built-in, predefined name). Therefore, you will need to create it (Figure 13.27).

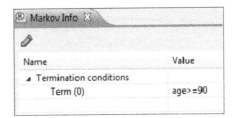

Figure 13.26   Setting the Termination Conditions for the Markov Model

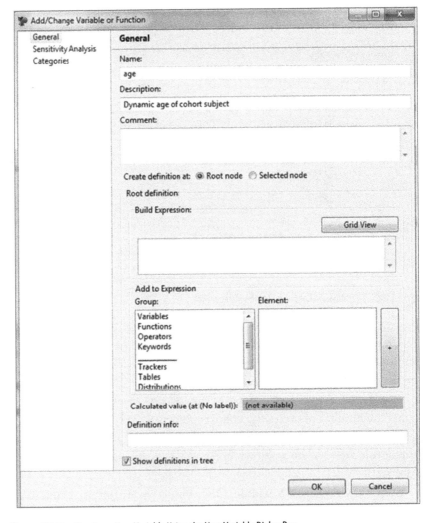

Figure 13.27   Creating a New Variable Using the New Variable Dialog Box

Enter a variable description in the description box. This can be in free text and may include spaces between words. In this case, type in "Dynamic age of cohort subject." This definition will help anyone looking at the model's parameters to understand their function. Click OK to save the name in the tree. This creates the variable but does not assign it a value or formula. We don't want to assign "age" a fixed numeric value (e.g., at the root node)—rather, it should be a dynamic value that represents the advancing age of the cohort, or a cohort subject. IMPORTANT! The "Name" of a variable cannot be a numeric value or have spaces between the words.

Step 12. Defining a Variable. To assign a value (or in our case, a formula) to the new variable called "age," choose Values > Variables and Tables . . . (or click on the big V= toolbar button). Figure 13.28 illustrates how to do this using the menu toolbar.

In the Variables List, select the variable "age." From the Root Definition column select the formula button on the right. Under Build Expression, type_stage*5, as shown in Figure 13.29. Click OK to save the definition. (And click "No" if you are asked if you want to edit another variable. This will return you to the model.)

During analysis, age will equal the value of the built-in _stage counter multiplied by 5 (since each cycle is five years long).

During the initial cycle, the cohort age is 0, because the _stage counter starts at 0. Prior to the start of the next cycle, _stage increments to 1 and age will equal 5. When _stage increments to 18, having completed 18 cycles of rewards and transitions, then the cohort age will equal $18 \times 5 = 90$, and the termination condition will cause the Markov analysis to stop. By setting a termination condition, the simulation will end; otherwise, it will continue until all the patients end up in the absorbing state (Dead).

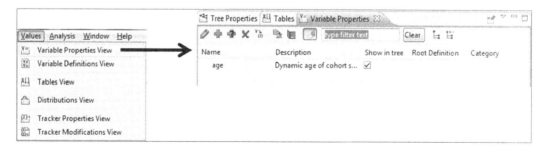

Figure 13.28   Assigning a Value to the Variable "age"

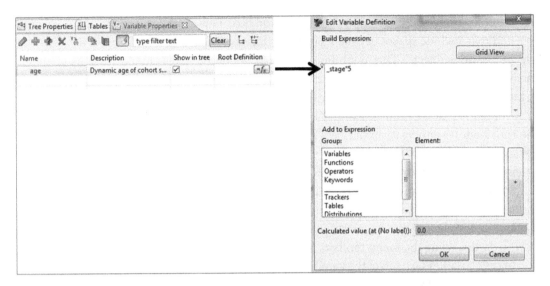

Figure 13.29   Defining the Variable "age"

The expression "_stage*5" could have been used directly in the Markov termination condition, but using a separate variable like age allows us to make the model both more transparent and easier to modify. For example, to start everyone at age 65 instead of birth, we could change the definition of age to "65 + _stage*5," or even better "startAge + _stage*5" where startAge is another user-defined variable.

Step 13. Transition Probabilities. Enter event probabilities in the branches to the right of the Alive state. We will specify the probability of dying during each cycle (i.e., five-year age range) and make survival equal to the remainder.

So enter a number sign ("#") under the Survive branch to tell the model to always assign the remainder here, that is: 1 − (probability of death).

At the transition node to Dead, type the expression tdead2000[age] in the transition probability box below the branch (Figure 13.30). During analysis, TreeAge Pro will look up the probability in a user-defined table called tdead2000, using the value of the variable age as an index, in order to pick the appropriate row.

After inputting the probabilities for the Survive and Die branches, an Add/Change Table window will appear. This window will allow you to provide a description of the table that was defined earlier as tdead2000, which is a user-defined table. Click on OK.

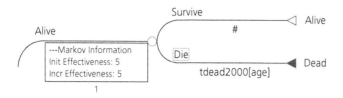

Figure 13.30   Setting the Probability of Die as tdead2000[age], Which Is Derived from an $n \times 2$ Matrix Table

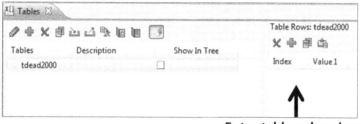

Enter table values here

Figure 13.31   Layout for Entering Values for a User-Defined Table

Step 14. Creating a Table. Click outside the probability box to save your changes. At this time, you will learn to create a table that TreeAge Pro will use in the model you are building. Go to the Values tab at the top of the menu bar, and select "Tables View." You will see a window for Tables. There should be an entry for "tdead2000" that you created earlier. To the right of it, there is another section called "Table Rows: tdead2000." This is where you will enter the values for the table (Figure 13.31).

Step 15. Entering Table Values. Now you can set up the table data in Excel and copy it into the empty TreeAge Pro table (Figure 13.31). (Make sure you also copy the headers.) An example set of Year 2000 age-specific mortality probabilities is provided for you in an Excel file ("tDead2000.xls") (Figure 13.32). Column B provides the five-year probabilities of dying for the corresponding age groups in Column A.

For example, a newborn has a 0.8 percent probability of dying by age five. The five-year mortality decreases to 0.08 percent for five-year-olds, but then increases at each age interval after that.

Although it does not affect us yet, TreeAge Pro will, by default, use linear interpolation to fill in missing rows/indexes in a table. For example, in a model with a one-year cycle length, the probability returned for `age=8` would be about 0.09 percent.

TIPS AND TRICKS

Advanced Tip: To get the age-specific probabilities, work from life tables. If you want to enter more recent values, U.S. Life Tables are available at:

> http://www.cdc.gov/nchs/
> deaths.htm

and international tables are available at either:

> http://www.census.gov/ipc/
> www/idb/

or

> http://www.who.int/research/en/

The 1999 WHO tables are put together in a nice document available at:

> http://whqlibdoc.who.int/hq/
> 2001/a78629.pdf

Life tables may be abridged (like ours, using age groups larger than one year, stating the number starting in an age group interval that die during that interval). *If your life table intervals do not match your cycle length, be sure to convert—for example, 5- or 10-year probabilities into 1-year probabilities.* Dividing is okay for small probabilities, but less accurate for larger probabilities.

After entering the table in Excel, copy the table, then switch back to the TreeAge Pro window.

Before entering the values from Excel into `tdead2000`, make sure that you select the data and copy it. Go to Values > Tables View, and click on the icon "Paste headers and rows." The values will automatically populate the columns "Index" and "Value1" (Figure 13.33).

Step 16. Numeric Format. Now, we want to tell the model how to present its output. In this case, the model is evaluating life expectancy (in years), not costs, so we will want to make sure that it gives us the proper units on expected values. From the Edit menu, choose "Numeric Formatting" (Figure 13.34).

In the Numeric Formatting settings in the Cost panel, change the Units to Currency. In the Effectiveness panel, change the units to Custom suffix, and type the word `Years` in the Suffix box (Figure 13.35).

Now, click OK to return to the tree. It should look like Figure 13.36.

Step 17. Rollback Analysis. Save the tree first. Then select the Analysis > Roll Back command. (Alternatively, you can click on the beach ball icon in the toolbar.)

A window will appear indicating that the willingness to pay is set to 0. Click OK. The tree should assume the appearance represented by Figure 13.37.

	A	B
1	Index	Value1
2	0	0.00823
3	5	0.00082
4	10	0.00104
5	15	0.00341
6	20	0.00479
7	25	0.00494
8	30	0.00578
9	35	0.00806
10	40	0.01182
11	45	0.01773
12	50	0.02576
13	55	0.03968
14	60	0.06133
15	65	0.09217
16	70	0.13838
17	75	0.20557
18	80	0.31503
19	85	0.46111
20	90	0.61506
21	95	0.75434
22	100	0.999

Figure 13.32   An Excel Table with the Probabilities of Death Associated with Each Age

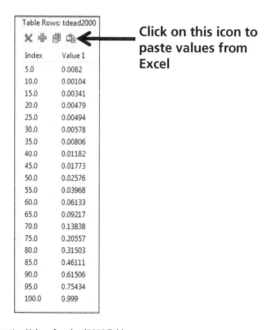

Click on this icon to paste values from Excel

Table Rows: tdead2000	
Index	Value 1
5.0	0.0082
10.0	0.00104
15.0	0.00341
20.0	0.00479
25.0	0.00494
30.0	0.00578
35.0	0.00806
40.0	0.01182
45.0	0.01773
50.0	0.02576
55.0	0.03968
60.0	0.06133
65.0	0.09217
70.0	0.13838
75.0	0.20557
80.0	0.31503
85.0	0.46111
90.0	0.61506
95.0	0.75434
100.0	0.999

Figure 13.33   Entering Values for tdead2000 Table

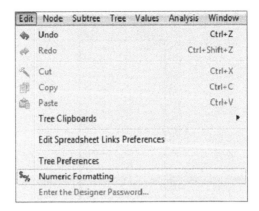

Figure 13.34   Selecting the Numeric Formatting Preferences from the Edit Menu

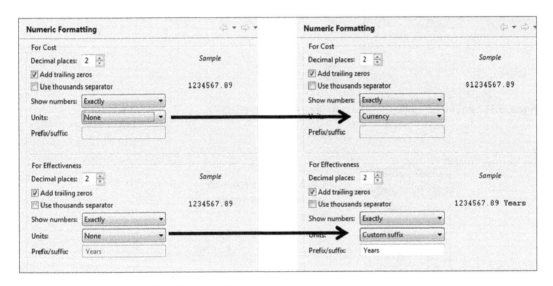

Figure 13.35   Changing the Payoff Units for Cost and Effectiveness

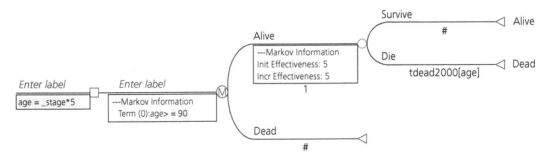

Figure 13.36   Overall Illustration of the Markov Model After Parameter Inputs and Unit Changes

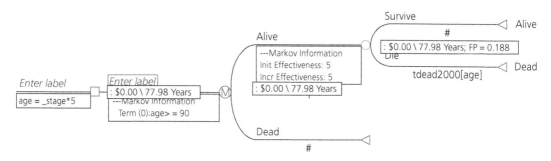

Figure 13.37   Results of the Rollback Analysis for the Markov Model

Congratulations! You have estimated the life expectancy of your cohort. You should have a life expectancy of 78 years. If you did not get the same answer, try checking your work to make sure everything was inputted correctly. Troubleshooting a model is just as important as constructing one, so practice going over your model periodically.

Summary. Let's briefly review what happened here. While a Markov cohort analysis doesn't really involve any hypothetical subjects, it may be easier to think of it this way initially. At time 0, 100 percent of the cohort begins in the Alive state, receiving the Initial state reward of five corresponding to the first five-year cycle. Subjects are then exposed to an age-specific risk of death. The small fraction that dies will be absorbed by the Dead state in the next cycle, finishing with an accumulated life expectancy of five.

The majority that survive will start another cycle in the Alive state, effectively having their age incremented to five years, and accumulate an incremental state reward of another five years. They are then exposed to an age-specific risk of death. The fraction that dies will be absorbed by the Dead state in the next cycle, finishing with a life expectancy of 10 years. This repeats until the termination condition is met (when the population reaches 90 years or greater). Figure 13.38 is a transition state diagram of the Markov model we just constructed.

At each cycle, the percentage in the Alive state (starting at 1 and eventually approaching 0) is multiplied by the state reward for that cycle, and this product is added to the total reward in order to calculate expected values for the process (e.g., expected survival and/or expected lifetime costs).

The reported expected value of 78 years therefore approximates the average life expectancy for a population based on the five-year mortality risks found in the life table when the surviving population age reaches 90 years or greater. While we simply chose to reward the surviving cohort members with life-years each cycle, we'll see later that they can also accrue

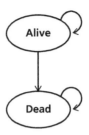

Figure 13.38   Transition State Diagram of a Markov Model with Alive and Dead States

costs or other values that you, the omnipotent researcher and modeler, deem necessary.

What's next? First, we'll refine the termination condition and rewards. Then we'll learn how to build upon this basic tree to answer critical research questions you might be facing.

Laboratory Exercise Two: Comparing Interventions

In Laboratory Exercise One, you learned how to build a basic Markov cycle tree that calculates life expectancy. In this exercise, we will refine the life expectancy calculation, and then add a comparison intervention to the tree. Now that you have the hang of the program, we'll move from a slow, click-by-click approach to a faster trip through the modeling process.

Step 1. Refining the Model. Before we make changes, save your existing model and then use File > Save As . . . to create a new copy (e.g., "Exercise #2.trex").

Now let's tell TreeAge Pro to show us a bit more of the model. Go back to Edit > Numeric Formatting, as you did in Step 16 of the previous exercise. Where it asks for Decimal places, at the top of the dialog box, make sure that the number "2" is entered for Costs, Effectiveness, and Cost-Effectiveness (if you haven't done so already). That allows reporting to be accurate to a tenth of a year. If you roll back the tree again, you'll see the more precise reporting of life expectancy for the model, 77.98 years (Figure 13.39).

Step 2. Adjusting Parameters. The last rollback estimates year 2000 life expectancy as about 78 years. While we're close to the life table, which reports 76.9 years (Figure 13.40), we should look at why we have overestimated.

Markov cohort analysis deals with discrete time advances and normally assumes that changes in state (i.e., jumps from Alive to Dead) occur at the end of a cycle. Our model assigns a reward of five to the proportion of the cohort that starts each cycle in Alive, some of whom will die at the cycle.

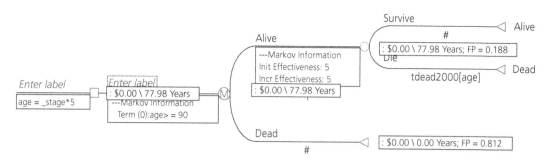

Figure 13.39 Results of Rollback Function

Age (x)	Life Expectancy at Age (x)	Number Surviving to Age (x)
0-1	76.9	100, 000
1-5	76.4	99, 307
5-10	72.5	99, 177
10-15	67.6	99, 095
15-20	62.6	98, 992
20-25	57.8	98, 654
25-30	53.1	98, 181
30-35	48.3	97, 696
35-40	43.6	97, 132
40-45	38.9	96, 349
45-50	34.4	95, 210
50-55	30.0	93, 522
55-60	25.7	91, 113
60-65	21.6	87, 498
65-70	17.9	82, 131
70-75	14.4	74, 561
75-80	11.3	64, 244
80-85	8.6	51, 037
85-90	6.3	34, 959
90-95	4.7	18, 839
95-100	3.5	7, 252
>100	2.6	1, 781

Figure 13.40 U.S. Life Table for Ages 0 to 100 and Over

However, in reality, deaths and other changes in state occur continuously throughout an interval, and therefore *on average about halfway* through an interval. This results in a cumulative overestimation of life expectancy of about half a cycle (e.g., 2.5 years in our model). Models often use a simple "half-cycle correction" to adjust for this fact, taking away half of the first cycle's worth of reward. To do this, double-click on the box directly below the Alive branch labeled "Markov Information" in Figure 13.41. Look for "Init Effectiveness" under the Rewards (Active Sets) section. Change the value from 5 to 5*(0.5). This will perform the half-cycle correction on the Initial Effectiveness only.

After you make the half-cycle correction, perform the rollback analysis again by clicking on the beach ball icon. This would reduce our life expectancy calculation to 75.48—now a little less than that of the life table (Figure 13.42).

Also remember that when we set the termination condition (Step 10 of the previous exercise), we had calculations stop at age >= 90 (e.g., without adding rewards for ages 90+). If you look again at the rollback results, note

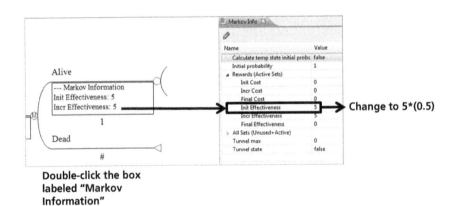

Double-click the box labeled "Markov Information"

Figure 13.41   Changing the Initial Cycle's Worth of Reward with the Half-Cycle Correction

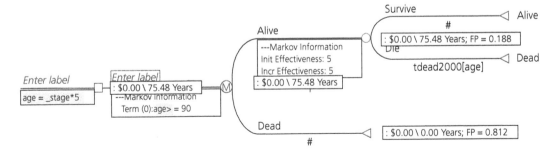

Figure 13.42   Rollback Results Using the Half-Cycle Correction on the Initial Effectiveness

the text "FP=0.188" next to the Alive state (Figure 13.42). This indicates that a large proportion (18.8 percent) of the cohort is still in the Alive state when the model stops after 18 cycles. This matches the life table in Figure 13.40 at age 90 (18,839/100,000).

TIPS AND TRICKS

Advanced Tip: To calculate life expectancy in your own models, you may have to extrapolate the probability of death for the older age intervals in your table. An *annual* probability of death could be calculated as 1/(life expectancy at age *x*). The termination age can be set to at least *x* + remaining life expectancy. If 100+-year-olds have a life expectancy of 2.6 years in the life table, the annual mortality rate is calculated as 1/2.6, or 0.38. The termination age should be set to at least $100 + 2.6 = 102.6$.

Because our model stops before counting future life expectancy of those living past age 90, we are ignoring the contribution to life expectancy made by nonagenarians (*underestimates* life expectancy).

(Note: TreeAge Pro will not extrapolate beyond the end of the table. If we let the analysis amble on long enough, it just continues to use the last probability of death entered into the tdead2000 table, for age 100. This would be more important to consider if using a life table ending at age 80, for example. In our case, the mortality probability of 0.999 would ensure that almost no one survives to age 105.)

Time to make our fixes and move on. First, let's implement the half-cycle correction for the Initial and Final states. Select the Alive state and open the Markov Information dialog box that you did earlier in Figure 13.41. Click in the Value field for "Init Effectiveness," then click on the little pencil icon on the top left-hand corner of the window (Figure 13.43). This will

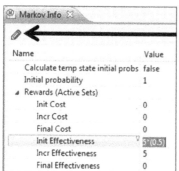

Click on the pencil icon

Figure 13.43   Opening the Define Initial Reward Window

open the Define Initial Reward window, where you can make adjustments to the amount of rewards in each health state.

Click on the Half-Cycle Correct button in the top right-hand corner of the window, as illustrated in in Figure 13.44.

To accomplish this same outcome you could just type "2.5." The impact is made in _stage 0, when the Initial reward is cut in half. (The Final reward component of the correction only has an impact in models that terminate before most of the cohort is dead.)

We also noted that age 90 is a little early to stop counting contributions to life expectancy. We'll set the termination condition to occur after life expectancy for 100-year-olds (i.e., 102.6), using a rule of age >= 105 years. This means the calculations stop before accruing rewards or transitions for 105-year-olds. Most everyone will be dead at 105 anyway, because of the 99.9 percent probability of mortality above age 100. To accomplish this change, double-click the Markov Information box below the Markov node and change age >= 90 to age >= 105 (Figure 13.45).

Click on the Half-Cycle Correct box

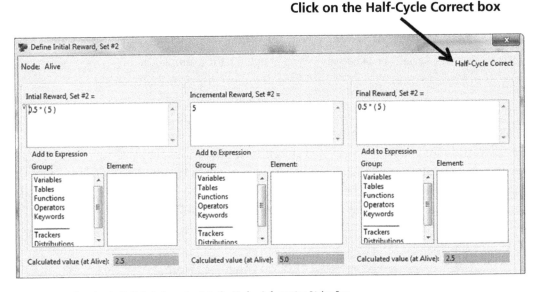

Figure 13.44   Entering the Half-Cycle Correction into the Markov Information Dialog Box

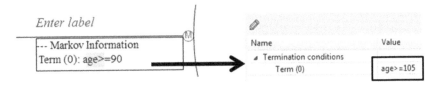

Figure 13.45   Defining the Termination Condition to an Age That Is 105 Years or Older

Try the rollback again, and see if you hit the 76.9 nail on the head. (You should if you have followed the preceding steps.) Verify your answer with Figure 13.46.

Let's move on, and try adding a comparison strategy with an impact on mortality.

Step 3. Copy Subtree. Click on the root, decision node, go to the Subtree menu and Select Subtree (shortcut = Control + B). Now go to the Edit menu and Copy. This will store a copy of the Markov subtree (including the Markov node) (Figure 13.47).

Step 4. Paste Subtree. Make sure the decision node is highlighted by clicking on it again, then go to the Edit menu and Paste to add a second copy of the Markov arm. If you did everything correctly, it should look like Figure 13.48.

Step 5. Decision Analysis. Now you have the basis for comparing just about any two interventions over a lifetime. We could compare two drugs or surgical procedures. Let's consider this possibility for a moment. (Here, hypothetical data are used.)

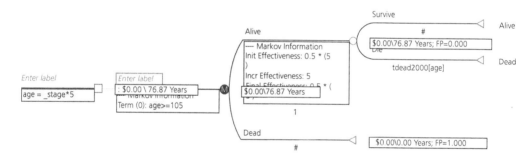

Figure 13.46   Rollback Analysis with Half-Cycle Correction and Life Cycle Greater Than 105 Years

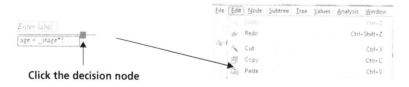

After copying the subtree, click on the decision node once again

Click the decision node

Figure 13.47   Selecting and Copying the Subtree

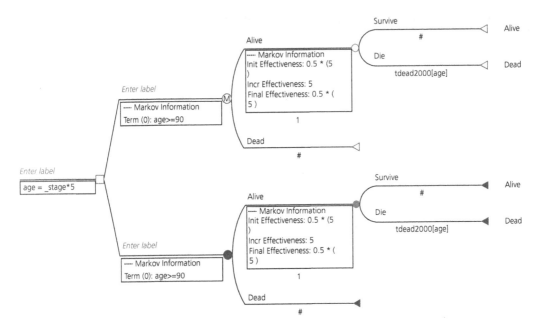

Figure 13.48   Adding a Second Subtree to the Decision Node

Suppose that you are comparing treatments for a congenital heart valve defect affecting some newborns, which can be corrected using one of two surgical procedures. The first is called the *Filmore* procedure (after Ignacious Danenhousen Filmore) and does a pretty good job of fixing the problem at no initial risk to the infant to speak of. However, each year the person will have approximately 25 percent higher than normal mortality due to this procedure.

Recently, Ludviga Elmore Reinkenshein modified the Filmore procedure so that it completely fixes the heart defect, with little or no excess mortality. However, she patented her *Reinkenshein* surgical technique, requiring a hospital to fork over $10,000 to her every time it's used. Let's have a look at these two procedures in terms of effectiveness alone.

First, rename the branches to reflect our current modeling problem. Make Filmore the top arm and Reinkenshein the bottom arm.

Next, we'll want to modify the mortality probability in the top, Filmore, branch to increase the mortality probability (currently "tDead2000[ ]") by a factor of 1.25 to reflect the increased mortality risk associated with the Filmore treatment. (See Figure 13.49 to see how to do this.) Multiplying probabilities (unless they are very small) can sometimes be tricky. One way to model this without resulting in probability errors is by multiplying against a *rate* or an *odds*. TreeAge Pro has functions to do this, including `ProbFactor(prob; odds_factor)` and `ProbTo-Prob(prob; rate_factor)`. Although you could experiment with the differences, we'll try something with more brute force: Multiplying the probability, but using the `Min( )` function to cap the probability at 1. `Min()`, returns the lowest value in its semicolon-separated list.

Before performing the rollback analysis, let's change the calculation method from a cost-effectiveness to a simple analysis. Recall that in Laboratory Exercise One you set up your model to be a cost-effectiveness analysis. Here, we want to look only at the Effectiveness payoff. In order to change from a cost-effectiveness to a simple analysis, click on Edit > Tree Preferences. Select "Calculation Method" and select "Simple" (Figure 13.50).

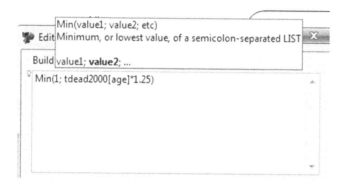

Figure 13.49   Multiplying Mortality Probability by a Factor of 1.25 and Capping It at 1

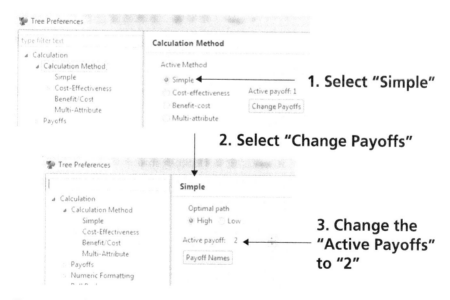

Figure 13.50   Changing Calculation Method from Cost-Effectiveness to Simple Analysis

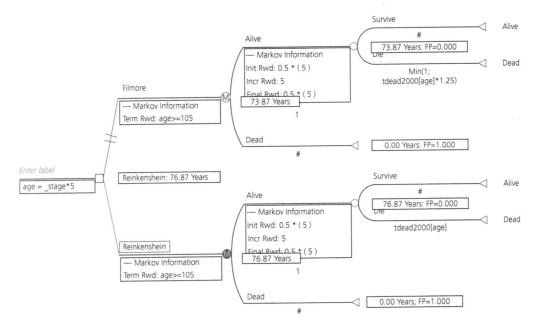

Figure 13.51   Results of Rollback Between Filmore and Rinkenshein Procedures

Select "Change Payoffs" and then change the "Active payoff" to "2," as in Figure 13.50. Then click OK.

Time to roll back again: Click the little beach ball in the toolbar, and compare expected values (Figure 13.51).

So we expect a population born with the disease and given the new Rinkenshein procedure to live about three years longer on average than a population given the older Filmore modification (76.87 – 73.87 = 3 years).

Step 6. Cost-Effectiveness. Now, let's take into account costs. Rinkenshein charges anyone who does the procedure $10,000, on top of the usual costs of the procedure. We'll assume we can ignore all other costs because they are equal in the two strategies.

Our objective is to evaluate the cost-effectiveness of the new, more expensive, more effective intervention. We'll examine the one-time *incremental* cost of the new surgical procedure, relative to its average incremental gain in survival. First, switch the model to a cost-effectiveness calculation method.

a.   *Make sure the tree is not rolled back,* then go to the Edit menu and Tree Preferences, select Calculation Method, and then select Cost-Effectiveness. Click on the Change Payoffs button and make sure that the Cost payoff is set to "1," and the Effectiveness payoff is set to "2" (Figure 13.52). *This is important!* (Why? Because we will need to

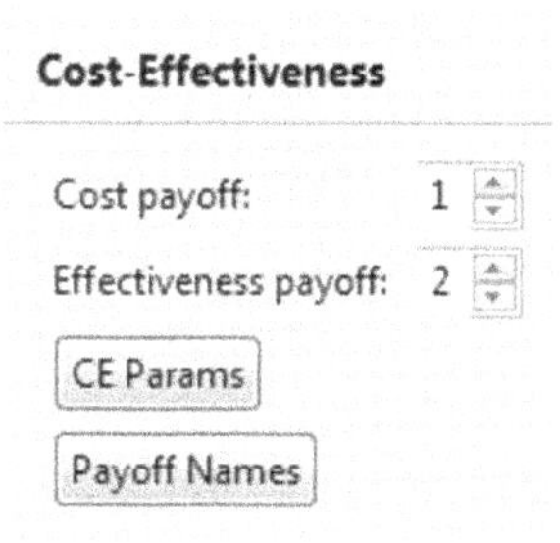

Cost-Effectiveness

Cost payoff: 1 ⏶⏷

Effectiveness payoff: 2 ⏶⏷

CE Params

Payoff Names

Figure 13.52   Modifying the Payoff for a Cost-Effectiveness Analysis

calculate incremental cost-effectiveness ratios. Cost needs to be in the numerator and Effectiveness needs to be in the denominator.)

b. Click on the CE Params button, under the Tree Preferences > Calculation Method > Cost-Effectiveness category. Entering a Willingness to pay (or threshold ICER) value or expression here will help pick an optimally cost-effective strategy during rollback. For example, entering a threshold of 40,000 (units might be $/year gained or $/QALY gained) will result in rollback selecting the most effective strategy with an ICER of 40,000 or less (Figure 13.53). (There are additional parameters at the bottom of the dialog box that instruct TreeAge Pro to invert, or minimize, the "effectiveness" measure, when necessary. This is not a feature that we will use in this model, but it may be required in other models that you build.)

c. Click OK to save the preferences.

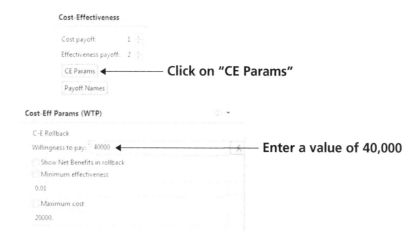

Figure 13.53   Entering a Willingness to Pay of $40,000 per Life-Year Gained

d. With the change to the calculation method, you will need to edit each Markov node's termination condition to confirm you still want the stopping rule to be age >= 105.

e. The $10K charge must be added in the Rinkenshein procedure arm. For now, the base costs of surgery will be ignored, assuming the costs and their timing are the same for both strategies (and would cancel each other out in the incremental analysis). Double-click the Markov Information box at the bottom of the Alive state for the Rinkenshein strategy. Under the Rewards (Active Sets) category, enter 10,000 in the Init Cost field (Figure 13.54). Make sure that you add only the value to the Initial reward box, since this operation happens once, after birth. (If we enter this in the Incremental box by accident, then 10,000 will be charged every year.)

f. No changes need be made in the top branch. Although the Filmore is not free, we only model the excess cost (of the Rinkenshein) where the strategies diverge.

Step 7. Rollback. If your tree looks right, calculate the tree using rollback (Figure 13.55). If the units are wrong (e.g., life expectancy = $75), make the fixes in Edit > Numeric Formatting.

Note, however, that what we really want the analysis to tell us—incremental costs divided by the incremental effectiveness, or the ICER—is not reported in the rollback display. We'll need a different analysis command for that information.

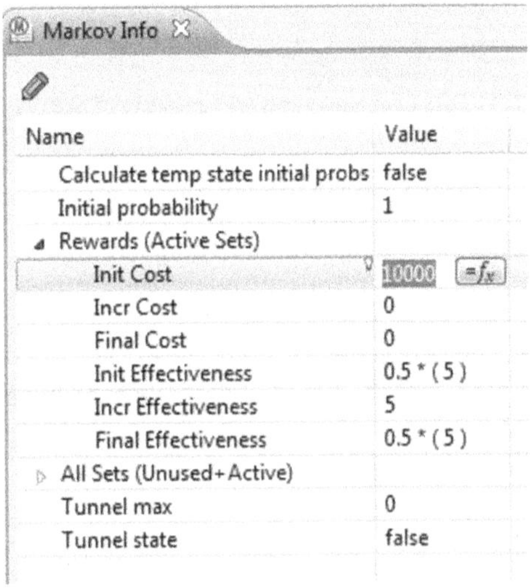

Name	Value
Calculate temp state initial probs	false
Initial probability	1
⊿ Rewards (Active Sets)	
Init Cost	10000
Incr Cost	0
Final Cost	0
Init Effectiveness	0.5 * (5)
Incr Effectiveness	5
Final Effectiveness	0.5 * (5)
▷ All Sets (Unused+Active)	
Tunnel max	0
Tunnel state	false

Figure 13.54   Defining the Reward Set in the Initial Stage of the Markov Model

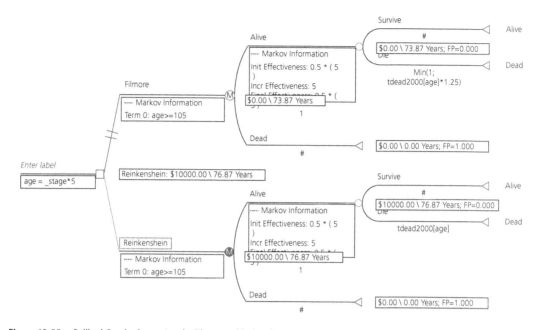

Figure 13.55   Rollback Results Comparing the Filmore and Rinkenshein Procedures

Step 8. CEA Rankings. Turn off rollback the same way you turned it on (e.g., by clicking the little beach ball). Click on the blue decision node to set the context for a new analysis, then choose Analysis > Rankings (Figure 13.56).

A rankings text report is generated, with the lowest cost strategy listed in the first row followed by the next lowest cost strategy (Figure 13.57). There are several different categories in the Rankings report, but this time they all provide the same information. (If there were more than three strategies, then the output would report which ones were eliminated by extended dominance.) The category that is most important for the current analysis is highlighted in Figure 13.57.

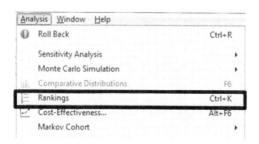

Figure 13.56   Selecting the Rankings from the Analysis Tab

The ICER is $3,329 per additional year of life gained (Table 13.1). In other words, the Rinkenshein procedure will cost an additional $3,329 to realize one additional life-year gained compared to the Filmore procedure.

So there you have it! Despite Rinkenshein's patent charges, her procedure costs just $3,329 per year of life gained. A true bargain in most health systems. (Of course, institutions with annual health budgets averaging a few dollars per person would present a different perspective. Note that we haven't tried to estimate the cost-effectiveness of the Filmore procedure relative to a "do nothing" strategy in this model.)

What's next? Having performed your first cost-effectiveness analysis, you may be feeling fairly sophisticated. You haven't seen anything yet. In the next lab, we will calculate the cost-effectiveness of health insurance in the United States!

Cost-Effectiveness Rankings

Category	Strategy	Cost	Incr Cost	Eff	Incr eff	Incr C/E (ICER)	NMB	C/E
◢ Excluding dominated								
undominated	Filmore	0.00		73.87			2954721.50	0.00
undominated	Reinkenshein	10000.00	10000.00	76.87	3.00	3329.08	3064874.80	130.09
◢ All								
undominated	Filmore	0.00		73.87			2954721.50	0.00
undominated	Reinkenshein	10000.00	10000.00	76.87	3.00	3329.08	3064874.80	130.09
◢ All referencing common baseline								
undominated	Filmore	0.00		73.87			2954721.50	0.00
undominated	Reinkenshein	10000.00	10000.00	76.87	3.00	3329.08	3064874.80	130.09
◢ All by Increasing effectiveness								
undominated	Filmore	0.00		73.87			2954721.50	0.00
undominated	Reinkenshein	10000.00		76.87			3064874.80	130.09

Figure 13.57 Rankings Output Comparing the Cost-Effectiveness of Rinkenshein and Filmore Procedures

Table 13.1 Results of the Base-Case Analysis

Strategy	Cost	Incremental Cost	Effectiveness	Incremental Effectiveness	Incremental C/E (ICER)
Filmore	$0K		73.9 years		
Rinkenshein	$10K	$10K	76.9 years	3.0 years	**$3,329**

Laboratory Exercise Three: The Cost-Effectiveness of Health Insurance

In this lab, we will (more or less) replicate a published CEA model that calculates the cost-effectiveness of providing health insurance to the uninsured in the United States. This model and the influenza model from the book will be used for all subsequent lab exercises.

The point of this exercise is not for you to learn how to gather the data but, rather, how to become comfortable with Markov models, working with tables, and calculating changes in life expectancy.

The assumption is that you have the basics of the TreeAge Pro program down. You should now be able to add the necessary structure, formulas, mortality tables, conditionals, and so forth. Ready to dive in?

Step 1. Background. Read the article "The Cost-Effectiveness of Health Insurance, by P. Muennig, P. Franks, and M. R. Gold (*American Journal of Preventive Medicine,* 2005, 28: 59–64).

Step 2. New Tree. Save the changes you've made to the Exercise Two model, your Filmore-versus-Rinkenshein decision tree. Then use File > Save As . . . to create a new copy (e.g., "Exercise #3.trex"), to which we'll make extensive changes.

Rename the competing alternatives (decision node's branches) to read "Insurance" and "No Insurance." In the "Insurance" strategy, take out the part of the probability expression reflecting the adjusted mortality risk of treating the congenital heart valve disease population with the Filmore procedure (i.e., delete the "1.25 *" factor in front of the tDead2000[age] table reference). Your model should look like Figure 13.58.

Step 3. Age-Indexed Tables. The cost and effectiveness values from Table 2 in the article must be entered in age-indexed tables for use in the tree (Table 13.2). The tree will be comparing "Insurance" (the Predicted column) against "No Insurance" (the Uninsured column).

Important: *The annual costs of insuring the uninsured, along with their health-related quality of life, can be found in the last column, "Predicted," in Table 13.2.* How does this work? The uninsured population tends to be less healthy than the general/insured population. Providing health insurance to the uninsured will not suddenly raise their health to the level of the insured population, however.

The researchers calculated the "Predicted" group's resulting higher-than-average health expenditures, for example, by taking a regression analysis that examines expenditures among the *already insured* (i.e., column

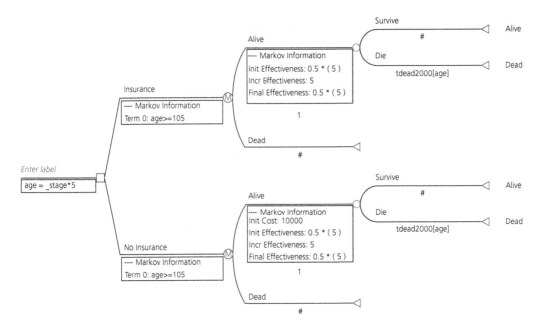

Figure 13.58   Insurance Versus No Insurance Competing Alternatives Model

1 in Table 13.2), and entering the sociodemographic characteristics of the *uninsured* population.

For example, the expenditures of the insured can be thought of as:

$$\text{Expenditures} = \beta 1 * \text{income} + \beta 2 * \text{region of residence}$$
$$+ \beta 3 * \text{marital status} + \beta 4 * \text{self-rated health}$$
$$+ \beta 5 * \text{race} + \beta 6 * \text{gender}$$
$$+ \beta 7 * \text{age} + \beta 8 * \text{education} \qquad (13.1)$$

Changing these characteristics to those of the uninsured (save for health insurance status) gives the predicted expenditures among the previously uninsured once they have health insurance. As you can see from Table 13.2, predicted expenditures tend to be higher than those of the already insured, particularly as you look at older age groups.

The HRQL health quality scores were obtained in a similar way. Average health quality tends to decrease as individuals age, but it declines more slowly in the insured, and is predicted to do so in the newly insured. (Remember that one year lived with an HRQL score of 0.8 is treated as equivalent to 0.8 year of life lived in perfect health.) Our tree will thus be calculating quality-adjusted life expectancy (based on QALYs), rather than simple life expectancy.

Table 13.2   Age-Indexed Tables for Use in the New Tree

	Age Group	Insured (1)	Uninsured (2)	Predicted (3)
Expenditures	25-34	$1,169	$326	$1,193
	35-44	$1,543	$519	$1,613
	45-54	$1,935	$742	$2,219
	55-64	$2,820	$2,280	$3,385
HRQL score	25-34	0.92	0.88	0.88
	35-44	0.9	0.84	0.86
	45-54	0.87	0.79	0.83
	55-64	0.84	0.73	0.78
Mortality	25-34	0.001	0.002	0.001
	35-44	0.002	0.003	0.002
	45-54	0.006	0.009	0.006
	55-64	0.012	0.02	0.013

Source: Muennig, et al. (2005).

Also note the predicted improvements in the two-year mortality risks. Rather than worry about using the actual mortality values presented in Table 13.2, however, we will use an age-adjusted hazard rate that reflects the data in the table.

Let's create some tables now. The first table is cInsurance[ ], for predicted costs of providing health insurance, and the second is cNoinsurance[ ], for healthcare costs of the uninsured. The third table is uInsurance[ ], for health utility among the newly insured, and the forth is uNoinsurance[ ]. To add tables, go to the Values menu and Tables View (Figure 13.59). Click on the green cross button ("Add new table") and type in the name of the third table "uInsurance" (Figure 13.60).

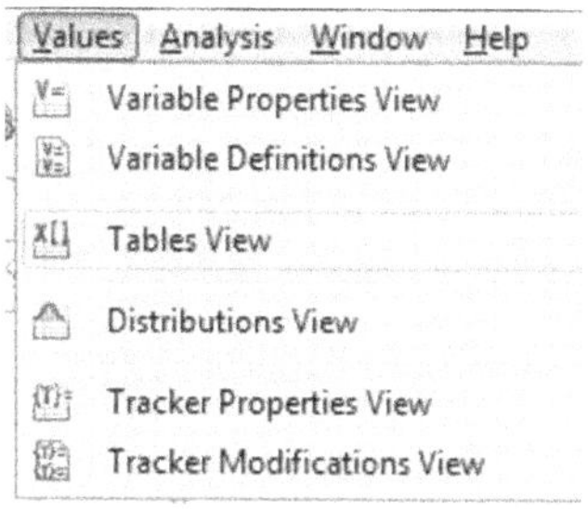

Figure 13.59   Adding Tables Under the Tables View Option

1. Select "Add new table"

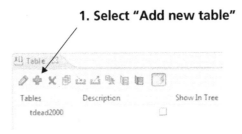

2. Enter name of the new table, "uInsurance"

Figure 13.60   Adding a New Table Under the Add/Change Box

When you click OK, the new table name appears in the Tables window along with `tdead2000` (Figure 13.61).

For missing rows, we want TreeAge Pro to use linear interpolation, which is the default setting. This tells TreeAge Pro to basically draw a linear function between existing table rows when looking up ages not explicitly listed in the index column.

TreeAge does not accept a range of age indexes for each row, but requires a single numeric index. In this case, you should use the average age in the range of ages from a row in Table 13.2. The interpretation is that the midpoint age is associated with the cost or utility value in the

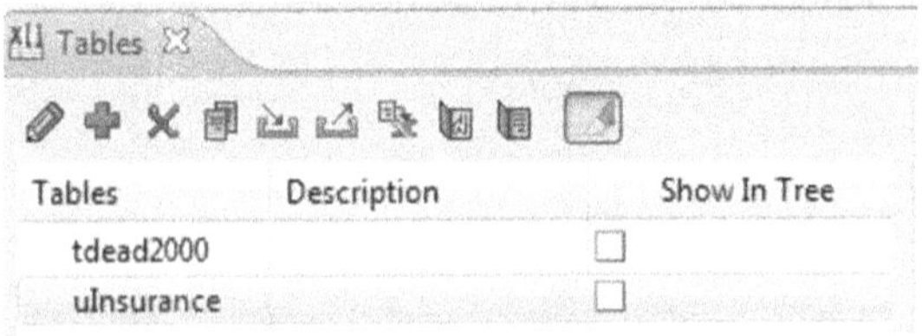

Figure 13.61   The New Table, cInsurance, Is Not Listed in the Tables Window

table, and ages found between two midpoints (i.e., missing rows) will use linear interpolation. Thus, the first entry for the uInsurance table should use an Index of 30 (the average age in the 25–34 age group) with a Value of 0.88 (the average HRQL for this group). Click on the green cross button on the "Table Rows: uInsurance" panel to the right of the Tables window (Figure 13.62). Input the index age of 30 and the value of 0.88. Repeat this process for the other age categories, as demonstrated in Figure 13.63.

The four tables will look like Figure 13.63.

Step 4. Numeric Format. Before we forget, we should update the tree preferences to present effectiveness output in terms of HRQL. From the Edit menu, choose "Numeric Formatting." Go to the "For Effectiveness" panel and change the Units to "Custom suffix" and in the Prefix/suffix settings enter "QALYs" (Figure 13.64).

Step 5. Hazard Ratio. Now let's create a variable called "HR," which stands for the mortality *hazard ratio* of having "No Insurance" relative to "Insurance." This is equal to 1.66, which we get from Table 4 in the Muennig et al. article (and which looks like what is reflected in Table 13.2, as well). Where does this go in the model? The risk of mortality for the uninsured is higher than that predicted for the newly insured. Therefore, we'll use it as some kind of multiplier for the mortality in the *uninsured branch* (like the "1.25" factor in Exercise Two).

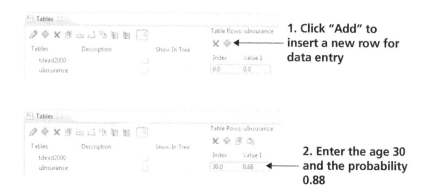

1. Click "Add" to insert a new row for data entry

2. Enter the age 30 and the probability 0.88

Figure 13.62 Including Values for a User-Defined Table

Table Rows: cInsurance		Table Rows: cNoInsurance		Table Rows: uInsurance		Table Rows: uNoInsurance	
Index	Value 1	Index	Value 1	Index	Value 1	Index	Value 1
30.0	1,193.0	30.0	326.0	30.0	0.88	30.0	0.88
40.0	1,613.0	40.0	519.0	40.0	0.86	40.0	0.84
50.0	2,219.0	50.0	742.0	50.0	0.83	50.0	0.79
60.0	3,385.0	60.0	2,280.0	60.0	0.78	60.0	0.73

Figure 13.63 Completed Tables for Costs and HRQL for Those Who Are Insured and Not Insured

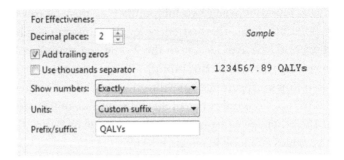

Figure 13.64   Changing the Effectiveness Units to "QALYs"

Take a moment to think about this approach. We are not using mortality data from Table 13.2. Rather, we are using mortality data for the U.S. population in general, which consists of both insured and uninsured persons. Because the uninsured were just 15 percent of the population in 2000, this approach is good enough to generate an estimate, but we would want to compare the actual uninsured population with the actual insured population before publishing this work.

A hazard ratio is technically a rate ratio, to be multiplied against a baseline rate rather than a probability. Rather than the brute force Min() function, let's use the ProbToProb() function this time. It converts a given probability to a rate, multiplies that by a given factor, and converts back to a probability. This is important with larger probabilities, such as the five-year mortality probabilities for older age groups. The new probability expression should be:

```
ProbToProb(tDead2000[age]; HR)
```

TIPS AND TRICKS

To accomplish this change you cannot simply paste this new function over the old one. Think about what you are trying to accomplish and remember that, unlike the last example in Laboratory Exercise Two, the top branch has unchanged mortality and the lower branch is the intervention leading to increased comparative mortality. Therefore, this function should be copied into the "Die" branch of the Uninsured Markov subtree

To create a new variable, go to the Values tab and select "Variables Properties View." This opens the Variables Properties window that contains all the variables in your model. Click on the green cross button ("Add/Change Variable"). The Add/Change Variable window appears, where you can enter the name, description, and values for the variable. Name the variable "HR" and enter the value "1.66," as shown in Figure 13.65. (You can also enter a short description

1. Enter the name and description

2. Enter the value 1.66

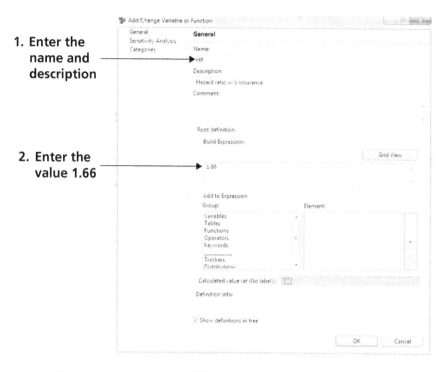

Figure 13.65   Creating a New Variable Called "HR" and Defining Its Value

of the variable, "Hazard ratio w/o insurance." It's helpful for keeping track of all the variables in the model.)

Step 6. Next, let's add references to the various tables in the right places. To make things easier on whoever may look at our model, let's use a few more variables this time. Remember from Laboratory Exercise One that we defined a formula for the "age" variable, using the Values > Variable Properties window. Let's go back to that dialog (Figure 13.66). In the Variables Properties window highlight "age" and click on the pencil icon ("Edit"). You can create formulas in the Build Expression dialog box. We will create new variables with formulas using the Build Expression dialog box.

In the Variables List, click on the green cross button ("Add new variable/function") to create four new variables: "cInsurance5yr," "cNoInsurance5yr," "uInsurance5yr," and "uNoInsurance5yr." The definitions to enter into the Build Expression dialog box are illustrated in Figure 13.67.

Our cycle length in each Markov subtree is five years—remember, the mortality table gave five-year mortality probabilities. The cost and utility tables, however, give one-year averages. So we must set the cost reward expressions to be "5*(age-specific cost)," for example. By

1. Click on the pencil icon

2. Change the formula here

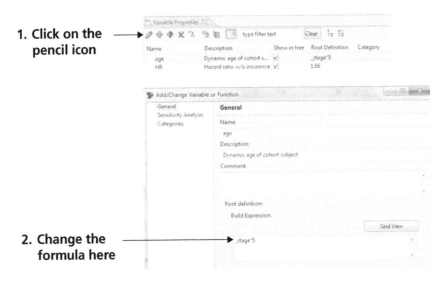

Figure 13.66   Defining the Value for "age" Under the Variables Properties Window

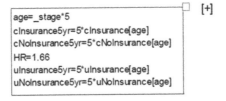

```
age=_stage*5
cInsurance5yr=5*cInsurance[age]
cNoInsurance5yr=5*cNoInsurance[age]
HR=1.66
uInsurance5yr=5*uInsurance[age]
uNoInsurance5yr=5*uNoInsurance[age]
```

[+]

Figure 13.67   Formula for the Four New Variables

multiplying inside the variable formulas, we will avoid cluttering the Markov state reward information with these extra details.

Once we use these variable names in the tree, their formulas will be recalculated many times during an analysis, as required by the Markov state reward calculations. Utilities will decrease and costs will increase as the _stage counter increments and the population ages.

Now go to each Markov subtree's "Alive" state, and edit the state reward information. We need to make very certain that each strategy uses the appropriate variable/table, of course. Similar to Laboratory Exercise Two, we can enter unit cost and utility reward expressions in the "Incremental" reward box, and click the "Half-Cycle Correct" button (Figure 13.68). You will need to first complete this step for the Insured Markov subtree and then repeat it for the Uninsured Markov subtree using the cNoInsurance5yr and uNoInsurance5yr variables. (Remember to click on the pencil icon to open the Define Reward Set for the Alive state.)

Step 7. Test the Model. WOW! That was easy. Anyone can become a super modeler. See how easy it was in the end? Your tree should look like Figure 13.69. (If you don't get the same results and your tree looks exactly

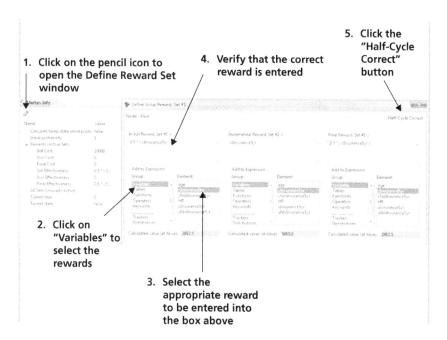

1. **Click on the pencil icon to open the Define Reward Set window**

4. **Verify that the correct reward is entered**

5. **Click the "Half-Cycle Correct" button**

2. **Click on "Variables" to select the rewards**

3. **Select the appropriate reward to be entered into the box above**

Figure 13.68 Adding the Half-Cycle Correction Factor for the Initial and Final Stages

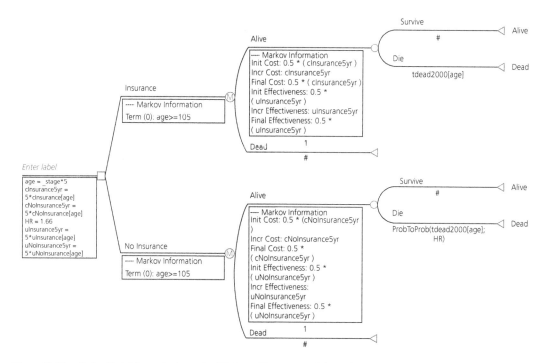

Figure 13.69 Markov Model Comparing Insured and Uninsured Strategies with the Updated Variables and Tables

like the one in Figure 13.69, check your tables to make sure the data is correctly entered.)

Step 8. Now let's evaluate the tree. Instead of clicking on the little beach ball, make sure to select "Rankings" from the Analysis menu. TreeAge provides an output that is similar to the one in Laboratory Exercise Two (Figure 13.70). (Also as in Exercise Two, the output provides the same answers because there are only two comparators.)

Table 13.3 is the CEA text report with base-case results.

Not a bad deal! Pay $14K for each year of life gained? I'm in. (Since this is quality adjusted, it means per year of perfect health, really. It would translate to *less* than $14K per year of average HRQL.)

As you might have suspected after reading the article, we are not done yet.

Step 9. Discounting values. Recall that all future values in a CEA should be discounted to their present value. As the Markov process moves into the future, we want to discount all costs and effectiveness values back to present values, at 3 percent per year. There is a built-in discounting

Cost-Effectiveness Rankings

Category	Strategy	Cost	Incr Cost	Eff	Incr eff	Incr C/E (ICER)	NMB	C/E
⏴ Excluding dominated								
undominated	No Insurance	63951.99		58.26			2266428.23	1097.71
undominated	Insurance	156605.90	92653.91	64.65	6.39	14501.67	2429341.80	2422.41
⏴ All								
undominated	No Insurance	63951.99		58.26			2266428.23	1097.71
undominated	Insurance	156605.90	92653.91	64.65	6.39	14501.67	2429341.80	2422.41
⏴ All referencing common baseline								
undominated	No Insurance	63951.99		58.26			2266428.23	1097.71
undominated	Insurance	156605.90	92653.91	64.65	6.39	14501.67	2429341.80	2422.41
⏴ All by Increasing effectiveness								
undominated	No Insurance	63951.99		58.26			2266428.23	1097.71
undominated	Insurance	156605.90		64.65			2429341.80	2422.41

Figure 13.70   Rankings Output Comparing Insurance to No Insurance

Table 13.3   Base-Case Results for the Markov Model

Strategy	Cost	Incremental Cost	Effectiveness	Incremental Effectiveness	Incremental C/E (ICER)
Uninsured	$64K		58.3 QALYs		
Insured	$157K	$93K	64.6 QALYs	6.4 QALYs	$14,502

Note: "Eff" and "Incr Eff" are rounded based on tree's numeric formatting.

function in TreeAge Pro called, appropriately enough, Discount. It takes the syntax "Discount(value_to_discount; rate; years)."

No changes need to be made directly to the Markov states, since we encapsulated the reward expressions in the four variables earlier. Only the definitions need to be changed (Figure 13.71). Compare this to Figure 13.67.

To accomplish these changes you have to also define "rate" as a new variable equal to .03. Once you have created the new variable "rate," you can review all the variables in the Markov model in the Variable Properties window (Figure 13.72).

Now select Analysis > Rankings and see what you get for discounted cost-effectiveness. Table 13.4 summarizes the base-case results for the Markov model after applying a 3 percent discount rate. (The TreeAge Pro output is omitted for this analysis.)

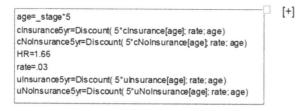

```
age=_stage*5
cInsurance5yr=Discount( 5*cInsurance[age]; rate; age)
cNoInsurance5yr=Discount( 5*cNoInsurance[age]; rate; age)
HR=1.66
rate=.03
uInsurance5yr=Discount( 5*uInsurance[age]; rate; age)
uNoInsurance5yr=Discount( 5*uNoInsurance[age]; rate; age)
```
[+]

Figure 13.71   Tree Properties with the Addition of a Discount Rate

Variable Properties

Name	Description	Show in tree	Root Definition
age	Dynamic age of cohort s...	✓	_stage*5
cInsurance5yr		✓	Discount(5*cInsurance[age]; rate; age)
cNoInsurance5yr		✓	Discount(5*cNoInsurance[age]; rate; age)
HR	Hazard ratio w/o insurance	✓	1.66
rate	Discount rate	✓	0.03
uInsurance5yr		✓	Discount(5*uInsurance[age]; rate; age)
uNoInsurance5yr		✓	Discount(5*uNoInsurance[age]; rate; age)

Figure 13.72   All the Variables That Are Used in the Current Markov Model

Table 13.4   Base-Case Results After Applying a 3 Percent Discount Rate

Strategy	Cost	Incremetal Cost	Effectiveness	Incremental Effectiveness	Incremental C/E (ICER)
Uninsured	$16K		24.8 QALYs		
Insured	$46K	$30K	25.7 QALYs	1.0 QALYs	**$30,386**

Note: "Eff" and "Incr Eff" are rounded based on the tree's numeric formatting.

What does this mean relative to the undiscounted results? In the discounted CEA, we are more heavily weighting *early* life expectancy gains (reduced mortality in the young), and also more heavily weighting costs that we can't put off far into the future.

Overall, insurance is still a good deal. Boom! You're done. You may still be wondering, however, why you got $30K per QALY gained rather than the $35K per QALY gained in the Muennig et al. article. There are a number of reasons for this. First, in the exercise we did not use age-specific mortality rates from the uninsured and predicted insured population (we just added an HR to the overall mortality in the general U.S. population). Second, we did not make little adjustments, such as adding the predicted administrative costs associated with health insurance. Rather, we just used actual expenditures at the doctor's office. Finally, the model here contains an error related to the study population—we'll deal with this last issue in the next exercise.

Laboratory Exercise Four: Sensitivity Analysis

At the end of the last lab, your discounted CEA rankings looked like Table 13.4.

We ended Laboratory Exercise Three by telling you that the model contained a small error related to the study population. The error is that we did not address the demographics of the cohort.

Step 1. Final Adjustments. The missing demographic piece of information was the *subjects' age*. As it stands, the model estimates lifetime costs and QALYs, starting from birth, and the Insured strategy assumes insurance is paid for from birth until death. What we actually want to do is model 25-year-olds and insure them up to their sixty-fifth birthday. Most people stay on their parents' insurance until reaching adulthood. Later in life, at age 65, Medicare coverage kicks in. We want to model this critical window of time when many people are uninsured, from age 25 to age 65.

So where to begin? Recall that the variable age was set equal to the _stage counter times the cycle length of five (years). To start off at age 25, we can change it to: age = 25 + _stage*5. Figure 13.73 illustrates how to do this.

Now our subjects will enter the model at age 25 (when _stage=0). They will be exposed to the costs within the 25–35 age category first. The tables that you created have rows for ages 30, 40, and so on. Since we have turned on linear interpolation, the costs will be gradually increased as they age (every one cycle or five years), while the HRQL score table will interpolate downward. But what happens when subjects pass age 65? At that point,

1. Select the definition   **2. Enter the new definition**

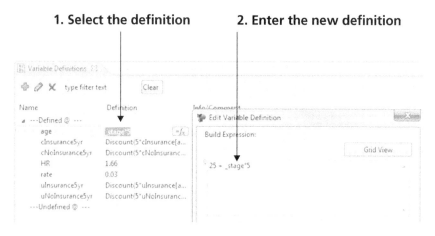

Figure 13.73   Changing the Start Age at the Decision Node

they go merrily on, tabulating the costs and HRQL of 65-year-olds (only their mortality goes up).

The simplest way to fix the problem in our model is to terminate calculations when subjects hit age 65. Change the termination condition at both Markov nodes to "age > 65," as illustrated by Figure 13.74.

Determine the incremental cost-effectiveness ratio by highlighting the blue decision node and going to Analysis > Ranking. You should get the results presented in Table 13.5.

Note that these cost and effectiveness values are still discounted—undiscounted, the gain in effectiveness is more like 2.5 QALYS, in other words, equivalent years of perfect health. Also note that such an

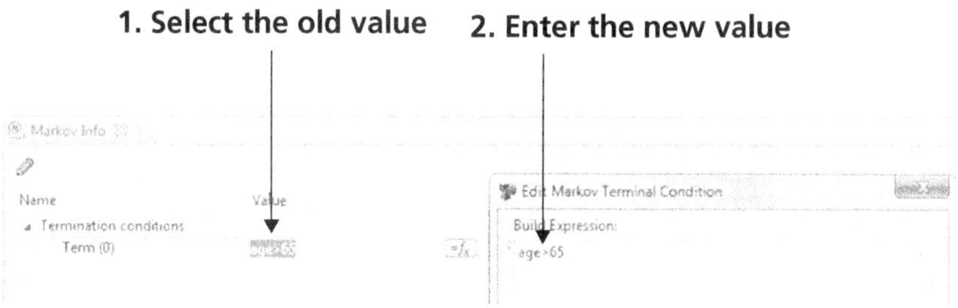

1. Select the old value   **2. Enter the new value**

Figure 13.74   Changing the Termination Conditions for the Insurance and No Insurance Arms of the Markov Model

Table 13.5   Results After Terminating Calculations at Age 65 or Older

Strategy	Cost	Incremental Cost	Effectiveness	Incremental Effectiveness	Incremental C/E (ICER)
Uninsured	$9K		9.2 QALYs		
Insured	$22K	$13K	9.7 QALYs	0.5 QALYs	$26,631

intervention would get some of the credit for improved mortality and morbidity *after* age 65.

Now let's get on with our model.

Step 2. Sensitivity Analysis Variables. Before starting, let's think about which tree variables are actually parameter uncertainties/unknowns, and what happens when we change our assumptions about the value of the uncertainties:

Age. Generally, sensitivity analysis variables are going to be defined as simple numbers; "age" has a formula. We are not concerned with error or uncertainty in age, per se. (In a different sense, we might be interested in what happens to the cost-effectiveness of providing health insurance to the uninsured as the starting age for initiation of coverage is increased. For example, it is the older age groups—e.g., starting with 50-year-olds—that will need and benefit most from things like cancer screening, antihypertensive medications, treatments for type II diabetes, cholesterol-lowering drugs, and so forth. In a different exercise, we could use a variable startAge in place of a fixed value of 25.)

Discount rate. Although this looks like a sensitivity analysis variable with its numeric definition, we are not concerned with error in this parameter. However, it is an important assumption, and it can be interesting and useful to see what happens to the ICER when the discount rate is varied. (Some people argue that discounting should be done at a rate greater than 0.03. Try asking someone if they would prefer to pay you $100 now or $103 a year from now. Chances are, they'll wait to pay unless you increase the rate past their personal discount rate. Others may argue that discounting is unnecessary.)

Hazard ratio. This looks like a candidate for sensitivity analysis, because it is defined numerically. With the HR, there is room for both random and nonrandom error. Nonrandom error includes variables that we did not foresee and control for in our survival analysis. Random error is also likely, given that we obtained the ratio from a subsample of the population. This will be our first clear parameter uncertainty.

Cost of insurance. As with the hazard ratio, there is likely both random and nonrandom error. Since it is an age-dependent function (in a table), sensitivity analysis is a little complicated. We could make a new multiplier variable, with a base value of 1, which could be used to vary cost assumptions proportionally across all age groups.

HRQL. This information is subject to the same kinds of error as costs. There may also be error introduced by the complicated interactions between the components of this measure—for example, age and quality of life. Like costs, this is a function within a table, making sensitivity analysis somewhat complicated.

tDead2000. The mortality rates can contain some error as well. Life expectancy in the United States is generated from death certificate data. Some folks get buried in the backyard without a certificate, while others go home to their country of birth for the big end. It's also the case that there are bureaucratic errors, and so forth. We can take a look at the effects of varying this if we wish, but chances are it won't make much of a difference since it affects both arms of the analysis equally. (This may be true of other mentioned parameters, as well.)

Step 3. One-Way Sensitivity Analysis. To conduct an analysis for the tree, first select the decision node (the blue box), and then choose Analysis > Sensitivity Analysis > 1-Way. The One-Way Sensitivity Analysis Setup window appears (Figure 13.75).

Let's take a look at what happens when we vary the mortality hazard ratio (for the uninsured) between 1.25 and 1.8 (Figure 13.76). Use the dropdown arrow and highlight "HR" from the variables list, then enter the value range in the relevant boxes. (Don't worry about the Intervals option at this point.)

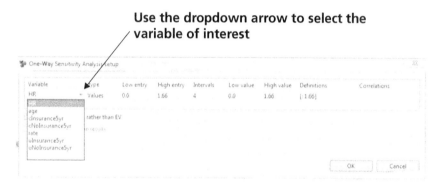

Use the dropdown arrow to select the variable of interest

Figure 13.75   One-Way Sensitivity Analysis Setup Window

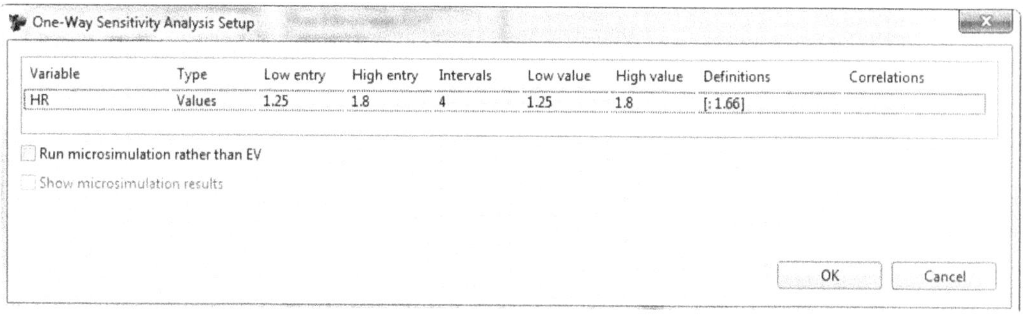

Figure 13.76   Defining Low and High Values for the HR Parameter

Click OK to begin the analysis. Once the recalculations (five of them in this case, if you specified four intervals) are complete, you will be presented with a cost-effectiveness sensitivity analysis output window with a bunch of different options (Figure 13.77). Most of these options we can ignore, but in complex cases they may be useful.

We are primarily interested in the graph of incremental cost-effectiveness (ICERs) at this point (look under "Graph Reports"). If you don't know why, stop! It is critical that you understand this point. Everything we do in CEA is based on comparing how much more effective one intervention is relative to another and how much more you have to pay for the gains. This entails obtaining the incremental cost divided by the incremental effectiveness (ICER).

Two other sensitivity analysis graph options, incremental costs and incremental effectiveness, separately are useful for thinking about the different ways that error/uncertainty in a variable might affect the analysis.

Before we begin, let's explicitly ask: Will the HR have much of an effect on the incremental cost of insuring the uninsured?

If you answered "not much," you were right. Let's take a look at the three incremental functions now. (The graphs can be exported into Excel using the icon in the upper right-hand corner of the graphical output.) (See Figure 13.78.)

The hazard ratio is the driving force behind differences in effectiveness, of course. The only influence it has on costs is to reduce the lifespan of subjects in the Uninsured arm of the analysis. In other words, the HR is greatly increasing the effectiveness of insurance. It is also driving down the costs of the No Insurance option slightly because it is killing people off at a young age.

Sensitivity Cost Effectiveness Analysis

HR	Strategy	Cost	Incr cost	Eff	Incr Eff	ICER	NMB	C/E	Dominance	Actions
▲ 1.25										──── Graph Reports ────
	No Insurance	9048.10	0.00	9.31	0.00	0.00	363387.50	971.78		
	Insurance	21632.78	12584.68	9.65	0.34	36867.12	364457.22	2241.22		Net Benefits (CE Thresholds)
▲ 1.3875										Cost-Effectiveness (animated)
	No Insurance	8944.36	0.00	9.26	0.00	0.00	361549.24	965.67		Cost-Effectiveness (animated, axes inverted)
	Insurance	21632.78	12688.42	9.65	0.39	32542.22	364457.22	2241.22		x vs Avg. Cost
▲ 1.525										x vs Incremental Cost
	No Insurance	8842.71	0.00	9.21	0.00	0.00	359738.89	959.65		
	Insurance	21632.78	12790.07	9.65	0.44	29220.30	364457.22	2241.22		x vs Avg. Eff.
▲ 1.6625										x vs Incremental Eff.
	No Insurance	8743.12	0.00	9.17	0.00	0.00	357955.28	953.71		x vs ICER (Incremental C-E)
	Insurance	21632.78	12889.66	9.65	0.48	26588.37	364457.22	2241.22		x vs Avg. C-E
▲ 1.8										
	No Insurance	8645.51	0.00	9.12	0.00	0.00	356198.49	947.86		
	Insurance	21632.78	12987.26	9.65	0.53	24451.42	364457.22	2241.22		

Figure 13.77   Cost-Effectiveness Sensitivity Analysis Output Window

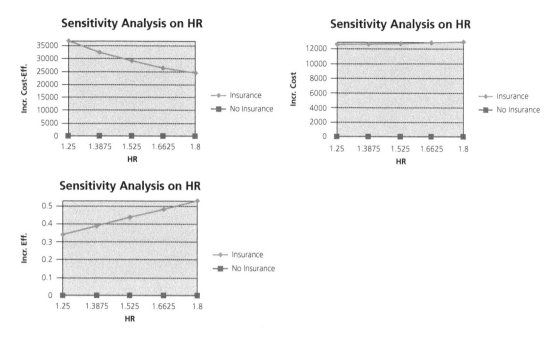

Figure 13.78   Results of the One-Way Sensitivity Analyses

Step 3. Set Up Tables for Sensitivity Analysis. What about the tables we included to estimate costs, utility, and baseline mortality? One way to conduct a one-way analysis on table values is to simply multiply the table lookup by an error term. If you create a variable called `cError`, for example, you can multiply the cost table references by the error term.

For instance, the cost of health insurance becomes:

```
Discount(5*cInsurance[age]*cError; rate; age)
```

and `cError` assumes a range of high and low percentile differences for `cInsurance`. For instance, if you think that the highest plausible value of `cInsurance` is 15 percent higher than the values you calculated, then `cError` has a high value of 1.15. Let's assume that the low value is about 85 percent of the baseline value. Give this a try.

Doing this with the HRQL tables is more complicated. For example, multiplying a utility of .92 by 115 percent would give a value greater than 1 (better than perfect). That is not our intent. What would make more sense would be to change the expressions a little, in order to multiply the *disutility* by the multiplier, and then subtract from 1. For example:

```
Discount(5*(1-((1-uInsurance[age])*uError)); rate; age)
```

Click on the green cross icon to open the "Add/Change Distribution" window

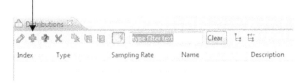

Figure 13.79 Creating a New Distribution Variable

Another way of dealing with table sensitivity analysis is to create more complex tables with high and low value columns for each parameter/age group.

Step 4. Probabilistic Sensitivity Analysis. In Chapter 9, you learned that each parameter estimate is associated with a probability distribution of values. Suppose that you conducted an analysis that required medical costs to be included. If the most likely real-world cost of a medical visit was obtained from MEPS, it will be associated with random error that is most likely normally distributed around a mean. Thus, if the value is $75 and the standard deviation is $15, there is only a 5 percent chance of observing a value as low as $45 or as high as $105.

In a second-order Monte Carlo simulation, TreeAge Pro samples parameter values from every distribution you use in tree formulas. Before you start, though, you will need to tell TreeAge Pro what you want these distributions to look like.

To define a distribution for the hazard ratio parameter, click on the decision node where HR is defined. Go to Values > Distributions View. Create a new distribution by clicking on the green cross icon. The "Add/Change Distribution" window appears (Figure 13.79).

First, enter a name for the distribution, "`dist_HR`" for the hazard ratio distribution. Then select a distribution from the list in Figure 13.80. In the Distribution list, select the "Triangular" distribution type for now (a more realistic HR distribution might be "Lognormal," but we'll keep it simple for this exercise).

Enter the familiar values already associated for the HR variable (min=1.25, mode=1.66, max=1.8). Click OK. Then click Values > Variable Properties, and edit the HR variable. In the Build Expression panel, delete the value that's there (1.66) and replace it with the distribution "`dist_HR`," just as in Figure 13.81.

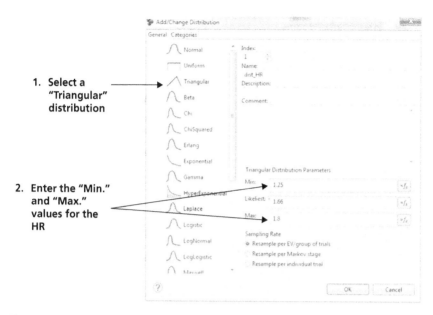

1. Select a "Triangular" distribution

2. Enter the "Min." and "Max." values for the HR

Figure 13.80   Add/Change Distribution Window

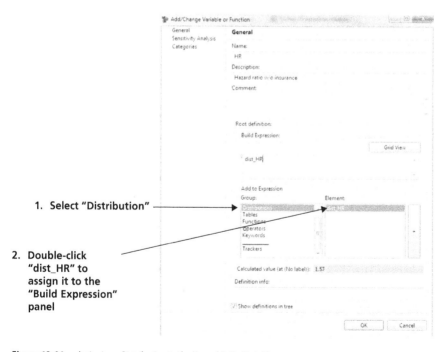

1. Select "Distribution"

2. Double-click "dist_HR" to assign it to the "Build Expression" panel

Figure 13.81   Assigning a Distribution to the Hazard Ratio Variable

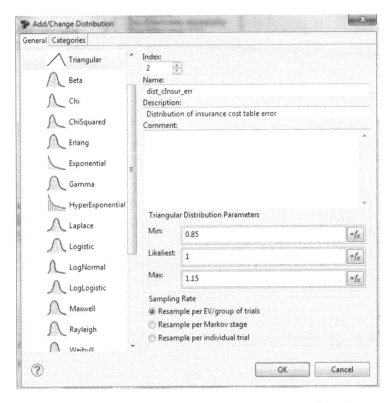

Figure 13.82   Creating Another Distribution Called "dist_cInsur_err" Using a Triangular Distribution

We have just told TreeAge Pro to assign a value to HR of no less than 1.25, no more than 1.8, and most likely around 1.66, our baseline estimate. Note that the Triangular mean value is not going to be 1.66, but is (min + mode + max)/3, or about 1.56.

Now let's move on and do something similar for other uncertain parameters in the model. So we don't want to do this with age or with rate, but we can do it for any table error terms in the model (Figure 13.82). For example, cError might be a symmetric Triangular distribution between 0.85 and 1.15.

Let's create another new distribution called "dist_cInsur_err" for the error associated with the costs of the Insurance group. Go to Values > Distribution View and click on the green cross icon to bring up the Add/Change Distribution window. In the name field, enter "dist_cInsur_err" and then select the "Triangular" distribution. Then enter the "Min" as 0.85, the "Max" as 1.15, and the "Likeliest" as 1.0 (Figure 13.83).

Do this for another distribution and name it "dist_cNoInsur_err" using the same values. When you are finished, there should be three distributions in the "Distributions" window (Figure 13.83).

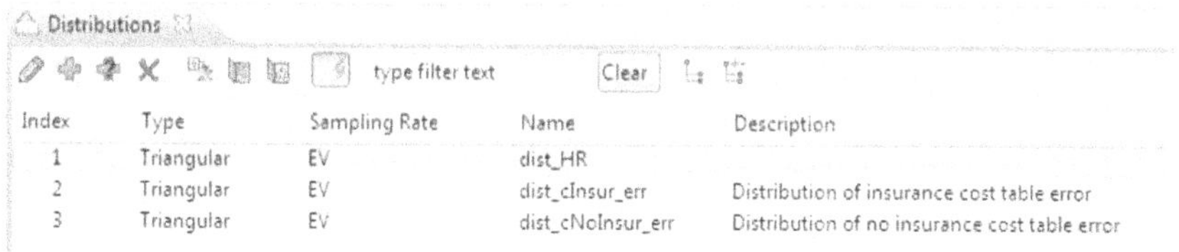

Figure 13.83   Distributions for Three Variables (HR, cInsur, and cNoInsur) in the Model

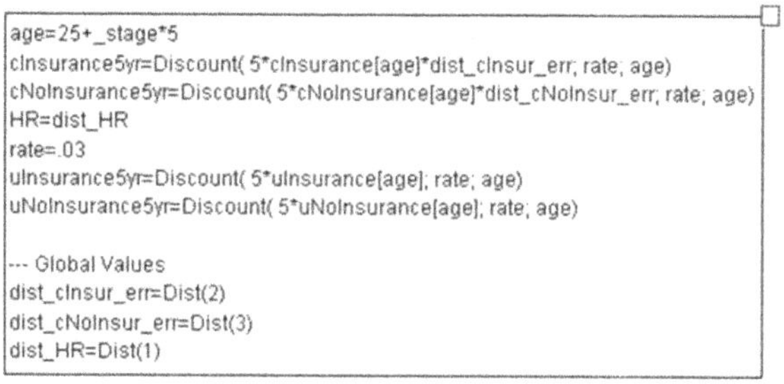

```
age=25+_stage*5
cInsurance5yr=Discount( 5*cInsurance[age]*dist_cInsur_err; rate; age)
cNoInsurance5yr=Discount( 5*cNoInsurance[age]*dist_cNoInsur_err; rate; age)
HR=dist_HR
rate=.03
uInsurance5yr=Discount( 5*uInsurance[age]; rate; age)
uNoInsurance5yr=Discount( 5*uNoInsurance[age]; rate; age)

--- Global Values
dist_cInsur_err=Dist(2)
dist_cNoInsur_err=Dist(3)
dist_HR=Dist(1)
```

Figure 13.84   Tree Properties with the Inclusion of Distributions

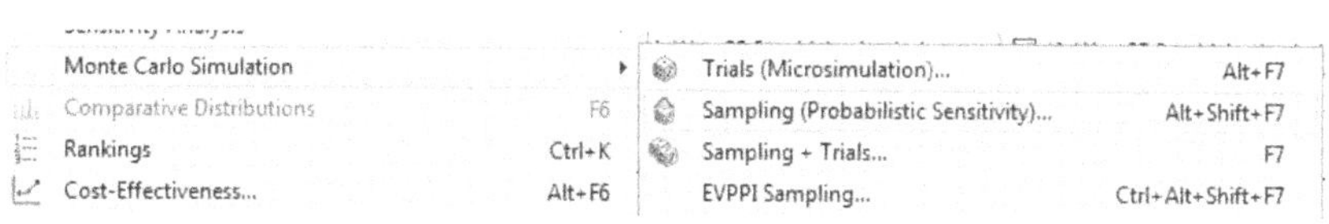

Figure 13.85   Selecting the Probabilistic Sensitivity Analysis

When all is said and done, the tree's parameters might look like Figure 13.84.

Now for the big moment.

Go to Analysis > Monte Carlo > Sampling (Probabilistic Sensitivity) . . . (Figure 13.85).

The simulation setup dialog appears at right. Use the default settings generally, but change the Number of samples from 1,000 to 10,000. Click Begin, and the analysis should complete quickly (Figure 13.86).

Each time you run the simulation, you'll get slightly different statistics because we are getting a random set of samples.

The simulation output includes an overwhelming number of graphs and reports to choose from. We can ignore most of them for now. On the right side of the output, there is a list of "Actions" that can be selected. Go to Charts > Output Distributions > . . . ICER (Figure 13.87). Expand the . . . ICER dropdown arrow and select "Insurance v. No Insurance." A window will appear asking "How many bars approximately do you want to graph?" Enter "1."

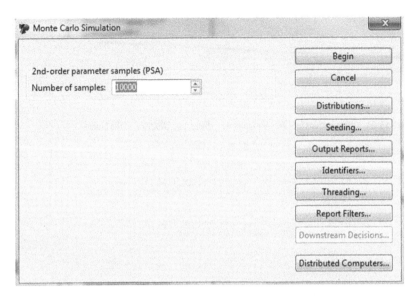

Figure 13.86   Monte Carlo Simulation Options Window

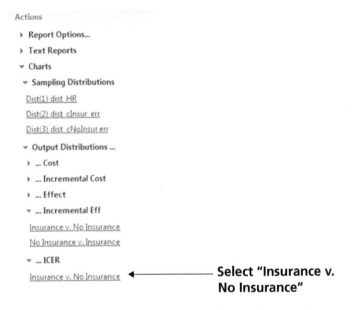

Figure 13.87   Selecting Incremental CE Ratio Output from the Monte Carlo Simulation Results Window

The probabilistic sensitivity analysis run only on the distributions of the hazard ratio and the cost error terms should look something like Figure 13.88.

Let's plot the ICER on the cost-effectiveness plane. This will provide more information about the scatterplots of ICER across the different quadrants. Go back to the Monte Carlo Simulations tab and to the Actions

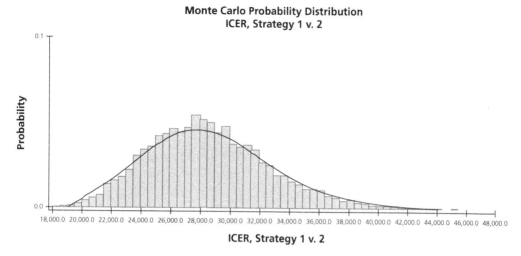

Figure 13.88   Distributions of ICERs Comparing Insurance Versus No Insurance Varying the Hazard Ratio and Cost Error Terms

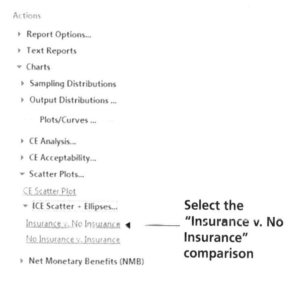

Figure 13.89   Selecting the ICER Scatterplot Comparing Insurance to No Insurance

window. Go to the Plots/Curves … and select Scatter Plots … > ICE Scatter + Ellipses …, and choose "Insurance v. No Insurance" (Figure 13.89).

Leave the willingness to pay as $40,000 per QALYs gained, and start from "1" and end at "1000." The ICER scatterplots are mostly below the willingness-to-pay threshold of $40,000 per QALY gained (Figure 13.90). This is an indication that Insurance is cost-effective up to a willingness-to-pay threshold of $40,000 per QALY gained.

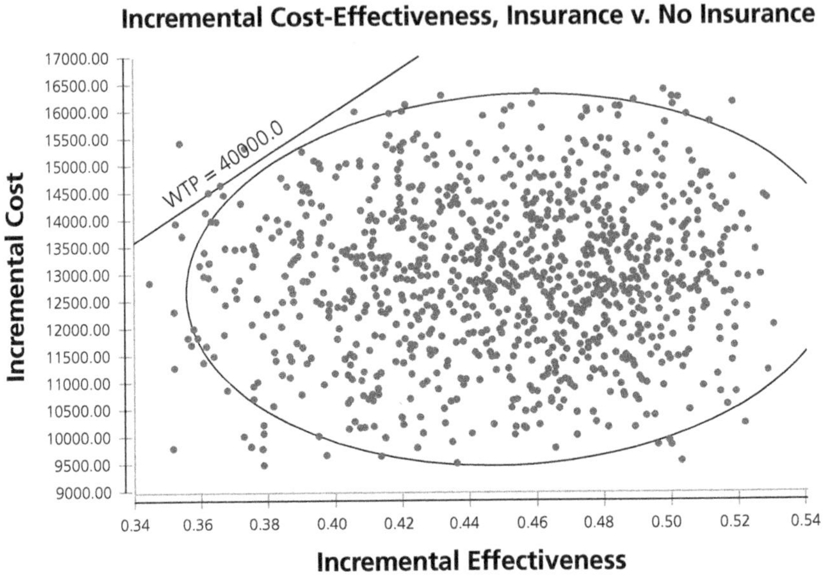

Figure 13.90   ICER Scatterplot Comparing Insurance to No Insurance

Incremental CE Plot Report

COMPONENT	QUADRANT	INCREFF	INCRCOST	INCRCE	FREQUENCY	PROPORTION
C1	IV	IE>0	IC<0	Superior	0	0
C2	I	IE>0	IC>0	ICER<40000.0	9,938	0.9938
C3	III	IE<0	IC<0	ICER>40000.0	0	0
C4	I	IE>0	IC>0	ICER>40000.0	62	0.0062
C5	III	IE<0	IC<0	ICER<40000.0	0	0
C6	II	IE<0	IC>0	Inferior	0	0
Indiff	origin	IE=0	IC=0	0/0	0	0

Figure 13.91   Proportion of ICER Scatterplots Below the Willingness-to-Pay Threshold of $40,000 per QALY Gained

Go to the Reports panel and click on "ICE Report." This will give you the proportion of ICER scatterplots that is below the willingness-to-pay threshold of $40,000 per QALY gained. According to the ICE Report, more than 99 percent of the ICER scatterplots were below the willingness-to-pay threshold (Figure 13.91).

Another graph that would be helpful is the Cost-Effectiveness Acceptability Curve. Return to the Monte Carlo Simulations tab and to the Actions window. Go to the Plots/Curves . . . and select CE Acceptability . . . > Acceptability Curve, and keep the default settings (Figure 13.92).

The Cost-Effectiveness Acceptability Curve shows two plots (Insurance and No Insurance). The two Cost-Effectiveness Acceptability Curves cross

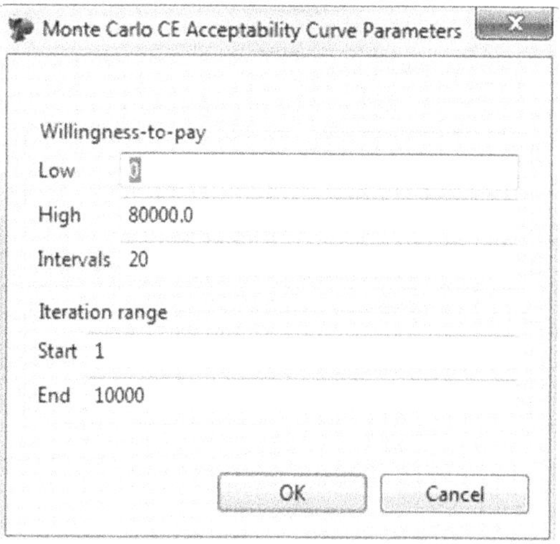

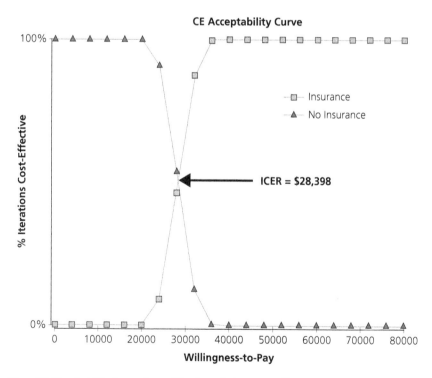

Figure 13.92   Cost-Effectiveness Acceptability Curve Parameter Window

CE Acceptability Curve

Figure 13.93   Cost-Effectiveness Acceptability Curves for Insurance and No Insurance

each other at 50 percent on the *y*-axis (Figure 13.93). The intersection on the *x*-axis is approximately at a willingness-to-pay level of $28,389, which is close to the ICER that was calculated in Table 13.5. (The ICER was determined by going to the Monte Carlo Simulation Report, then to the

Actions panel > CE Analysis > CE graph > Text Report.) Therefore, a consumer with a willingness to pay that is greater than $28,389 per QALY will consider Insurance cost-effective compared to No Insurance. That's because at a higher willingness to pay, you get the additional benefits of Insurance over No Insurance; however, this comes at a higher cost. If the consumer was not willing to spend a dime on Insurance, then forgoing insurance is a cost-effective strategy for that person.

You are encouraged to play around with the other graphing options, such as the ellipsoidal map of ICER points and Excel spreadsheet exports.

And that's it. You are done. You have now built and evaluated a Markov model.

Summary

In the laboratories in this chapter, you were introduced to TreeAge Pro and its many features. More important, the laboratories walked you through the development, construction, and analysis of two comparable treatments using a Markov model. Even though TreeAge Pro performs a lot of the heavy lifting, it is not a substitute for good research practice. A good cost-effectiveness analysis will contain lessons from this book, but it is up to you to make sure that you have a good scientific question, choose the best design for answering it, and then present your results to stakeholders. With practice, you will be able to submit your work to conferences and, eventually, for publication. We look forward to reading your future work.

ANSWER KEY TO EXERCISES

Chapter 1

1. The total cost of Staphbegone is $12,000 + $1,000/day × 5 days = $17,000. The total cost of Staphbeilln is $4,000 + $1,000/day × 10 days = $14,000. The incremental cost of Staphbegone is therefore $17,000 − $14,000 = $3,000.

2. The incremental cost is $17,000 − $14,000 = $3,000, and the incremental effectiveness is 35 QALYs − 34.5 QALYs = 0.5 QALYs. Therefore, the incremental cost-effectiveness is $3,000 ÷ 0.5 QALYs = $6,000 per QALY gained.

3. 1,000 ÷ 375 per QALY gained = 2.67 QALYs gained.

4. The mosquito net strategy will purchase $1,000 ÷ $846 per QALY gained = 1.18 QALYs. The measles strategy will purchase $1,000 ÷ $375 per QALY gained = 2.67 QALYs. The number of QALYs forgone is equal to 2.67 QALYs − 1.18 QALYs = 1.49 QALYs.

Chapter 2

1. To calculate the incremental cost-effectiveness ratio for oseltamivir relative to supportive care, the next most effective intervention is subtracted from the most effective intervention. The incremental cost-effectiveness of providing oseltamivir to persons with influenza is ($100 − $10)/(0.5 − 0.1) = ($90/0.4) = $225 per QALY gained.

2. To calculate the incremental cost-effectiveness ratio, the next most effective intervention is subtracted from the most effective intervention. The incremental cost-effectiveness of vaccination relative to treatment is thus ($150 − $100)/(0.75 − 0.5) = $200 per QALY gained.

3. This question will inform policymakers of the maximum possible benefit that would be realized by vaccinating everyone, with the caveat

that it is not likely that the goal will ever be achieved. It will be relevant in instances in which a law is passed requiring people to receive vaccination but will not have much relevance for a recommendation in favor of vaccination that produces only small increases in vaccination rates.

4. Any costs associated with long-term side effects of the vaccine that affect quality of life. If there is no vaccine-related morbidity that the insurance company might have to pay for, such as side effects from the vaccine, then no morbidity costs are included. However, it may or may not be relevant to include the monetary costs associated with medical care provided to treat minor or short-term side effects. Here, it is critical to distinguish pain and suffering caused by side effects (morbidity costs) from costs associated with medical care consumed secondary to the side effects (direct costs).

5. Rather than use an incremental cost-effectiveness ratio based on QALYs gained, you would need to base it on life-years gained. Costs associated with morbidity will need to be monetized. These costs will now be included in the numerator. In most cases, the time a patient spends ill with disease (for example, lost productivity and leisure time costs) is captured in the HRQL score. However, in this scenario, you will not include an HRQL score in your analysis because you are looking at life-years gained rather than QALYs gained. Therefore, you'll want to come up with some value for the time a patient spends while sick. There is no perfect way to measure such a subjective state, but a conservative approach is to include lost wages, which will go into the numerator of the incremental cost-effectiveness ratio.

Chapter 3

1. In this question, the critical decision you are asked to make is between what is currently thought to be the best practice and something that may or may not be better. Therefore, you want to know how the new drug compares to the antibiotic that most experts think is the optimal choice.

2. The payer perspective is mostly interested in direct costs. Therefore, costs related to the medical care (e.g., cost of vaccination, administration cost, storage, and delivery) and number of hospitalizations prevented should be included. Since this is from the payer's perspective, indirect costs are not measured. If the societal perspective was

used, indirect costs such as worker productivity costs lost due to illness would be used along with direct costs.

3. Vaccines can result in adverse events such as rash, pain at the injection site, and anaphylactic reactions. Some of these adverse events can have significant costs and health risks associated with them that would be of interest in a cost-effectiveness analysis. Events such as Guillain-Barré syndrome can have significant costs and a decrease in health benefits associated with vaccination. One possible sketch would include a pathway for severe adverse reactions associated with vaccination.

Chapter 4

1. Hospitalization cost include many elements. The most common element is the cost for an inpatient stay. This cost includes the resources used to care for the patient during the hospitalization. Nurse's time to administer medication and the physician's time treating the patient may also be included as part of the hospitalization costs. Medications and special procedures are important elements of a hospitalization and should be accounted for.

    If we are looking at this from the patient's perspective, we need to consider other costs.

    First, there is the cost of the patient's time. If the patient spends 10 days in the hospital, the value of his or her time can be quite high. Second, there is the cost of transportation to the hospital. This can be high if the patient was brought in an ambulance, for example. Finally, we might think of home care and so on for someone who was sick enough to be hospitalized. There is no 100 percent right answer to this question; it is designed to help you identify some of the costs associated with each event in an event pathway.

2. Using 2012 data, you should have obtained a mean charge of around $29,000 for influenza virus infection, ICD-9 code 487. The design of this web site changes frequently, and hospitals may have been added, so the number you get may differ slightly.

3. This exercise asks you to place a value on the patient's time and add it to the hospital charge you calculated in Exercise 2. To solve this problem, you will need to figure out the number of days a person spends in the

TIPS AND TRICKS

At the time of the printing of this book in 2015, the United States was still using ICD-9 codes for most public datasets. The rest of the world is mostly using ICD-10 codes.

hospital due to an influenza infection. Using the HCUP data, you can figure this out. Repeat the above exercise but change the "Outcomes and Measures" by clicking on "Length of Stay." Again, the numbers you calculate may have changed slightly, but if you got 4.5 days, then the patient time costs are:

$$4.5 \text{ days} \times \$100 \text{ per day} = \$450.$$

4. To calculate the cost-to-charge ratio, simply locate the Medicare reimbursement and then divide by the Covered Charges. For the DRG code 195, that would be:

$$\$428,954,775 \div \$2,065,184,954 = 0.21.$$

5. Use the HCUP data to figure out the charge for bacterial pneumonia. Use the same process for Exercise 2. The average charge is approximately $31,000 (Don't worry if this is not exactly what you see. As long if it's in the ballpark, the calculation shouldn't change too much).

The Cost-to-Charge ratio is 0.21. Therefore, the total cost for bacterial pneumonia is:

$$\text{Charge} \times \text{Cost-to-Charge Ratio} = \$30,000 \times 0.21 = \$6,300.$$

6. In the following table, we see how costs are inflated from year to year. Note that the correct answer depends on when the original cost of $100 was incurred. If it occurred in January 2011, we would want to inflate the base figure by the 2010 rate of inflation. But here we'll assume it occurred at the end of the year. The cost is $108.84 in 2014 $US after adjusting for inflation.

Year	Percentage Change	
2011		$100
2012	3.7 percent	$100 + (\$100 \times 0.037) = \$103.70$
2013	2.5 percent	$103.70 + (\$103.70 \times 0.025) = \$106.29$
2014	2.4 percent	$106.29 + (\$106.29 \times 0.024) = \$108.84$

Chapter 5

1. Assuming that you only get supportive care if you do not receive a vaccine, the cost of illness is $84. However, if you receive a vaccine, the cost of illness is only $38.

Using these pieces of information, we can estimate the costs of supportive care and vaccination strategies.

The cost of supportive care strategy = 0.01 × $84 = $0.84, or about $1. We can't forget to include the cost of the vaccine, which is $10. The cost of vaccination strategy is about $10 + 0.01 × $38 = $10.30, or about $10.

2. The expected probability can be derived using the probabilities in Figure 5.9. The probability of becoming ill is 0.30, the probability of seeing a doctor is 0.20, and the probability of being hospitalized is 0.01. Therefore, the expected probability is 0.30 × 0.20 × 0.01 = 0.0006 or 0.06%.

3. If that person sees a doctor, she will incur a cost of $12 plus $110 (for the medical visit). This is represented in the Sees Doctor arm as "Cost = Cost + $110." Because the cost up to that point is $12, the variable Cost assumes a total value of $110 + $12 = $122 at this point in the tree. Finally, we must add the cost of hospitalization to this running total. The total value of Cost at the end of this pathway is $12 + $110 + $5,000 = $5,122.

4. The expected cost of a person who received a vaccine and remains well is $9.70 = (0.97 × $10).

In Figure 5.10, the probability of being ill after receiving a vaccination is 3%. The cost of vaccination is $10. Since the person does not experience any illness, then they do not incur the additional costs associated with illness. Therefore, the only costs that incurred is the vaccination costs.

Since we're interested in the expected costs of the average person who received a vaccine and remains well, we use the probability of remaining well multiplied by the total costs for being well.

5. (Refer to Figure A.1). In order to calculate the expected cost and outcomes at node A, we will need to figure out the expected costs and outcomes for nodes C and D. We will go through these step by step. (Some of the decimal values are very long, so make sure to get these right!)

Step 1. At node D, the expected costs and outcomes are: $137 [(0.999 × $132) + (0.001 × $5132)] and 0.003 [(0.999 × 0.002997) + (0.001 × 0.0000003)].

Step 2. At node C, the expected costs and outcomes are: $33.5 [(0.90 × $22) + (0.10 × $137)] and 0.025 [(0.90 × 0.027) + (0.10 × 0.003)].

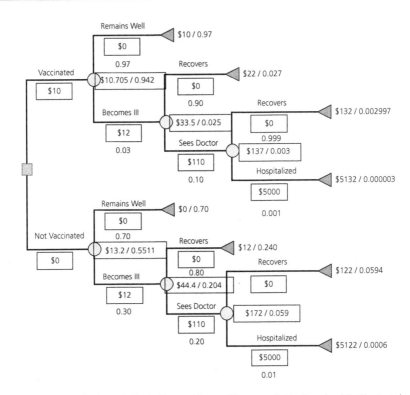

Figure A.1 The Rollback Results for the Expected Costs and Outcomes for Vaccinated and Not Vaccinated Strategies

Step 3. At node A, the expected costs and outcomes are: $10.705 [(0.97 × $10) + (0.03 × $33.5)] and 0.942 [(0.97 × 0.97) + (0.03 × 0.025)].

6. Similar to the way we calculated node A, node B requires us to also calculate the expected costs and outcomes for the nodes associated with Not Vaccinated. Fortunately, one of the nodes has been calculated in the book for us. Therefore, we just need to calculate the expected costs and outcomes for node E in order to solve for node B.

Step 1. At node E, the expected costs and outcomes are: $44.4 [(0.80 × $12) + (0.20 × $174.2)] and 0.204 [(0.80 × 0.240) + (0.20 × 0.059)].

Step 2. At node B, the expected costs and outcomes are: $13.2 [(0.70 × $0) + (0.30 × $44.4)] and 0.5511 [(0.70 × 0.70) + (0.30 × 0.204)].

Table A.1   Comparison Between Vaccinated and Not Vaccinated Strategies

	Cost	Incremental Costs	Effectiveness	Incremental Effectiveness	ICER
Not Vaccinated	13.2	—	0.5511	—	—
Vaccinated	10.705	−2.495	0.942	0.3909	Dominant

7. The cost-effective strategy is the one that provides us with the most "bang for our buck." Therefore, we want to select the strategy that yields the best outcomes relative to the costs. In this example, we are looking at the cost of Vaccinated per person relative to the cost of Not Vaccinated per person.

    There are two ways to do this:

    • First method: Look at the rollback results. The Vaccinated arm has an expected cost and outcome of $10.705 and 0.942. Dividing $10.705 by 0.942 yields the cost per patient, which is $11.36. For the Not Vaccinated arm, the cost per patient is $23.95. The Vaccinated arm costs less compared to the Not Vaccinated arm.

    • Second method: Calculate the incremental cost-effectiveness ratio (ICER). The expected costs and outcomes for Vaccinated are $10.705 and 0.942. The expected costs and outcomes for Not Vaccinated are $13.2 and 0.5511. Therefore, the ICER is −$6.38 per patient ($10.705 − $13.2) ÷ (0.942 − 0.5511). Because the incremental cost is negative and the incremental unit of effectiveness (patient) is positive, the Vaccinated strategy is dominant over the Not Vaccinated strategy. (Refer to Table A.1.)

Chapter 6

1. Figure A.2 is a sketch of the Markov model from Exercise 1 in Chapter 6. The transition probabilities have been included for each transition branch. Students should be able to sketch something resembling this illustration.

2. At the end of 10 weeks, the number of patients remaining in the Healthy state is 75. However, there are 855 patients who were sick and then recovered. These should also be included. Therefore, the

Table A.2 Markov Model Using a Vaccine Effectiveness of 75 Percent

Week	Healthy	Sick	Recovered	Dead
1	1000	0	0	0
2	750	250	0	0
3	563	188	238	13
4	422	141	416	22
5	316	105	549	29
6	237	79	649	34
7	178	59	725	38
8	133	44	781	41
9	100	33	823	43
10	75	25	855	45

final number of patients who are healthy at the end of 10 weeks is 930. The spreadsheet file with the calculations can be downloaded from the following link: http://www.wiley.com/WileyCDA/WileyTitle/productCd-1119011264.html.

3. Figure A.3 is the TreeAge Pro rollback results for the Markov model you created. Notice that the _stage = 9 because we had to include _stage = 0, which is week 1. Each FP provides the proportion for each

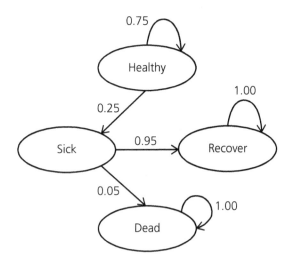

Figure A.2 Markov Model from Chapter 6, Exercise 1

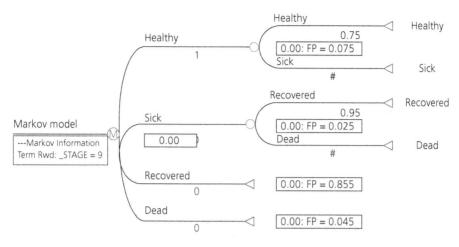

Figure A.3   A Tree Diagram with Rollback Results from TreeAge Pro

transition state. Therefore, you can multiply each FP by a hypothetical cohort of 1,000 patients to get the number of patients in each state at the end of 10 weeks. Similar to Exercise 2, the number of healthy patients (including those who recovered) is 930.

Chapter 7

1. There are three methods that have been introduced in the chapter: standard gamble, time trade-off, and rating scales. The preferred method is the standard gamble because it is grounded in the axioms of game theory developed by von Neumann and Morgenstern. However, the time trade-off is easier to use and is a good alternative if the other method is too difficult to apply. Rating scales have no basis on any utility or behavioral theory and should not be used as a method for estimating utility scores. However, in practice, you may need to use a rating scale due to convenience and availability.

2. The EuroQol instrument (EQ-5D) has five attributes or domains. They are: (1) mobility, (2) self-care, (3) usual activities, (4) pain/discomfort, and (5) anxiety/depression. The EQ-5D is a multiattribute health status classification system, which combines all the attributes (or domains) into a single utility score. Therefore, it is able to capture different attributes of a disease into a single HRQL score. The disadvantage with using a multiattribute health status instrument is the possibility that not all the critical attributes are captured, which would yield an HRQL score that is not accurate or reflective of the disease of interest.

3. The index value for a U.S. patient with a dimension score of 14213 is 0.706. A U.K. patient's index value is 0.623.

Chapter 8

1. You have been told that mortality is reduced by 50 percent. This is equivalent to a risk ratio of 0.5. In the life table, enter 0.5 where it says "Crude Risk Ratio." You will notice that life expectancy increases from 78.7 to 87.2 years, or a gain of 8.5 years.

2. The life table provides the average life expectancy for the average American (which is 78.7 years at birth and 23.1 years at age 60). On the spreadsheet, enter 1.1 in each cell for persons over the age of 60. You should see that life expectancy at birth changes to 77.9, and life expectancy at age 60 changes to 22.2. The life expectancy for the average person with diabetes is thus 22.2 years. Those receiving treatment have a 5 percent risk reduction from 1.1, or $1.1 \times 0.95 = 1.045$. Replacing the 1.1 values with 1.045, you end up with a life expectancy at age 60 of 22.7 years. Thus, your gain in life-years at age 60 is $22.7 - 22.2 = 0.5$ years of life.

3. First, calculate QALY for persons at age 60 who are receiving current practice. Enter 1.1 in every risk ratio cell starting at age 60. Next, enter 0.7 in every HRQL score cell beginning at age 60. The QALE at birth should be 72.0 QALYs, and the QALE at age 60 should be 15.5 QALYs. You have a 10 percent improvement in HRQL with treatment, so the mean HRQL among treated persons is $0.7 \times 1.1 = 0.77$. Don't forget to reenter 1.045 as the risk ratio for treated people (recall from Exercise 2 that the treatment reduces the risk of mortality by 5 percent, RR = 0.95). Your new QALE at age 60 is 17.5. Thus, your gain in QALYs is $17.5 - 15.5 = 2.0$ QALYs gained at age 60.

4. The answer varies depending on your country of origin and demographics.

5. Over the one year of operation, you spend $100,000 on program costs. However, you are also preventing HIV cases. For every HIV case you prevent, you will save $1,000 per year for the rest of each patient's life. Therefore, future HIV costs prevented must be considered over the remaining life of each patient. For instance, preventing a single HIV-positive case who has five years of life remaining would reduce future (undiscounted) costs by $15 \times \$1,000 = \$15,000$.

6. HIV-positive people live 15 years. If these 100 cases had become positive, they would have cost $1,000 × 15 years each. This amounts to $15,000 × 100 = $1,500,000 over their lifetimes. Thus, you have saved $1.5 million in future medical costs.

7. Remember to discount the $1,000 "$t$" years into the future using the formula: $1,000/(1.03)^t$. Thus, year 5 values are $1,000/(1.03)^5$. Savings per patient over 15 years are as follows:

Year	Base Savings	Discounted Savings
1	$1,000	$1,000 ($1000/1.03^0)
2	$1,000	$971 ($1000/1.03^1)
3	$1,000	$943 ($1000/1.03^2)
4	$1,000	$915 ($1000/1.03^3)
5	$1,000	$888 ($1000/1.03^4)
6	$1,000	$863 ($1000/1.03^5)
7	$1,000	$837 ($1000/1.03^6)
8	$1,000	$813 ($1000/1.03^7)
9	$1,000	$789 ($1000/1.03^8)
10	$1,000	$766 ($1000/1.03^9)
11	$1,000	$744 ($1000/1.03^10)
12	$1,000	$722 ($1000/1.03^11)
13	$1,000	$701 ($1000/1.03^12)
14	$1,000	$681 ($1000/1.03^13)
15	$1,000	$661 ($1000/1.03^14)
Sum	$15,000	$12,296

Thus, the total savings are 100 × $12,296 = $1,229,600.

8.

Year	QALYs	Discounted QALYs
1	0.6	0.6 (6/1.03^0)
2	0.6	0.58 (6/1.03^1)
3	0.6	0.57 (6/1.03^2)
4	0.6	0.55 (6/1.03^3)
5	0.6	0.53 (6/1.03^4)
6	0.6	0.52 (6/1.03^5)
7	0.6	0.50 (6/1.03^6)
8	0.6	0.49 (6/1.03^7)
9	0.6	0.47 (6/1.03^8)
10	0.6	0.46 (6/1.03^9)
11	0.6	0.45 (6/1.03^10)
12	0.6	0.43 (6/1.03^11)
13	0.6	0.42 (6/1.03^12)
14	0.6	0.41 (6/1.03^13)
15	0.6	0.40 (6/1.03^14)
Sum	9.00	7.38

9. The incremental gain in discounted QALYs is 3.69 QALYs (11.07 QALYs – 7.38 QALYs).

	HIV-Positive		HIV-Negative	
Year	QALYs	Discounted QALYs	QALYs	Discounted QALYs
1	0.6	0.6	0.9	0.9 (0.9/1.03^0)
2	0.6	0.58	0.9	0.87 (0.9/1.03^1)
3	0.6	0.57	0.9	0.85 (0.9/1.03^2)
4	0.6	0.55	0.9	0.82 (0.9/1.03^3)
5	0.6	0.53	0.9	0.80 (0.9/1.03^4)
6	0.6	0.52	0.9	0.78 (0.9/1.03^5)
7	0.6	0.50	0.9	0.75 (0.9/1.03^6)
8	0.6	0.49	0.9	0.73 (0.9/1.03^7)
9	0.6	0.47	0.9	0.71 (0.9/1.03^8)
10	0.6	0.46	0.9	0.69 (0.9/1.03^9)
11	0.6	0.45	0.9	0.67 (0.9/1.03^10)
12	0.6	0.43	0.9	0.65 (0.9/1.03^11)
13	0.6	0.42	0.9	0.63 (0.9/1.03^12)
14	0.6	0.41	0.9	0.61 (0.9/1.03^13)
15	0.6	0.40	0.9	0.60 (0.9/1.03^14)
Sum	9.00	7.38	13.50	11.07

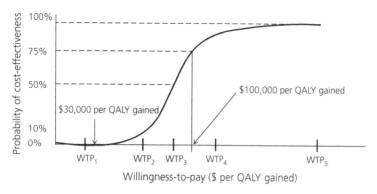

Figure A.4   Cost-Effectiveness Acceptability Curve Showing Where the 75 Percent Probability of Cost-Effectiveness Is in Relation to the Willingness-to-Pay Axis

Chapter 9

1. $20.92 and $41.82.

2.   Using the cost-effectiveness acceptability curve in Figure 9.16, the probability that the new drug, Expensive, is cost-effective compared to the competing alternative is approximately 75 percent. (See Figure A.4.)

3.   Since the payer's willingness-to-pay is $30,000 per QALY gained, the probability that the new drug, Expensive, is cost-effective compared to the competing alternative is 0 percent.

Chapter 11

1.   The cumulative incidence of death for Hospital A is 36 per 1,000 surgical patients, and the cumulative incidence for Hospital B is 156 per 1,000 surgical patients.

2.   Since there are 1,000 surgical patients in the ICU ward, then there should be 500 surgical patients in the non-ICU ward (1,500 – 1,000 = 500) for Hospital A. In Hospital B, there are 500 surgical patients in the ICU ward and 500 surgical patients in the non-ICU ward (1,000 – 500 = 500). The ICU-specific mortality rate is calculated by multiplying the number of deaths by the number of surgical patients in each location of the hospital (ICU and non-ICU). In Hospital A, the ICU-specific mortality rate is 50 per 1,000 surgeries $\left(\frac{50}{1000} \times 10^3\right)$. The following completed table has the answer:

| | Hospital A | | | Hospital B | | |
Location	Deaths	Number of Surgeries	Deaths per 1,000	Deaths	Number of Surgeries	Deaths per 1,000
ICU	50	1,000	50	100	500	200
Non-ICU	4	500	8	56	500	112

3. The standard population sizes for the ICU and non-ICU wards are determined from Hospital A and Hospital B. For the ICU ward, the standard population size is 1,500 (1,000 + 500), and for the non-ICU ward, the standard population size is 1,000 (500 + 500). The following completed table has the answer:

| | Hospital A | Hospital B | Standard Population Size |
Location	Number of Surgeries (1)	Number of Surgeries (2)	(1) + (2)
ICU	1,000	500	1,500
Non-ICU	500	500	1,000

4. The expected number of deaths is determined by multiplying the mortality rate by the standard population size for the ICU and non-ICU locations. Therefore, the expected number of deaths in Hospital A in the ICU is 75 (0.50 × 1,500). The total number of deaths in each hospital is the sum of the deaths in the ICU and non-ICU locations. Therefore, the total number of expected deaths in Hospital A is 83 (75 + 8), and the total number of expected deaths at Hospital B is 412 (300 + 112). The answers are listed in following completed table:

| | Hospital A | | | Hospital B | | |
	ICU	Non-ICU	Total	ICU	Non-ICU	Total
Mortality rate per 1,000	50	8	58	200	112	312
Standard population size	1,500	1000	2,500	1,500	1000	2500
Expected number of deaths	75	8	83	300	112	412

5. The ICU-adjusted mortality rate for Hospital A is calculated as 33.2 deaths per 1,000 surgeries. The ICU-adjusted mortality rate for Hospital B is calculated as 164.8 deaths per 1,000 surgeries.

$$\text{Hospital A} = \frac{83}{2,500} \times 10^3 = 33.2 \text{ deaths per 1,000 surgeries}$$

$$\text{Hospital B} = \frac{412}{2,500} \times 10^3 = 164.8 \text{ deaths per 1,000 surgeries}$$

6. If you averaged the probability of cure over the three studies, you would get a probability of 0.594 ((0.750 + 0.200 + 0.833) ÷ 3). By estimating the probability of cure with this method, you are assigning equal weights to each study. We know from the exercise that each study had different sample sizes. Therefore, we need to apply different weights to each one.

    Using the following table, the weights for each study were obtained.

	No. Cured	No. of Patients	Probability Cured
Trial 1	15	20	0.750
Trial 2	2	10	0.200
Trial 3	5	6	0.833
Average	7.33	12	0.594

    The weight for Trial 1 is the size of the trial, which is 20. Trial 2 is 10, and Trial 3 is 6. The weighted-average probability of cure is calculated as:

$$\frac{(20 \times 0.750) + (10 \times 0.200) + (6 \times 0.833)}{36} = 0.61.$$

We conclude that the probability of cure is 61 percent.

Chapter 12

1. The best dataset in which to find this information is the CDC's WONDER dataset. The web site is located at http://wonder.cdc.gov. Under the Mortality section, select Detailed Mortality. Agree to the terms and conditions. Under "Organize the table layout," group

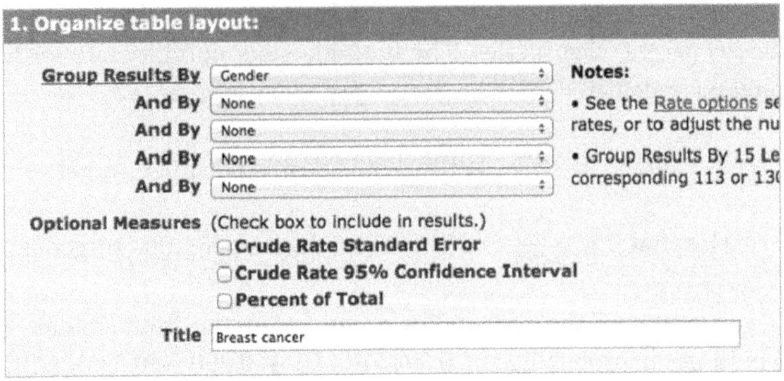

Figure A.5   Using the CDC's Wonder Mortality Database and Selecting Breast Cancer

results by gender. Under the Title field, type in "Breast cancer." See Figure A.5.

Make sure the entire United States is selected in the "Select location" section. There's no need to make any adjustments to the "Demographics" section. Select 2011. Under cause of death, use the search tab and type in "breast" as a search term. Select ICD-10 code C50 (Malignant neoplasm of breast). See Figure A.6.

Make sure the "Show Totals" selection is checked. Click on Send. The total number of breast cancer-related deaths in 2011 is 41,374. See Figure A.7.

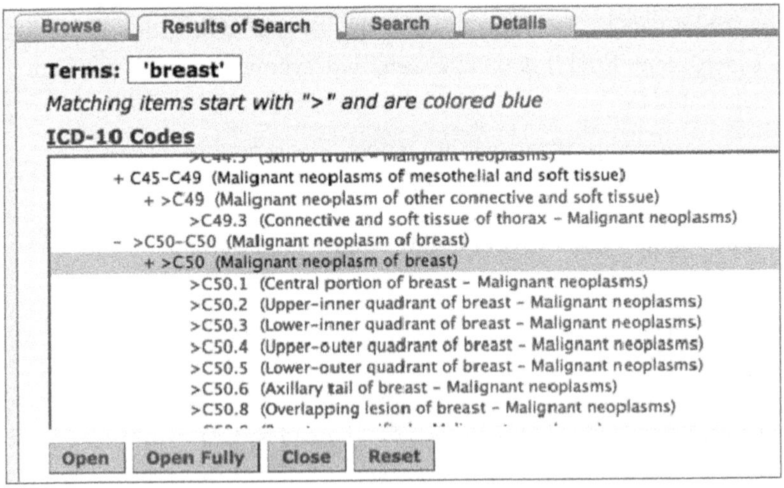

Figure A.6   Selecting the ICD-10 Code for Breast Cancer

Gender ⬇	➡ Deaths ⬆⬇
Female	40,931
Male	443
Total	**41,374**

Figure A.7   Results of the Breast Cancer Query Grouped by Gender for 2011

You can also use the SEER database to find the number of breast cancer deaths in the United States.

2. Since you grouped results by gender, you already have the number of male deaths due to breast cancer, which is 443.

3. Since this is from the payer's perspective, we are interested in direct costs. Therefore, we need to know the average hourly rate of a dermatologist's salary The U.S. Bureau of Labor and Statistics has this information (http://www.bls.gov/bls/blswage.htm). Under National Wage Data, select "For over 800 occupations." Select "Healthcare Practitioners and Technical Occupations." There is no occupational code for dermatologists. Since there is no specific code for dermatologists, you should look for the next reasonable occupation that comes close. Fortunately, there is an occupational cost for Family and General Practitioners, which is $84.87 per hour. Since a dermatologist spends 30 minutes with a patient, the average cost of seeing a dermatologist is approximately $42.44 dollars.

Although many dermatological conditions are seen by primary physicians, wages for this group are much lower than for dermatologists. Therefore, make sure to at least attempt an estimate of the proportion of cases seen by dermatologists and try to obtain an alternative estimate of such wages. Thus, if a dermatologist earns $175 per hour and sees 10 percent of the cases, then you would weight these wages 0.1 and the wage of primary care providers 0.9 to come up with your average.

LIFE EXPECTANCY AND QUALITY-ADJUSTED LIFE EXPECTANCY TABLES

Table B.1 Abridged Life Table for the Total Population, United States, 2011

Age (years)	Probability of Dying Between Ages X and $X+N$ (1)	Number Surviving to Age X (2)	Number Dying Between Ages X and $X+N$ (Col. 1 × Col. 2) (3)	Person-Years Lived Between Ages X and $X+N$ (4)	Total Number of Person-Years Lived Above Age X (Sum of Col. 4 Values) (5)	Expectancy of Life at Age X (Col.5/ Col. 2) (6)
0–1*	0.006058	100,000	606	99,472	7,969,412	79.7
1–5	0.001054	99,394	105	496,709	7,869,940	79.2
5–10	0.000603	99,289	60	496,298	7,373,231	74.3
10–15	0.000709	99,230	70	495,972	6,876,934	69.3
15–20	0.002438	99,159	242	495,192	6,380,962	64.4
20–25	0.004296	98,917	425	493,525	5,885,770	59.5
25 30	0.004824	98,493	475	491,275	5,392,245	54.7
30–35	0.005638	98,017	553	488,705	4,900,970	50.0
35–40	0.006985	97,465	681	485,622	4,412,265	45.3
40–45	0.010006	96,784	968	481,499	3,926,643	40.6
45–50	0.016018	95,816	1,535	475,241	3,445,144	36.0
50–55	0.024459	94,281	2,306	465,639	2,969,904	31.5
55–60	0.035105	91,975	3,229	451,802	2,504,265	27.2
60–65	0.049332	88,746	4,378	432,785	2,052,463	23.1

(*Continued*)

Table B.1 Abridged Life Table for the Total Population, United States, 2011 *(Continued)*

Age (years)	Probability of Dying Between Ages X and X + N (1)	Number Surviving to Age X (2)	Number Dying Between Ages X and X + N (Col. 1 × Col. 2) (3)	Person-Years Lived Between Ages X and X + N (4)	Total Number of Person-Years Lived Above Age X (Sum of Col. 4 Values) (5)	Expectancy of Life at Age X (Col.5/Col. 2) (6)
65–70	0.07331	84,368	6,185	406,377	1,619,678	19.2
70–75	0.110896	78,183	8,670	369,239	1,213,301	15.5
75–80	0.172915	69,513	12,020	317,514	844,061	12.1
80–85	0.274093	57,493	15,758	248,069	526,547	9.2
85–90	0.429792	41,735	17,937	163,830	278,478	6.7
90–95	0.617599	23,797	14,697	82,244	114,648	4.8
95–100	0.787828	9,100	7,169	27,577	32,404	3.6
100 and over	1	1,931	1,931	4,827	4,827	2.5

*The Person-Years Lived Between Ages 0–1 was determined using a separation factor of 0.128. Formula: [(0.128*100,000) + ((1 − 0.128)*99,394)].
Source: Centers for Disease Control and Prevention, National Center for Health Statistics, and Agency for Health Research and Quality.

Table B.2 Abridged Quality-Adjusted Life Table for the Total Population, United States, 2011

Age (years)	Probability of Dying Between Ages X and X + N (1)	Number Surviving to Age X (2)	Number Dying Between Ages X and X + N (Col. 1 × Col. 2) (3)	Person-Years Lived Between Ages X and X + N (4)*	HRQL Score[a] (5)	Quality-Adjusted Person-Years Lived Between Ages X and X+N (6)	Total Number of Quality-Adjusted Person-Years Lived Above Age X (Sum of Col. 6 Values) (7)	Quality-Adjusted Life Expectancy at Age X (Col.7/Col. 2) (8)
0–1	0.006058	100,000	606	99,472	0.94	93,504	6,541,244	65.4
1–5	0.001054	99,394	105	496,709	0.94	466,907	6,447,740	64.9
5–10	0.000603	99,289	60	496,298	0.93	461,557	5,980,833	60.2
10–15	0.000709	99,230	70	495,972	0.93	461,254	5,519,276	55.6
15–20	0.002438	99,159	242	495,192	0.92	455,576	5,058,022	51.0
20–25	0.004296	98,917	425	493,525	0.89	439,237	4,602,446	46.5
25–30	0.004824	98,493	475	491,275	0.84	412,671	4,163,209	42.3

(Continued)

Table B.2 *(Continued)*

Age (years)	Probability of Dying Between Ages X and $X + N$ (1)	Number Surviving to Age X (2)	Number Dying Between Ages X and $X + N$ (Col. 1 × Col. 2) (3)	Person-Years Lived Between Ages X and $X + N$ (4)*	HRQL Score[a] (5)	Quality-Adjusted Person-Years Lived Between Ages X and $X + N$ (6)	Total Number of Quality-Adjusted Person-Years Lived Above Age X (Sum of Col. 6 Values) (7)	Quality-Adjusted Life Expectancy at Age X (Col.7/Col. 2) (8)
30–35	0.005638	98,017	553	488,705	0.84	410,513	3,750,538	38.3
35–40	0.006985	97,465	681	485,622	0.84	407,922	3,340,025	34.3
40–45	0.010006	96,784	968	481,499	0.84	404,459	2,932,103	30.3
45–50	0.016018	95,816	1,535	475,241	0.84	399,202	2,527,644	26.4
50–55	0.024459	94,281	2,306	465,639	0.79	367,855	2,128,442	22.6
55–60	0.035105	91,975	3,229	451,802	0.73	329,815	1,760,587	19.1
60–65	0.049332	88,746	4,378	432,785	0.73	315,933	1,430,772	16.1
65–70	0.07331	84,368	6,185	406,377	0.73	296,655	1,114,839	13.2
70–75	0.110896	78,183	8,670	369,239	0.73	269,545	818,184	10.5
75–80	0.172915	69,513	12,020	317,514	0.65	206,384	548,639	7.9
80–85	0.274093	57,493	15,758	248,069	0.65	161,245	342,255	6.0
85–90	0.429792	41,735	17,937	163,830	0.65	106,489	181,010	4.3
90–95	0.617599	23,797	14,697	82,244	0.65	53,458	74,521	3.1
95–100	0.787828	9,100	7,169	27,577	0.65	17,925	21,063	2.3
100 and over	1	1,931	1,931	4,827	0.65	3,138	3,138	1.6

[a] HRQL scores obtained from Medical Expenditure Panel Survey. Scores for subjects aged 0 to 18 from Erickson P., R. Wilson, and L. Shannon. (1995). Years of Healthy Life. *Healthy People 2000 Stat Notes* (7): 1–15.
Source: Centers for Disease Control and Prevention, National Center for Health Statistics, and Agency for Health Research and Quality.

EQ-5D-5L HEALTH QUESTIONNAIRE (ENGLISH VERSION FOR THE UNITED STATES)

Under each heading, please check the ONE box that best describes your health TODAY.

MOBILITY

I have no problems in walking about ☐

I have slight problems in walking about ☐

I have moderate problems in walking about ☐

I have severe problems in walking about ☐

I am unable to walk about ☐

SELF-CARE

I have no problems washing or dressing myself ☐

I have slight problems washing or dressing myself ☐

I have moderate problems washing or dressing myself ☐

I have severe problems washing or dressing myself ☐

I am unable to wash or dress myself ☐

(Continued)

USUAL ACTIVITIES (e.g., work, study, housework, family, or leisure activities)

I have no problems doing my usual activities ☐

I have slight problems doing my usual activities ☐

I have moderate problems doing my usual activities ☐

I have severe problems doing my usual activities ☐

I am unable to do my usual activities ☐

PAIN/DISCOMFORT

I have no pain or discomfort ☐

I have slight pain or discomfort ☐

I have moderate pain or discomfort ☐

I have severe pain or discomfort ☐

I have extreme pain or discomfort ☐

ANXIETY/DEPRESSION

I am not anxious or depressed ☐

I am slightly anxious or depressed ☐

I am moderately anxious or depressed ☐

I am severely anxious or depressed ☐

I am extremely anxious or depressed ☐

- We would like to know how good or bad your health is TODAY.

- This scale is numbered from 0 to 100.

- 100 means the best health you can imagine. 0 means the worst health you can imagine.

- Mark an X on the scale to indicate how your health is TODAY.

- Now, please write the number you marked on the scale in the box below.

Your Health Today: _____

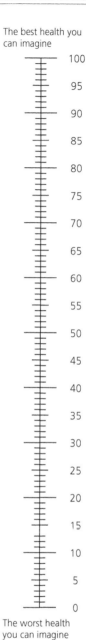

The best health you can imagine

The worst health you can imagine

DIAGNOSIS, CHARGES, MEDICARE REIMBURSEMENT, AVERAGE LENGTH OF STAY, AND COST-TO-CHARGE RATIO BY DIAGNOSIS-RELATED GROUPS, 2011

	1	2	3	4	5	6	7
DRG Code	Total Charges	Coveraged Charges	Medicare Reimbursement	Total Days	Number of Discharges	AVG Total Days	Cost-to-Charge Ratio
1	$1,438,849,607	$1,388,494,856	$337,259,832	67,403	1,745	38.6	0.24
2	$217,693,541	$213,341,162	$45,776,248	8,869	447	19.8	0.21
3	$12,001,344,356	$11,740,191,911	$2,697,138,414	915,820	25,943	35.3	0.23
4	$7,878,897,492	$7,701,082,127	$1,800,641,007	781,109	28,251	27.6	0.23
5	$574,914,064	$558,332,567	$106,798,735	27,195	1,213	22.4	0.19
6	$104,129,379	$102,214,523	$14,835,995	3,639	404	9	0.15
7	$293,416,163	$286,548,777	$48,912,058	12,519	667	18.8	0.17
8	$164,682,709	$157,241,513	$18,566,550	5,747	500	11.5	0.12
10	$22,648,368	$21,896,400	$3,020,263	891	105	8.5	0.14
11	$322,669,648	$320,169,812	$71,403,534	33,150	2,224	14.9	0.22
12	$243,575,372	$240,595,616	$52,852,720	25,667	2,531	10.1	0.22

	1	2	3	4	5	6	7
DRG Code	Total Charges	Coveraged Charges	Medicare Reimburse-ment	Total Days	Number of Dis-charges	AVG Total Days	Cost-to-Charge Ratio
13	$75,587,605	$74,567,267	$14,489,284	8,146	1,243	6.6	0.19
14	$261,111,804	$238,702,533	$67,854,821	20,859	800	26.1	0.28
15	$394,957,195	$388,063,473	$102,477,876	42,500	2,247	18.9	0.26
20	$458,533,725	$451,795,514	$94,877,531	29,249	1,662	17.6	0.21
21	$111,995,080	$110,128,805	$22,886,576	7,852	572	13.7	0.21
22	$22,434,967	$22,085,103	$3,786,985	1,396	167	8.4	0.17
23	$978,573,636	$963,358,578	$196,187,811	71,497	6,429	11.1	0.20
24	$258,901,945	$253,350,838	$50,440,807	17,158	2,574	6.7	0.20
25	$2,337,602,393	$2,319,504,393	$507,679,229	194,146	18,502	10.5	0.22
26	$1,112,903,264	$1,104,837,747	$221,211,829	91,946	13,390	6.9	0.20
27	$968,391,979	$958,808,585	$174,755,529	55,766	15,087	3.7	0.18
28	$386,324,508	$381,843,722	$83,000,693	33,472	2,569	13	0.22
29	$395,416,448	$390,996,913	$79,014,110	31,806	4,841	6.6	0.20
30	$201,318,140	$199,209,867	$37,148,634	13,864	4,281	3.2	0.19
31	$194,376,622	$192,385,245	$44,271,312	20,390	1,694	12	0.23
32	$167,261,880	$165,268,501	$33,453,746	16,265	3,029	5.4	0.20
33	$144,214,651	$143,687,718	$26,252,831	9,577	3,694	2.6	0.18
34	$122,456,017	$118,204,781	$22,730,261	8,505	1,157	7.4	0.19
35	$198,992,917	$194,381,187	$35,920,870	10,407	3,232	3.2	0.18
36	$328,272,536	$322,361,612	$57,467,056	11,187	7,233	1.5	0.18
37	$566,272,229	$544,480,782	$110,559,003	53,555	6,308	8.5	0.20

	1	2	3	4	5	6	7
DRG Code	Total Charges	Coveraged Charges	Medicare Reimbursement	Total Days	Number of Discharges	AVG Total Days	Cost-to-Charge Ratio
38	$759,127,925	$740,589,728	$120,230,305	60,050	16,966	3.5	0.16
39	$1,471,306,136	$1,443,683,453	$212,315,342	81,913	49,939	1.6	0.15
40	$653,214,634	$645,339,995	$143,582,229	78,460	6,239	12.6	0.22
41	$516,702,913	$505,989,203	$100,810,676	61,027	9,063	6.7	0.20
42	$191,995,337	$180,062,825	$32,306,153	13,443	4,009	3.4	0.18
52	$95,426,081	$93,136,952	$24,346,518	19,248	1,923	10	0.26
53	$20,722,688	$18,147,117	$4,025,182	6,406	712	9	0.22
54	$493,708,902	$489,141,899	$102,692,634	74,606	12,493	6	0.21
55	$417,138,440	$413,931,200	$78,488,823	64,590	14,000	4.6	0.19
56	$724,432,438	$711,182,739	$182,571,832	169,304	16,627	10.2	0.26
57	$2,322,538,158	$2,209,371,215	$669,025,094	836,092	89,214	9.4	0.30
58	$55,161,419	$54,227,457	$13,036,066	9,801	1,242	7.9	0.24
59	$133,239,698	$120,574,971	$24,817,485	28,130	4,354	6.5	0.21
60	$107,697,094	$98,446,909	$18,081,839	19,719	4,539	4.3	0.18
61	$363,214,830	$360,468,910	$68,746,486	34,226	4,331	7.9	0.19
62	$394,363,700	$390,183,200	$66,224,066	36,417	6,948	5.2	0.17
63	$96,844,176	$96,130,544	$14,670,964	7,562	2,074	3.6	0.15
64	$4,373,891,349	$4,341,987,240	$900,849,892	608,054	89,053	6.8	0.21
65	$4,571,401,680	$4,541,873,495	$861,075,367	714,349	150,931	4.7	0.19
66	$2,003,684,240	$1,988,131,794	$321,429,807	281,025	87,550	3.2	0.16
67	$64,880,450	$64,534,907	$12,006,175	8,594	1,580	5.4	0.19

	1	2	3	4	5	6	7
DRG Code	Total Charges	Coveraged Charges	Medicare Reimbursement	Total Days	Number of Discharges	AVG Total Days	Cost-to-Charge Ratio
68	$296,133,543	$284,309,469	$46,235,189	37,656	11,710	3.2	0.16
69	$2,479,918,433	$2,347,349,346	$351,605,612	309,590	118,991	2.6	0.15
70	$733,831,988	$726,612,749	$169,745,948	120,658	16,562	7.3	0.23
71	$555,765,604	$547,644,457	$116,749,464	107,567	20,867	5.2	0.21
72	$165,521,763	$159,897,555	$26,506,723	25,431	7,916	3.2	0.17
73	$396,398,908	$380,876,750	$86,378,365	65,768	11,268	5.8	0.23
74	$956,813,439	$924,445,878	$171,816,267	161,184	40,110	4	0.19
75	$98,070,709	$97,485,009	$17,832,136	13,709	1,939	7.1	0.18
76	$21,886,732	$21,738,591	$3,586,873	3,430	879	3.9	0.17
77	$99,738,645	$98,734,319	$21,688,101	13,423	2,148	6.2	0.22
78	$87,582,336	$86,931,921	$15,674,292	13,240	3,251	4.1	0.18
79	$23,068,018	$22,738,969	$3,787,131	3,243	1,140	2.8	0.17
80	$83,077,810	$81,786,088	$16,766,028	13,587	2,545	5.3	0.20
81	$175,467,164	$171,363,767	$34,483,358	32,845	9,120	3.6	0.20
82	$209,694,137	$208,265,561	$46,020,208	21,872	3,711	5.9	0.22
83	$144,102,469	$141,692,470	$27,476,580	18,353	3,673	5	0.19
84	$90,104,384	$89,345,703	$15,800,665	10,076	3,459	2.9	0.18
85	$668,368,153	$656,795,983	$147,672,151	91,900	11,883	7.7	0.22
86	$668,884,865	$663,478,120	$133,807,928	97,864	21,054	4.6	0.20
87	$396,365,324	$393,151,380	$71,007,517	53,077	18,488	2.9	0.18
88	$48,840,380	$48,466,631	$9,242,907	6,087	1,152	5.3	0.19

	1	2	3	4	5	6	7
DRG Code	Total Charges	Coveraged Charges	Medicare Reimbursement	Total Days	Number of Discharges	AVG Total Days	Cost-to-Charge Ratio
89	$109,070,703	$107,028,064	$18,270,219	13,427	3,923	3.4	0.17
90	$62,672,575	$60,218,937	$8,858,901	6,323	2,905	2.2	0.15
91	$600,633,272	$587,210,450	$131,471,901	92,918	13,520	6.9	0.22
92	$651,587,847	$631,082,387	$127,967,658	116,008	26,077	4.4	0.20
93	$321,302,285	$311,119,431	$52,506,785	47,400	16,314	2.9	0.17
94	$206,366,642	$204,788,355	$47,748,275	29,405	2,096	14	0.23
95	$121,831,421	$121,106,093	$23,697,215	16,127	1,780	9.1	0.20
96	$43,797,066	$43,598,842	$7,438,559	4,666	764	6.1	0.17
97	$164,766,089	$163,598,095	$34,248,641	21,697	1,803	12	0.21
98	$79,159,512	$77,100,074	$16,078,761	14,629	1,495	9.8	0.21
99	$24,852,280	$24,664,544	$4,209,792	3,580	692	5.2	0.17
100	$1,125,254,785	$1,108,720,071	$230,748,397	157,767	26,651	5.9	0.21
101	$1,511,458,015	$1,492,230,914	$269,506,334	232,950	70,272	3.3	0.18
102	$51,953,549	$50,660,095	$9,929,414	7,574	1,808	4.2	0.20
103	$341,303,466	$329,821,600	$50,185,259	49,170	17,412	2.8	0.15
113	$47,770,177	$47,202,552	$9,811,818	4,573	819	5.6	0.21
114	$16,709,787	$16,050,881	$2,583,472	1,543	530	2.9	0.16
115	$39,997,730	$39,337,881	$7,599,014	4,810	1,092	4.4	0.19
116	$24,112,224	$23,823,391	$4,569,729	2,774	571	4.9	0.19
117	$12,958,136	$12,224,622	$2,171,934	1,297	609	2.1	0.18
121	$25,488,585	$25,267,956	$5,263,334	5,107	1,002	5.1	0.21

	1	2	3	4	5	6	7
DRG Code	Total Charges	Coveraged Charges	Medicare Reimbursement	Total Days	Number of Discharges	AVG Total Days	Cost-to-Charge Ratio
122	$10,624,184	$10,543,676	$2,029,378	2,456	647	3.8	0.19
123	$92,084,949	$89,047,825	$12,674,711	10,668	3,984	2.7	0.14
124	$38,177,595	$37,518,888	$7,983,679	5,986	1,146	5.2	0.21
125	$108,504,109	$105,567,743	$19,099,786	19,556	5,749	3.4	0.18
129	$137,662,108	$135,640,187	$29,115,498	11,126	2,105	5.3	0.21
130	$55,412,688	$53,910,493	$9,473,313	4,053	1,405	2.9	0.18
131	$105,411,062	$103,681,549	$20,340,398	8,951	1,553	5.8	0.20
132	$36,371,201	$34,590,013	$6,444,834	2,423	948	2.6	0.19
133	$162,641,478	$159,068,116	$32,474,172	17,372	3,059	5.7	0.20
134	$85,026,529	$78,462,377	$11,940,605	6,484	3,007	2.2	0.15
135	$30,819,156	$30,195,800	$5,746,329	3,058	518	5.9	0.19
136	$12,132,176	$11,810,655	$1,888,625	818	362	2.3	0.16
137	$42,340,792	$41,183,478	$8,183,333	5,729	1,147	5	0.20
138	$23,030,641	$21,618,016	$3,836,240	2,345	999	2.3	0.18
139	$40,781,961	$38,154,503	$5,780,248	2,506	1,478	1.7	0.15
146	$68,857,643	$68,139,195	$16,124,805	10,788	993	10.9	0.24
147	$61,829,827	$60,726,638	$12,767,251	10,570	1,754	6	0.21
148	$15,252,493	$14,674,555	$3,189,947	2,471	730	3.4	0.22
149	$783,465,486	$762,951,199	$114,292,378	107,205	43,083	2.5	0.15
150	$58,249,199	$57,738,074	$12,090,375	8,877	1,664	5.3	0.21
151	$119,772,607	$118,652,320	$21,939,084	21,159	7,631	2.8	0.18

	1	2	3	4	5	6	7
DRG Code	Total Charges	Coveraged Charges	Medicare Reimburse-ment	Total Days	Number of Dis-charges	AVG Total Days	Cost-to-Charge Ratio
152	$102,716,442	$101,028,583	$20,285,718	17,010	3,766	4.5	0.20
153	$341,053,540	$336,168,413	$58,289,251	61,389	20,047	3.1	0.17
154	$130,575,107	$128,817,070	$28,196,662	20,849	3,377	6.2	0.22
155	$188,865,257	$186,717,245	$35,614,590	31,943	7,802	4.1	0.19
156	$73,995,479	$72,567,893	$12,185,499	12,160	4,318	2.8	0.17
157	$84,030,846	$83,229,041	$18,831,650	12,915	1,861	6.9	0.23
158	$120,630,438	$118,372,666	$23,657,164	20,973	5,025	4.2	0.20
159	$33,276,101	$32,192,825	$5,356,416	5,393	2,051	2.6	0.17
163	$2,232,255,600	$2,213,932,534	$459,396,639	231,294	16,795	13.8	0.21
164	$1,645,867,848	$1,634,250,057	$318,460,852	165,751	23,815	7	0.19
165	$700,461,763	$693,993,339	$124,854,607	59,285	14,196	4.2	0.18
166	$3,246,629,619	$3,142,573,040	$706,476,577	419,640	28,892	14.5	0.22
167	$1,152,360,828	$1,142,386,059	$225,929,629	148,973	21,371	7	0.20
168	$178,157,082	$174,742,768	$30,146,099	20,114	4,941	4.1	0.17
175	$879,251,367	$873,118,112	$175,381,887	144,447	21,802	6.6	0.20
176	$1,411,731,162	$1,400,592,558	$265,388,087	246,029	54,109	4.5	0.19
177	$4,948,214,875	$4,896,680,156	$1,110,536,946	836,777	92,343	9.1	0.23
178	$2,859,211,402	$2,834,639,621	$645,718,070	532,649	80,356	6.6	0.23
179	$462,396,092	$458,703,556	$104,298,638	94,536	20,113	4.7	0.23
180	$1,282,830,736	$1,271,241,177	$252,990,341	199,204	27,090	7.4	0.20
181	$977,277,097	$967,692,465	$183,871,814	156,169	29,810	5.2	0.19

	1	2	3	4	5	6	7
DRG Code	Total Charges	Coveraged Charges	Medicare Reimbursement	Total Days	Number of Discharges	AVG Total Days	Cost-to-Charge Ratio
182	$74,860,225	$73,889,898	$12,784,509	11,668	3,350	3.5	0.17
183	$150,351,822	$148,822,529	$30,562,771	24,539	3,931	6.2	0.21
184	$206,737,687	$204,778,515	$34,971,327	31,835	7,634	4.2	0.17
185	$55,063,773	$53,978,410	$8,536,883	8,677	2,985	2.9	0.16
186	$534,117,621	$530,428,460	$109,763,615	87,147	13,254	6.6	0.21
187	$379,927,330	$377,281,710	$72,000,906	62,160	13,300	4.7	0.19
188	$76,521,358	$75,341,227	$13,967,421	12,898	3,908	3.3	0.19
189	$5,679,054,737	$5,471,379,752	$1,223,957,505	1,043,810	142,477	7.3	0.22
190	$6,053,707,755	$6,003,900,816	$1,213,413,021	1,086,087	199,865	5.4	0.20
191	$4,791,141,837	$4,745,322,353	$938,290,673	880,025	200,584	4.4	0.20
192	$2,900,618,480	$2,871,221,763	$547,961,788	576,248	167,874	3.4	0.19
193	$6,288,546,827	$6,233,596,391	$1,297,860,766	1,083,045	167,089	6.5	0.21
194	$6,650,709,392	$6,600,553,971	$1,391,493,737	1,287,734	273,721	4.7	0.21
195	$2,082,079,378	$2,065,184,954	$428,954,775	440,135	124,884	3.5	0.21
196	$404,136,894	$401,146,545	$80,763,888	66,959	9,393	7.1	0.20
197	$231,685,809	$229,916,065	$45,060,745	39,057	8,005	4.9	0.20
198	$75,741,752	$75,050,316	$14,458,728	13,108	3,706	3.5	0.19
199	$250,814,442	$249,651,308	$50,791,233	42,171	5,272	8	0.20
200	$304,445,719	$301,986,976	$57,120,314	51,456	11,578	4.4	0.19
201	$70,259,256	$69,360,957	$13,125,991	13,368	3,987	3.4	0.19
202	$1,180,433,566	$1,164,063,534	$215,298,420	214,370	53,399	4	0.18

	1	2	3	4	5	6	7
DRG Code	Total Charges	Coveraged Charges	Medicare Reimbursement	Total Days	Number of Discharges	AVG Total Days	Cost-to-Charge Ratio
203	$581,833,902	$573,663,430	$97,103,691	114,890	37,687	3	0.17
204	$563,536,757	$545,103,792	$94,992,914	83,653	29,497	2.8	0.17
205	$415,291,715	$405,559,549	$81,999,385	62,338	10,435	6	0.20
206	$547,162,025	$530,441,167	$94,154,455	83,869	25,999	3.2	0.18
207	$10,015,799,324	$9,678,098,021	$2,305,123,759	1,333,992	61,746	21.6	0.24
208	$6,051,277,017	$5,982,999,908	$1,205,993,756	708,482	96,076	7.4	0.20
215	$93,829,580	$93,185,175	$19,813,091	3,508	239	14.7	0.21
216	$3,355,325,294	$3,331,011,751	$716,518,213	211,040	12,791	16.5	0.22
217	$1,336,539,076	$1,331,116,944	$269,890,789	78,634	7,614	10.3	0.20
218	$205,605,145	$204,327,175	$35,682,840	10,810	1,387	7.8	0.17
219	$4,043,179,933	$4,023,645,728	$879,906,819	237,005	18,961	12.5	0.22
220	$3,438,939,290	$3,425,757,959	$678,165,185	182,580	24,204	7.5	0.20
221	$686,465,179	$682,458,806	$124,846,752	33,536	5,762	5.8	0.18
222	$580,106,187	$576,514,756	$117,045,189	30,518	2,512	12.1	0.20
223	$556,332,148	$553,086,499	$113,633,181	20,568	3,443	6	0.21
224	$698,402,355	$694,348,750	$139,663,642	34,213	3,378	10.1	0.20
225	$688,863,099	$685,409,987	$139,668,125	22,846	4,548	5	0.20
226	$1,270,088,608	$1,259,631,431	$264,811,813	64,334	7,293	8.8	0.21
227	$3,804,835,355	$3,747,247,822	$772,798,560	92,062	29,159	3.2	0.21
228	$583,298,987	$580,504,935	$117,197,651	37,788	2,741	13.8	0.20
229	$416,064,053	$414,315,956	$77,765,606	25,943	3,183	8.2	0.19

	1	2	3	4	5	6	7
DRG Code	Total Charges	Coveraged Charges	Medicare Reimbursement	Total Days	Number of Discharges	AVG Total Days	Cost-to-Charge Ratio
230	$94,052,336	$93,170,386	$15,376,286	5,032	882	5.7	0.17
231	$354,944,079	$353,334,710	$66,327,240	19,959	1,623	12.3	0.19
232	$234,845,374	$233,925,416	$40,317,684	13,151	1,460	9	0.17
233	$3,560,800,263	$3,537,857,063	$658,374,876	246,600	18,422	13.4	0.19
234	$3,912,572,546	$3,889,798,742	$656,338,495	261,479	29,860	8.8	0.17
235	$1,816,534,346	$1,806,611,065	$351,618,962	124,871	11,592	10.8	0.19
236	$2,973,652,702	$2,960,394,869	$521,661,906	189,333	29,055	6.5	0.18
237	$4,325,829,869	$4,294,838,273	$886,684,937	292,821	29,292	10	0.21
238	$4,195,525,588	$4,171,292,918	$778,154,672	200,034	50,226	4	0.19
239	$1,390,566,955	$1,371,574,281	$321,461,678	183,819	12,471	14.7	0.23
240	$799,152,964	$793,519,504	$167,260,313	117,411	12,600	9.3	0.21
241	$68,664,970	$68,291,615	$13,178,893	11,071	1,903	5.8	0.19
242	$2,127,792,184	$2,109,929,273	$447,602,190	179,344	22,903	7.8	0.21
243	$3,023,523,952	$2,994,589,286	$600,346,347	212,994	45,448	4.7	0.20
244	$2,349,954,743	$2,313,578,568	$430,427,282	126,463	44,870	2.8	0.19
245	$429,461,009	$413,573,023	$85,158,335	16,516	3,936	4.2	0.21
246	$3,690,843,963	$3,616,789,483	$651,091,359	204,887	39,853	5.1	0.18
247	$9,665,996,555	$8,969,146,625	$1,306,024,914	372,209	157,336	2.4	0.15
248	$1,589,056,993	$1,573,774,364	$285,570,675	113,143	17,768	6.4	0.18
249	$2,716,171,806	$2,619,773,578	$387,605,997	136,808	47,912	2.9	0.15
250	$993,438,436	$985,236,124	$186,457,009	77,672	10,927	7.1	0.19

	1	2	3	4	5	6	7
DRG Code	Total Charges	Coveraged Charges	Medicare Reimbursement	Total Days	Number of Discharges	AVG Total Days	Cost-to-Charge Ratio
251	$2,641,884,654	$2,501,572,649	$373,447,534	123,300	41,740	3	0.15
252	$3,957,843,229	$3,889,430,840	$858,682,441	374,473	47,387	7.9	0.22
253	$3,669,602,767	$3,606,616,638	$675,006,919	321,188	54,066	5.9	0.19
254	$2,012,987,603	$1,902,653,223	$317,286,074	116,011	43,015	2.7	0.17
255	$186,555,310	$184,262,628	$43,910,136	28,521	2,960	9.6	0.24
256	$165,900,683	$164,449,077	$33,550,709	28,877	4,141	7	0.20
257	$12,069,581	$12,038,986	$2,387,902	2,189	513	4.3	0.20
258	$60,062,066	$59,299,845	$13,813,932	5,597	851	6.6	0.23
259	$212,034,198	$207,645,625	$41,579,948	14,210	4,418	3.2	0.20
260	$244,904,042	$240,760,673	$52,905,347	25,808	2,416	10.7	0.22
261	$206,235,045	$204,995,673	$39,978,992	19,876	4,527	4.4	0.20
262	$90,008,817	$88,884,683	$14,331,925	7,125	2,637	2.7	0.16
263	$26,765,718	$26,501,868	$5,345,683	3,157	549	5.8	0.20
264	$1,844,226,437	$1,791,999,775	$401,948,899	236,040	26,121	9	0.22
265	$110,742,176	$107,398,165	$20,465,303	6,214	1,719	3.6	0.19
280	$4,042,208,771	$4,012,277,613	$834,603,747	564,720	89,428	6.3	0.21
281	$1,894,193,153	$1,882,577,367	$354,881,113	258,980	64,717	4	0.19
282	$929,046,766	$922,602,288	$147,350,092	110,785	42,996	2.6	0.16
283	$754,103,281	$749,265,271	$148,572,950	79,510	15,396	5.2	0.20
284	$85,046,965	$84,664,336	$16,403,676	10,293	3,867	2.7	0.19
285	$22,867,912	$22,782,667	$3,843,503	2,776	1,603	1.7	0.17

	1	2	3	4	5	6	7
DRG Code	Total Charges	Coveraged Charges	Medicare Reimbursement	Total Days	Number of Dis-charges	AVG Total Days	Cost-to-Charge Ratio
286	$2,031,930,560	$2,011,221,809	$375,957,892	224,312	33,512	6.7	0.19
287	$5,212,175,302	$5,127,031,046	$754,870,401	478,356	153,640	3.1	0.15
288	$282,820,707	$277,858,808	$68,063,224	49,553	3,625	13.7	0.24
289	$81,746,762	$80,844,555	$18,022,707	16,074	1,619	9.9	0.22
290	$9,111,260	$8,992,623	$1,990,354	1,764	283	6.2	0.22
291	$9,115,171,056	$9,025,786,290	$1,907,000,542	1,478,263	240,609	6.1	0.21
292	$7,320,787,734	$7,247,458,848	$1,510,597,152	1,367,505	298,253	4.6	0.21
293	$2,203,284,363	$2,173,035,663	$423,171,499	419,659	133,344	3.1	0.19
294	$33,817,386	$33,280,521	$7,544,796	7,420	1,435	5.2	0.23
295	$8,423,042	$8,363,930	$2,028,097	2,542	644	3.9	0.24
296	$114,383,867	$113,626,672	$18,475,636	8,539	3,015	2.8	0.16
297	$17,245,527	$17,181,517	$2,917,519	1,488	935	1.6	0.17
298	$6,689,630	$6,636,412	$1,182,238	689	544	1.3	0.18
299	$1,044,273,880	$1,031,890,671	$225,488,696	182,112	27,922	6.5	0.22
300	$1,475,100,546	$1,461,323,523	$306,997,623	296,237	61,292	4.8	0.21
301	$582,021,420	$574,679,675	$108,760,463	121,841	35,893	3.4	0.19
302	$211,637,967	$207,654,101	$43,789,458	33,648	7,958	4.2	0.21
303	$835,900,885	$815,247,172	$138,125,192	128,627	52,303	2.5	0.17
304	$111,082,815	$109,720,718	$20,857,037	17,518	3,951	4.4	0.19
305	$772,592,239	$757,532,470	$120,076,652	119,522	45,491	2.6	0.16
306	$140,538,445	$139,110,657	$36,303,438	22,600	4,103	5.5	0.26

	1	2	3	4	5	6	7
DRG Code	Total Charges	Coveraged Charges	Medicare Reimburse- ment	Total Days	Number of Dis- charges	AVG Total Days	Cost- to- Charge Ratio
307	$161,246,888	$158,677,299	$33,116,314	27,343	7,681	3.6	0.21
308	$2,693,405,658	$2,670,951,196	$541,025,009	432,237	85,404	5.1	0.20
309	$2,955,806,064	$2,926,037,570	$551,162,051	486,420	140,743	3.5	0.19
310	$2,362,572,336	$2,328,999,697	$365,906,487	373,504	159,836	2.3	0.16
311	$242,042,407	$235,952,115	$36,107,528	38,208	17,607	2.2	0.15
312	$4,033,356,705	$3,833,950,558	$627,539,391	578,621	205,174	2.8	0.16
313	$3,188,942,716	$2,985,219,038	$419,678,053	385,579	193,646	2	0.14
314	$3,578,938,075	$3,451,095,370	$780,631,233	522,934	71,238	7.3	0.23
315	$903,654,643	$889,128,629	$176,547,320	146,065	35,633	4.1	0.20
316	$207,138,221	$202,336,650	$34,446,590	31,726	12,254	2.6	0.17
326	$2,158,578,509	$2,134,236,651	$474,829,019	226,204	14,563	15.5	0.22
327	$1,002,102,552	$989,685,176	$200,311,794	113,516	13,684	8.3	0.20
328	$534,894,371	$525,763,510	$92,482,880	45,360	13,327	3.4	0.18
329	$7,526,932,362	$7,459,191,487	$1,618,540,466	847,163	56,960	14.9	0.22
330	$4,955,263,190	$4,916,170,373	$977,007,149	657,476	76,219	8.6	0.20
331	$1,404,480,529	$1,395,635,575	$247,859,327	169,603	33,669	5	0.18
332	$232,457,922	$229,659,104	$48,390,504	26,575	1,961	13.6	0.21
333	$398,730,541	$395,396,782	$78,273,512	49,065	6,290	7.8	0.20
334	$175,258,647	$173,791,788	$30,411,782	18,866	4,105	4.6	0.17
335	$1,026,339,512	$1,018,554,295	$214,895,139	124,260	9,262	13.4	0.21
336	$1,018,043,494	$1,010,322,821	$199,534,303	142,066	16,833	8.4	0.20

	1	2	3	4	5	6	7
DRG Code	Total Charges	Coveraged Charges	Medicare Reimbursement	Total Days	Number of Discharges	AVG Total Days	Cost-to-Charge Ratio
337	$417,775,618	$412,964,489	$71,495,569	51,961	10,369	5	0.17
338	$141,353,725	$140,251,687	$28,094,638	16,292	1,654	9.9	0.20
339	$206,603,956	$205,336,956	$37,334,373	26,575	4,183	6.4	0.18
340	$135,272,491	$134,199,542	$22,497,323	15,062	4,170	3.6	0.17
341	$73,998,655	$73,385,004	$13,742,376	7,647	1,131	6.8	0.19
342	$139,011,746	$137,585,304	$22,126,705	13,866	3,756	3.7	0.16
343	$225,717,097	$222,721,542	$32,387,317	15,947	8,360	1.9	0.15
344	$107,039,410	$106,071,382	$21,890,933	13,563	1,169	11.6	0.21
345	$191,373,407	$189,453,484	$38,220,996	28,490	4,273	6.7	0.20
346	$108,123,820	$107,303,172	$20,114,104	15,624	3,584	4.4	0.19
347	$139,868,740	$137,758,775	$30,010,462	18,229	2,042	8.9	0.22
348	$206,106,014	$203,264,780	$39,059,959	30,096	5,639	5.3	0.19
349	$108,322,886	$104,403,709	$16,039,378	13,522	4,840	2.8	0.15
350	$142,338,477	$141,295,360	$29,386,828	16,643	2,146	7.8	0.21
351	$208,936,293	$205,769,689	$36,933,908	24,685	5,708	4.3	0.18
352	$188,713,501	$178,201,580	$26,448,273	17,858	7,611	2.3	0.15
353	$338,753,484	$335,470,155	$69,120,365	36,905	4,417	8.4	0.21
354	$538,842,432	$530,150,646	$95,586,601	63,050	12,793	4.9	0.18
355	$455,135,487	$428,883,301	$65,156,192	44,249	15,739	2.8	0.15
356	$1,062,662,579	$1,042,764,163	$237,657,387	129,870	10,144	12.8	0.23
357	$576,029,140	$568,959,388	$112,768,120	70,944	9,927	7.1	0.20

	1	2	3	4	5	6	7
DRG Code	Total Charges	Coveraged Charges	Medicare Reimburse-ment	Total Days	Number of Dis-charges	AVG Total Days	Cost-to-Charge Ratio
358	$99,089,697	$96,503,973	$15,753,315	10,449	2,621	4	0.16
368	$214,274,523	$211,299,253	$43,940,299	29,520	4,308	6.9	0.21
369	$200,068,328	$198,728,678	$37,279,065	29,926	7,121	4.2	0.19
370	$43,562,383	$42,894,257	$6,963,684	6,222	2,109	3	0.16
371	$1,611,943,625	$1,589,873,161	$379,070,179	283,543	30,963	9.2	0.24
372	$1,437,638,784	$1,424,272,010	$316,969,226	289,871	48,125	6	0.22
373	$316,552,740	$313,228,146	$65,538,601	67,255	15,709	4.3	0.21
374	$624,410,383	$619,496,223	$137,968,034	95,484	10,959	8.7	0.22
375	$764,585,907	$757,392,111	$154,279,819	127,068	22,586	5.6	0.20
376	$77,811,189	$75,756,437	$13,316,401	11,822	3,308	3.6	0.18
377	$3,092,909,807	$3,056,456,600	$653,359,278	430,933	68,364	6.3	0.21
378	$4,756,561,822	$4,711,307,382	$899,463,575	736,875	186,087	4	0.19
379	$1,055,605,436	$1,034,584,145	$179,593,358	168,100	59,385	2.8	0.17
380	$204,404,198	$201,313,398	$43,988,730	30,011	4,005	7.5	0.22
381	$219,875,453	$218,068,360	$41,885,362	34,497	7,550	4.6	0.19
382	$68,399,746	$67,124,540	$11,764,778	10,584	3,150	3.4	0.18
383	$52,768,955	$51,977,086	$9,346,844	8,100	1,482	5.5	0.18
384	$226,543,864	$222,228,400	$34,962,359	33,331	9,695	3.4	0.16
385	$140,273,536	$137,569,492	$29,596,369	23,667	2,721	8.7	0.22
386	$322,791,894	$317,999,042	$59,098,028	58,636	11,546	5.1	0.19
387	$117,054,801	$114,538,468	$20,356,318	21,671	5,685	3.8	0.18

	1	2	3	4	5	6	7
DRG Code	Total Charges	Coveraged Charges	Medicare Reimbursement	Total Days	Number of Discharges	AVG Total Days	Cost-to-Charge Ratio
388	$1,036,214,711	$1,023,941,120	$222,842,448	177,703	24,273	7.3	0.22
389	$1,676,610,180	$1,660,907,898	$321,800,635	321,980	71,084	4.5	0.19
390	$907,839,574	$899,235,768	$150,661,742	176,328	54,840	3.2	0.17
391	$2,045,317,530	$2,008,424,527	$407,944,373	339,065	63,876	5.3	0.20
392	$6,720,565,560	$6,493,079,261	$1,082,854,149	1,150,998	345,396	3.3	0.17
393	$1,430,898,584	$1,396,557,488	$312,985,386	228,220	30,073	7.6	0.22
394	$1,668,152,381	$1,638,777,023	$316,670,666	286,489	63,466	4.5	0.19
395	$484,165,248	$470,238,969	$76,004,046	78,260	26,403	3	0.16
405	$931,472,275	$920,021,513	$203,693,625	89,797	5,853	15.3	0.22
406	$559,913,672	$553,165,071	$117,009,788	54,811	6,982	7.9	0.21
407	$155,547,748	$153,481,421	$29,859,413	14,163	2,791	5.1	0.19
408	$177,862,181	$176,469,016	$38,243,341	20,847	1,621	12.9	0.22
409	$98,707,132	$98,008,768	$20,907,247	12,869	1,557	8.3	0.21
410	$27,293,652	$27,157,995	$4,803,906	3,173	561	5.7	0.18
411	$68,342,203	$67,547,500	$13,350,122	7,854	678	11.6	0.20
412	$57,242,528	$57,115,733	$10,731,066	6,822	838	8.1	0.19
413	$23,847,925	$23,680,223	$3,994,262	2,529	480	5.3	0.17
414	$506,085,957	$502,037,376	$104,544,271	58,383	5,369	10.9	0.21
415	$362,068,308	$360,532,539	$67,337,516	45,556	6,630	6.9	0.19
416	$165,483,875	$164,752,881	$27,903,171	19,962	4,606	4.3	0.17
417	$1,593,025,658	$1,580,408,552	$296,373,617	178,035	23,219	7.7	0.19

	1	2	3	4	5	6	7
DRG Code	Total Charges	Coveraged Charges	Medicare Reimbursement	Total Days	Number of Discharges	AVG Total Days	Cost-to-Charge Ratio
418	$1,672,897,709	$1,652,601,684	$279,124,072	181,766	35,958	5.1	0.17
419	$1,189,205,888	$1,152,948,923	$169,594,412	105,878	35,509	3	0.15
420	$86,457,286	$83,129,461	$16,595,138	9,713	762	12.7	0.20
421	$56,374,666	$55,164,853	$11,546,219	6,832	1,133	6	0.21
422	$10,650,666	$10,588,759	$1,805,184	1,088	267	4.1	0.17
423	$230,709,558	$227,060,282	$53,841,665	26,756	1,911	14	0.24
424	$62,350,398	$61,845,336	$12,502,761	7,926	947	8.4	0.20
425	$5,579,607	$5,488,046	$1,118,869	599	126	4.8	0.20
432	$672,659,252	$664,651,681	$143,299,541	93,810	14,738	6.4	0.22
433	$249,455,322	$246,774,158	$47,978,795	41,297	9,750	4.2	0.19
434	$8,142,237	$7,814,742	$1,357,316	1,576	463	3.4	0.17
435	$805,196,789	$799,331,312	$165,522,227	116,148	16,262	7.1	0.21
436	$527,133,709	$520,697,045	$99,441,158	84,330	16,189	5.2	0.19
437	$72,396,943	$71,235,768	$11,656,636	9,709	2,681	3.6	0.16
438	$1,005,407,775	$989,383,963	$216,934,667	153,023	19,847	7.7	0.22
439	$979,206,413	$968,929,753	$186,182,988	173,677	37,469	4.6	0.19
440	$512,282,185	$506,138,706	$84,288,526	92,025	27,939	3.3	0.17
441	$1,186,583,180	$1,171,657,762	$255,125,531	165,131	22,946	7.2	0.22
442	$666,590,569	$659,236,360	$133,545,772	114,124	25,715	4.4	0.20
443	$113,660,985	$111,040,600	$19,890,647	21,222	6,278	3.4	0.18
444	$720,498,355	$714,044,061	$141,731,916	103,939	16,508	6.3	0.20

	1	2	3	4	5	6	7
DRG Code	Total Charges	Coveraged Charges	Medicare Reimbursement	Total Days	Number of Discharges	AVG Total Days	Cost-to-Total Charge Ratio
445	$753,182,797	$744,118,016	$134,385,176	108,872	25,501	4.3	0.18
446	$336,571,690	$327,973,582	$51,013,780	46,830	15,997	2.9	0.16
453	$492,161,301	$488,230,775	$109,793,792	22,137	1,758	12.6	0.22
454	$912,029,397	$906,093,223	$192,801,788	29,130	4,593	6.3	0.21
455	$589,535,753	$585,930,962	$117,330,631	14,858	4,085	3.6	0.20
456	$406,622,569	$403,396,535	$92,208,498	20,650	1,589	13	0.23
457	$742,119,389	$739,931,054	$167,834,311	29,642	4,539	6.5	0.23
458	$256,433,296	$254,487,463	$57,530,247	8,140	2,161	3.8	0.23
459	$860,438,957	$857,690,135	$185,184,783	50,573	5,520	9.2	0.22
460	$8,016,257,431	$7,963,912,799	$1,655,279,631	319,332	86,852	3.7	0.21
461	$80,020,785	$77,862,200	$15,401,823	5,373	644	8.3	0.20
462	$1,063,382,042	$1,058,032,883	$212,227,424	51,929	13,440	3.9	0.20
463	$959,544,293	$940,149,785	$222,949,656	142,363	7,106	20	0.24
464	$825,847,449	$817,537,895	$170,371,303	103,665	11,097	9.3	0.21
465	$159,411,629	$157,025,743	$30,167,251	18,356	3,199	5.7	0.19
466	$583,375,777	$578,323,420	$125,907,464	43,552	4,919	8.9	0.22
467	$2,279,980,807	$2,268,693,640	$460,913,540	132,842	28,975	4.6	0.20
468	$1,391,679,154	$1,385,173,854	$268,914,134	72,329	21,806	3.3	0.19
469	$2,698,535,237	$2,682,820,883	$570,284,288	259,565	33,749	7.7	0.21
470	$27,843,133,978	$27,644,350,269	$5,328,112,349	1,952,592	561,799	3.5	0.19
471	$513,922,380	$510,886,846	$108,980,603	36,506	3,961	9.2	0.21

	1	2	3	4	5	6	7
DRG Code	Total Charges	Coveraged Charges	Medicare Reimbursement	Total Days	Number of Discharges	AVG Total Days	Cost-to-Charge Ratio
472	$939,942,486	$936,066,785	$184,120,642	47,409	12,771	3.7	0.20
473	$1,902,307,511	$1,892,631,777	$343,841,648	64,304	35,389	1.8	0.18
474	$354,553,304	$348,472,114	$79,434,236	49,531	3,853	12.9	0.23
475	$256,556,429	$254,143,610	$51,807,564	39,666	5,020	7.9	0.20
476	$42,065,109	$41,649,508	$7,544,434	6,205	1,535	4	0.18
477	$289,528,596	$285,951,030	$62,334,338	38,816	3,385	11.5	0.22
478	$566,702,482	$561,454,864	$109,698,306	66,507	9,662	6.9	0.20
479	$206,585,749	$203,044,893	$36,397,131	19,495	4,728	4.1	0.18
480	$2,428,103,325	$2,412,996,116	$522,159,999	274,588	32,232	8.5	0.22
481	$4,995,990,852	$4,966,929,885	$962,659,376	556,441	104,236	5.3	0.19
482	$1,531,377,948	$1,522,934,505	$282,817,018	167,948	38,995	4.3	0.19
483	$1,006,769,976	$1,002,318,273	$191,815,756	56,829	16,370	3.5	0.19
484	$1,433,253,268	$1,422,796,012	$255,969,208	58,638	28,382	2.1	0.18
485	$122,839,346	$122,500,518	$26,816,133	15,205	1,456	10.4	0.22
486	$182,924,827	$181,374,297	$35,635,507	23,334	3,357	7	0.20
487	$53,036,681	$52,690,253	$9,825,775	6,749	1,390	4.9	0.19
488	$198,196,474	$195,529,508	$38,396,167	20,062	4,571	4.4	0.20
489	$190,173,064	$181,974,131	$30,839,444	16,416	6,046	2.7	0.17
490	$1,255,599,575	$1,242,957,717	$233,116,281	113,720	25,346	4.5	0.19
491	$1,492,422,349	$1,439,409,436	$213,284,485	105,655	51,064	2.1	0.15
492	$582,142,694	$577,489,841	$120,836,634	61,016	7,305	8.4	0.21

	1	2	3	4	5	6	7
DRG Code	Total Charges	Coveraged Charges	Medicare Reimbursement	Total Days	Number of Discharges	AVG Total Days	Cost-to-Charge Ratio
493	$1,385,726,555	$1,369,605,350	$251,843,348	132,449	27,531	4.8	0.18
494	$1,148,260,609	$1,122,433,309	$188,314,128	96,942	31,821	3	0.17
495	$198,659,265	$194,896,452	$44,734,328	27,603	2,303	12	0.23
496	$292,289,471	$288,693,167	$57,746,918	35,284	6,616	5.3	0.20
497	$181,527,368	$178,510,756	$30,027,887	14,807	5,841	2.5	0.17
498	$112,284,453	$111,302,070	$23,439,661	14,501	1,899	7.6	0.21
499	$28,547,591	$28,089,392	$4,942,765	2,705	1,010	2.7	0.18
500	$251,919,226	$247,468,313	$57,354,591	36,317	2,792	13	0.23
501	$285,039,716	$280,822,486	$55,454,640	39,334	6,754	5.8	0.20
502	$191,323,459	$180,990,284	$31,524,970	19,025	6,762	2.8	0.17
503	$78,138,599	$77,470,930	$17,041,414	11,889	1,205	9.9	0.22
504	$160,589,922	$158,803,555	$31,197,103	23,920	3,939	6.1	0.20
505	$86,135,698	$84,610,844	$14,567,989	9,251	2,839	3.3	0.17
506	$30,209,231	$29,858,169	$5,306,005	3,457	885	3.9	0.18
507	$41,222,880	$40,909,439	$8,264,825	4,592	819	5.6	0.20
508	$30,458,024	$28,249,442	$5,634,849	2,019	938	2.2	0.20
509	$12,492,367	$11,958,984	$2,204,855	1,280	344	3.7	0.18
510	$85,878,393	$85,171,558	$16,221,071	8,986	1,431	6.3	0.19
511	$220,209,160	$216,904,959	$37,800,991	21,045	5,519	3.8	0.17
512	$261,446,576	$253,832,288	$39,247,090	19,064	8,677	2.2	0.15
513	$66,454,785	$66,015,815	$12,250,672	8,629	1,781	4.8	0.19

	1	2	3	4	5	6	7
DRG Code	Total Charges	Coveraged Charges	Medicare Reimbursement	Total Days	Number of Discharges	AVG Total Days	Cost-to-Charge Ratio
514	$28,490,041	$27,674,708	$4,321,147	3,116	1,210	2.6	0.16
515	$435,101,571	$430,053,138	$89,453,773	51,233	4,958	10.3	0.21
516	$668,887,516	$656,424,195	$125,927,668	74,225	13,060	5.7	0.19
517	$423,627,990	$406,033,940	$71,706,862	35,732	10,454	3.4	0.18
533	$36,852,432	$36,328,485	$8,643,945	6,571	1,025	6.4	0.24
534	$75,607,386	$74,833,420	$17,399,912	17,855	4,298	4.2	0.23
535	$315,379,710	$312,575,513	$71,890,156	56,800	10,051	5.7	0.23
536	$775,677,105	$769,220,392	$179,481,837	184,285	44,996	4.1	0.23
537	$25,746,306	$25,461,112	$4,703,208	4,696	1,150	4.1	0.18
538	$12,498,598	$12,292,843	$2,245,196	2,343	792	3	0.18
539	$494,281,214	$477,298,938	$127,755,886	122,965	6,528	18.8	0.27
540	$246,531,209	$243,753,100	$59,111,045	60,352	6,122	9.9	0.24
541	$42,161,417	$41,383,625	$9,462,306	10,885	1,560	7	0.23
542	$354,686,433	$350,044,912	$75,505,470	57,812	6,804	8.5	0.22
543	$592,501,340	$586,143,684	$118,855,698	107,156	19,659	5.5	0.20
544	$135,412,521	$133,115,262	$27,002,116	27,647	7,004	3.9	0.20
545	$327,176,147	$322,472,054	$76,690,111	43,787	4,839	9	0.24
546	$237,328,704	$232,940,407	$48,454,239	40,671	7,738	5.3	0.21
547	$81,597,624	$79,322,855	$14,689,193	14,574	4,050	3.6	0.19
548	$72,471,087	$71,651,915	$18,993,511	15,948	1,120	14.2	0.27
549	$67,203,323	$65,901,326	$15,377,850	15,956	1,891	8.4	0.23

	1	2	3	4	5	6	7
DRG Code	Total Charges	Coveraged Charges	Medicare Reimbursement	Total Days	Number of Discharges	AVG Total Days	Cost-to-Charge Ratio
550	$15,750,307	$15,415,720	$3,514,311	3,620	785	4.6	0.23
551	$659,102,076	$651,874,236	$141,117,143	108,241	15,837	6.8	0.22
552	$2,118,185,894	$2,042,378,010	$381,911,630	387,466	98,288	3.9	0.19
553	$122,576,697	$120,937,835	$28,868,669	19,962	3,411	5.9	0.24
554	$499,514,408	$489,698,962	$122,370,246	125,677	28,634	4.4	0.25
555	$132,141,126	$130,259,161	$26,144,584	20,846	4,017	5.2	0.20
556	$446,655,410	$430,798,785	$76,460,648	78,740	24,655	3.2	0.18
557	$248,368,068	$245,860,699	$54,661,080	45,424	6,108	7.4	0.22
558	$509,865,288	$503,330,221	$98,496,793	98,980	23,005	4.3	0.20
559	$322,835,516	$316,255,109	$79,863,934	75,782	4,797	15.8	0.25
560	$301,053,683	$296,347,272	$74,502,444	76,382	8,873	8.6	0.25
561	$115,706,591	$111,034,529	$25,595,166	24,627	6,659	3.7	0.23
562	$268,264,555	$265,190,775	$56,621,678	44,834	7,775	5.8	0.21
563	$732,276,525	$715,097,646	$135,440,353	143,300	39,991	3.6	0.19
564	$135,390,765	$132,415,822	$32,125,923	25,997	2,882	9	0.24
565	$148,954,048	$146,435,610	$30,997,872	31,004	5,692	5.4	0.21
566	$39,204,830	$37,862,601	$8,043,157	8,197	2,116	3.9	0.21
573	$736,696,925	$709,303,136	$182,984,893	151,956	7,100	21.4	0.26
574	$588,064,529	$578,314,811	$136,255,457	124,523	11,884	10.5	0.24
575	$116,286,110	$115,033,595	$22,565,400	22,988	4,216	5.5	0.20
576	$104,194,260	$102,141,511	$24,029,007	13,576	911	14.9	0.24

	1	2	3	4	5	6	7
DRG Code	Total Charges	Coveraged Charges	Medicare Reimbursement	Total Days	Number of Dis-charges	AVG Total Days	Cost-to-Charge Ratio
577	$161,353,616	$157,610,322	$31,565,712	18,847	3,110	6.1	0.20
578	$97,105,063	$92,932,126	$16,159,636	9,620	2,997	3.2	0.17
579	$533,690,647	$519,440,424	$121,728,914	87,443	6,296	13.9	0.23
580	$648,183,893	$633,416,047	$121,753,115	93,703	15,902	5.9	0.19
581	$388,285,554	$364,055,802	$53,354,094	34,242	13,758	2.5	0.15
582	$168,099,032	$166,482,685	$26,007,981	13,965	5,330	2.6	0.16
583	$207,420,827	$204,046,153	$28,646,451	13,810	8,216	1.7	0.14
584	$47,190,547	$46,717,677	$8,527,414	5,509	1,062	5.2	0.18
585	$61,285,935	$57,470,702	$8,627,514	4,094	1,886	2.2	0.15
592	$558,336,957	$535,555,149	$140,201,249	138,834	8,151	17	0.26
593	$417,719,858	$408,556,049	$101,962,193	113,494	13,910	8.2	0.25
594	$41,118,051	$40,677,696	$10,472,792	12,079	2,168	5.6	0.26
595	$77,109,087	$76,306,862	$17,809,462	12,556	1,510	8.3	0.23
596	$145,414,892	$142,609,536	$30,422,486	29,624	6,428	4.6	0.21
597	$38,787,234	$37,412,410	$8,276,518	7,388	818	9	0.22
598	$62,588,526	$62,045,352	$12,516,739	12,016	2,013	6	0.20
599	$4,139,365	$4,046,695	$1,004,565	886	260	3.4	0.25
600	$38,992,482	$38,616,608	$7,825,874	7,672	1,462	5.2	0.20
601	$16,843,094	$16,672,995	$3,472,349	3,814	1,104	3.5	0.21
602	$1,338,047,478	$1,324,878,121	$296,491,183	252,199	34,703	7.3	0.22
603	$3,829,036,499	$3,792,743,109	$785,382,908	853,275	192,912	4.4	0.21

	1	2	3	4	5	6	7
DRG Code	Total Charges	Coveraged Charges	Medicare Reimbursement	Total Days	Number of Discharges	AVG Total Days	Cost-to-Charge Ratio
604	$130,994,112	$128,132,430	$25,877,476	19,671	3,625	5.4	0.20
605	$492,319,756	$480,532,537	$85,916,369	81,079	25,249	3.2	0.18
606	$86,986,783	$84,069,258	$19,584,472	15,603	2,234	7	0.23
607	$169,349,691	$166,744,906	$34,110,076	35,895	9,546	3.8	0.20
614	$155,670,863	$154,301,502	$31,661,264	12,224	2,136	5.7	0.21
615	$77,699,492	$77,250,661	$12,646,057	4,973	1,770	2.8	0.16
616	$257,550,935	$253,972,875	$59,476,880	37,562	2,344	16	0.23
617	$540,176,633	$535,278,500	$108,959,613	84,574	10,836	7.8	0.20
618	$5,255,524	$5,233,027	$1,085,981	944	185	5.1	0.21
619	$101,668,393	$92,888,529	$21,325,288	7,663	1,051	7.3	0.23
620	$222,394,021	$206,788,110	$39,542,589	13,216	4,260	3.1	0.19
621	$576,047,653	$534,902,315	$94,524,063	26,314	14,086	1.9	0.18
622	$182,918,264	$180,090,671	$44,556,132	34,728	1,805	19.2	0.25
623	$208,117,967	$205,324,047	$47,174,902	40,443	3,899	10.4	0.23
624	$8,025,802	$7,982,829	$1,592,580	1,548	303	5.1	0.20
625	$102,603,142	$101,528,759	$20,062,383	10,365	1,464	7.1	0.20
626	$135,622,618	$134,252,009	$22,043,382	10,761	3,780	2.8	0.16
627	$348,988,265	$336,704,727	$45,100,553	19,484	14,071	1.4	0.13
628	$437,973,370	$426,514,409	$101,490,457	54,029	4,838	11.2	0.24
629	$395,372,334	$390,114,629	$82,717,745	56,017	7,008	8	0.21
630	$19,561,057	$18,467,608	$3,802,092	2,271	546	4.2	0.21

	1	2	3	4	5	6	7
DRG Code	Total Charges	Coveraged Charges	Medicare Reimbursement	Total Days	Number of Discharges	AVG Total Days	Cost-to-Charge Ratio
637	$1,101,617,881	$1,084,447,986	$236,348,635	183,029	28,525	6.4	0.22
638	$1,637,884,512	$1,614,096,230	$326,070,150	311,640	74,185	4.2	0.20
639	$452,473,757	$442,499,955	$78,253,984	86,092	31,669	2.7	0.18
640	$2,262,992,871	$2,225,761,937	$514,150,114	389,041	78,275	5	0.23
641	$3,649,518,906	$3,600,934,833	$715,433,080	724,780	213,028	3.4	0.20
642	$67,629,260	$59,268,034	$12,081,751	14,184	2,023	7	0.20
643	$377,584,532	$372,831,314	$84,049,196	62,187	8,701	7.1	0.23
644	$474,068,313	$469,039,637	$94,981,288	86,334	17,528	4.9	0.20
645	$163,823,879	$160,255,542	$27,883,890	29,022	8,526	3.4	0.17
652	$2,054,274,442	$2,028,908,140	$277,966,500	79,025	11,209	7.1	0.14
653	$360,668,891	$354,974,650	$78,081,215	36,427	2,286	15.9	0.22
654	$440,387,275	$435,980,827	$85,394,036	46,702	5,111	9.1	0.20
655	$116,277,425	$114,001,481	$20,244,417	10,573	1,893	5.6	0.18
656	$431,562,076	$428,561,090	$91,796,699	42,107	4,356	9.7	0.21
657	$638,344,672	$632,796,150	$117,906,889	63,141	11,639	5.4	0.19
658	$383,595,729	$378,325,944	$62,345,312	29,927	9,222	3.2	0.16
659	$484,769,986	$478,168,442	$112,837,388	56,833	5,125	11.1	0.24
660	$573,529,592	$566,697,101	$113,866,166	64,420	11,159	5.8	0.20
661	$201,777,925	$194,071,911	$31,935,713	14,800	5,356	2.8	0.16
662	$80,464,518	$78,406,275	$18,683,043	10,640	1,030	10.3	0.24
663	$89,160,642	$86,224,383	$16,494,597	11,445	2,278	5	0.19

	1	2	3	4	5	6	7
DRG Code	Total Charges	Coveraged Charges	Medicare Reimbursement	Total Days	Number of Discharges	AVG Total Days	Cost-to-Charge Ratio
664	$95,699,591	$87,041,321	$14,151,388	5,980	3,128	1.9	0.16
665	$62,007,753	$61,286,979	$11,756,684	9,511	779	12.2	0.19
666	$110,000,446	$108,883,646	$20,737,058	15,437	2,480	6.2	0.19
667	$58,722,833	$55,559,687	$7,950,972	6,183	2,525	2.4	0.14
668	$287,632,557	$285,272,582	$60,597,007	38,603	4,393	8.8	0.21
669	$691,554,689	$684,203,138	$118,011,938	83,415	19,992	4.2	0.17
670	$217,119,072	$201,915,458	$29,838,784	22,595	9,720	2.3	0.15
671	$37,528,281	$36,916,374	$7,419,379	4,929	937	5.3	0.20
672	$20,085,486	$18,985,538	$2,956,788	1,737	788	2.2	0.16
673	$1,187,070,509	$1,157,936,178	$258,761,914	146,317	14,371	10.2	0.22
674	$605,519,890	$595,766,997	$117,733,428	73,427	10,395	7.1	0.20
675	$96,462,530	$88,250,961	$15,088,731	6,137	2,514	2.4	0.17
682	$5,438,880,158	$5,367,039,553	$1,207,005,462	905,305	132,858	6.8	0.22
683	$5,053,460,362	$5,003,261,322	$1,001,020,983	938,667	201,108	4.7	0.20
684	$644,801,629	$634,476,021	$114,932,582	124,921	39,445	3.2	0.18
685	$77,002,354	$74,379,607	$16,480,280	12,340	3,572	3.5	0.22
686	$83,415,446	$82,890,487	$19,099,858	13,669	1,725	7.9	0.23
687	$116,124,293	$115,254,413	$23,875,061	20,787	4,132	5	0.21
688	$15,323,218	$14,725,964	$2,515,817	2,844	804	3.5	0.17
689	$2,690,074,730	$2,658,935,833	$596,233,581	525,609	92,030	5.7	0.22
690	$5,330,950,107	$5,269,269,045	$1,067,562,733	1,080,386	278,922	3.9	0.20

	1	2	3	4	5	6	7
DRG Code	Total Charges	Coveraged Charges	Medicare Reimbursement	Total Days	Number of Dis-charges	AVG Total Days	Cost-to-Charge Ratio
691	$49,297,033	$48,257,942	$9,267,099	4,999	1,266	3.9	0.19
692	$10,734,132	$9,760,418	$1,787,176	845	412	2.1	0.18
693	$110,110,472	$109,067,415	$20,047,010	15,267	2,897	5.3	0.18
694	$471,404,643	$457,986,762	$69,149,655	58,095	24,362	2.4	0.15
695	$57,581,090	$57,180,057	$11,824,584	9,764	1,798	5.4	0.21
696	$243,142,024	$237,492,441	$45,143,808	46,191	14,999	3.1	0.19
697	$14,845,241	$14,422,670	$2,450,529	2,120	690	3.1	0.17
698	$1,470,509,973	$1,443,661,698	$334,239,002	241,996	35,582	6.8	0.23
699	$1,061,230,881	$1,047,149,219	$225,369,193	181,356	40,304	4.5	0.22
700	$176,718,778	$172,985,915	$33,913,883	32,063	9,971	3.2	0.20
707	$359,494,965	$356,455,168	$59,264,179	28,761	7,090	4.1	0.17
708	$903,741,615	$896,105,482	$125,815,056	44,619	23,681	1.9	0.14
709	$57,793,093	$57,074,356	$11,647,893	6,744	1,007	6.7	0.20
710	$60,162,535	$53,853,190	$9,430,585	2,854	1,639	1.7	0.18
711	$48,722,912	$48,488,353	$9,219,177	7,366	912	8.1	0.19
712	$10,876,221	$10,286,366	$1,613,330	1,407	464	3	0.16
713	$363,106,542	$354,218,229	$59,251,780	44,676	10,574	4.2	0.17
714	$406,256,614	$375,478,305	$51,173,176	38,446	21,524	1.8	0.14
715	$33,208,504	$32,967,796	$6,042,100	4,185	635	6.6	0.18
716	$19,061,082	$17,930,137	$2,265,784	934	659	1.4	0.13
717	$50,182,194	$49,606,970	$10,171,281	7,180	1,045	6.9	0.21

	1	2	3	4	5	6	7
DRG Code	Total Charges	Coveraged Charges	Medicare Reimbursement	Total Days	Number of Discharges	AVG Total Days	Cost-to-Charge Ratio
718	$11,695,728	$11,341,347	$1,770,367	1,491	517	2.9	0.16
722	$33,009,483	$32,270,096	$7,309,311	6,210	736	8.4	0.23
723	$62,955,223	$62,241,936	$12,912,715	12,186	2,235	5.5	0.21
724	$5,475,947	$5,362,465	$920,907	902	323	2.8	0.17
725	$28,622,109	$28,487,402	$6,059,503	5,154	847	6.1	0.21
726	$99,135,083	$98,253,980	$18,180,382	18,380	5,493	3.3	0.19
727	$80,774,062	$79,821,188	$17,583,667	14,961	2,077	7.2	0.22
728	$160,693,918	$159,451,196	$29,154,625	32,628	8,190	4	0.18
729	$34,091,063	$33,483,658	$7,197,642	6,638	1,074	6.2	0.21
730	$5,875,226	$5,655,446	$1,109,317	1,007	357	2.8	0.20
734	$164,979,169	$163,065,038	$30,707,486	15,396	2,140	7.2	0.19
735	$58,359,741	$57,794,693	$8,653,085	3,756	1,616	2.3	0.15
736	$144,366,433	$144,109,126	$29,928,854	14,890	1,147	13	0.21
737	$232,481,109	$230,867,082	$43,878,964	26,184	4,093	6.4	0.19
738	$35,764,359	$35,620,497	$5,637,120	3,190	941	3.4	0.16
739	$111,987,625	$110,727,680	$23,760,044	10,825	1,142	9.5	0.21
740	$268,399,329	$266,132,882	$45,595,603	24,414	5,782	4.2	0.17
741	$230,199,148	$223,397,676	$32,238,518	14,393	6,646	2.2	0.14
742	$502,353,304	$493,498,535	$86,346,294	48,055	12,443	3.9	0.17
743	$868,294,021	$842,198,778	$116,708,685	61,391	31,989	1.9	0.14
744	$89,001,424	$87,714,323	$17,732,975	11,873	2,009	5.9	0.20

	1	2	3	4	5	6	7
DRG Code	Total Charges	Coveraged Charges	Medicare Reimbursement	Total Days	Number of Discharges	AVG Total Days	Cost-to-Charge Ratio
745	$32,193,661	$31,474,305	$4,920,573	2,828	1,300	2.2	0.16
746	$114,989,056	$113,964,937	$21,347,360	13,019	3,004	4.3	0.19
747	$191,525,443	$174,672,900	$25,737,253	13,033	7,723	1.7	0.15
748	$468,783,249	$443,972,553	$62,903,548	29,340	18,015	1.6	0.14
749	$98,547,192	$98,262,022	$19,230,595	12,161	1,359	8.9	0.20
750	$12,819,928	$12,440,863	$1,824,638	1,214	422	2.9	0.15
754	$86,790,466	$85,994,534	$20,110,525	14,649	1,580	9.3	0.23
755	$131,606,537	$130,203,478	$27,626,106	23,839	4,470	5.3	0.21
756	$8,506,617	$8,268,206	$1,787,805	1,639	517	3.2	0.22
757	$92,244,510	$90,974,741	$20,749,489	17,062	1,929	8.8	0.23
758	$84,752,996	$83,825,999	$18,043,408	16,804	2,937	5.7	0.22
759	$23,442,402	$23,188,211	$4,720,885	4,836	1,274	3.8	0.20
760	$62,726,014	$61,699,898	$12,289,049	10,299	2,845	3.6	0.20
761	$18,280,430	$17,685,937	$3,023,386	2,994	1,399	2.1	0.17
765	$116,085,054	$113,545,411	$29,305,213	20,727	4,313	4.8	0.26
766	$55,646,430	$54,854,004	$13,211,847	10,052	3,249	3.1	0.24
767	$5,632,040	$4,726,533	$1,277,448	1,057	334	3.2	0.27
768	$417,545	$417,545	$108,995	45	11	4.1	0.26
769	$5,902,568	$5,889,193	$1,845,809	673	136	4.9	0.31
770	$4,556,375	$4,219,586	$823,799	452	220	2.1	0.20
774	$35,128,625	$34,655,636	$8,729,138	7,229	2,173	3.3	0.25

	1	2	3	4	5	6	7
DRG Code	Total Charges	Coveraged Charges	Medicare Reimbursement	Total Days	Number of Dis-charges	AVG Total Days	Cost-to-Charge Ratio
775	$81,520,588	$80,701,741	$17,920,978	16,807	7,148	2.4	0.22
776	$16,681,191	$16,274,726	$3,851,148	3,545	874	4.1	0.24
777	$5,370,366	$5,284,056	$792,812	487	207	2.4	0.15
778	$6,014,308	$5,961,096	$1,384,933	1,592	524	3	0.23
779	$1,997,993	$1,822,540	$382,594	273	144	1.9	0.21
780	$272,935	$245,126	$41,322	62	54	1.1	0.17
781	$78,539,291	$76,567,047	$19,443,322	19,111	4,348	4.4	0.25
782	$2,465,775	$2,454,519	$583,888	598	225	2.7	0.24
790	$3,232,044	$2,990,547	$458,593	535	*	178.3	0.15
791	$169,368	$169,368	$80,725	179	*	179	0.48
793	$4,703	$4,703	$6,974	*	*	2	1.48
794	$30,744	$30,744	$10,686	*	*	6	0.35
799	$89,902,150	$89,631,573	$18,189,113	7,928	630	12.6	0.20
800	$54,243,623	$53,926,717	$10,603,730	5,460	764	7.1	0.20
801	$19,944,787	$19,913,497	$3,557,693	1,786	476	3.8	0.18
802	$109,862,088	$107,925,345	$25,206,553	13,166	1,118	11.8	0.23
803	$70,826,043	$70,088,225	$14,325,675	8,497	1,472	5.8	0.20
804	$28,504,251	$27,895,693	$4,158,498	2,617	863	3	0.15
808	$643,762,617	$636,370,356	$147,194,423	89,852	11,246	8	0.23
809	$586,052,481	$580,037,071	$121,194,494	89,757	18,376	4.9	0.21
810	$67,642,456	$67,051,261	$12,807,030	9,923	2,767	3.6	0.19

	1	2	3	4	5	6	7
DRG Code	Total Charges	Coveraged Charges	Medicare Reimbursement	Total Days	Number of Discharges	AVG Total Days	Cost-to-Charge Ratio
811	$1,378,949,540	$1,347,716,329	$287,334,747	214,865	42,076	5.1	0.21
812	$2,668,744,205	$2,573,953,445	$504,090,569	452,378	132,417	3.4	0.20
813	$707,587,097	$681,316,413	$144,686,237	66,448	13,285	5	0.21
814	$93,019,000	$91,629,193	$20,091,907	13,739	1,986	6.9	0.22
815	$126,816,652	$125,249,794	$24,135,077	20,742	4,657	4.5	0.19
816	$30,998,957	$30,555,300	$5,520,282	5,352	1,737	3.1	0.18
820	$271,063,910	$268,916,680	$59,456,376	27,711	1,622	17.1	0.22
821	$167,296,600	$165,872,284	$34,295,138	17,528	2,528	6.9	0.21
822	$72,964,821	$71,406,544	$12,474,728	5,793	2,013	2.9	0.17
823	$299,533,204	$296,846,448	$65,002,973	34,797	2,319	15	0.22
824	$239,621,084	$237,590,935	$46,204,683	29,462	3,657	8.1	0.19
825	$56,981,797	$55,778,804	$9,198,819	5,741	1,540	3.7	0.16
826	$111,272,774	$110,193,078	$24,308,778	11,329	820	13.8	0.22
827	$120,259,069	$118,837,225	$23,991,413	12,978	1,880	6.9	0.20
828	$50,272,910	$49,758,442	$9,147,157	4,427	1,218	3.6	0.18
829	$152,356,437	$150,470,664	$31,229,902	16,999	1,798	9.5	0.21
830	$18,853,536	$18,618,143	$3,227,875	1,709	523	3.3	0.17
834	$757,894,889	$746,689,590	$173,992,818	83,645	5,036	16.6	0.23
835	$248,386,270	$244,692,318	$60,840,430	33,532	3,887	8.6	0.25
836	$46,785,701	$45,730,008	$9,704,970	6,448	1,439	4.5	0.21
837	$370,228,704	$365,385,416	$94,385,658	45,268	2,015	22.5	0.26

	1	2	3	4	5	6	7
DRG Code	Total Charges	Coveraged Charges	Medicare Reimbursement	Total Days	Number of Discharges	AVG Total Days	Cost-to-Charge Ratio
838	$177,299,163	$173,636,044	$45,535,084	21,897	2,124	10.3	0.26
839	$68,914,153	$67,963,036	$15,991,145	10,505	1,868	5.6	0.24
840	$844,756,348	$834,863,569	$186,522,272	111,400	10,238	10.9	0.22
841	$583,213,339	$576,963,428	$119,118,943	84,831	13,052	6.5	0.21
842	$131,620,977	$129,385,788	$23,169,819	17,572	4,367	4	0.18
843	$106,240,732	$105,795,011	$22,511,877	16,619	2,100	7.9	0.21
844	$126,395,599	$125,581,827	$24,839,279	21,619	3,842	5.6	0.20
845	$20,661,172	$20,413,870	$3,589,897	3,400	868	3.9	0.18
846	$250,987,560	$247,741,583	$56,595,035	29,602	3,425	8.6	0.23
847	$870,222,618	$848,317,849	$160,701,954	94,099	26,581	3.5	0.19
848	$32,990,539	$32,219,816	$6,601,064	4,162	1,406	3	0.20
849	$47,999,419	$47,658,577	$9,555,095	7,768	1,078	7.2	0.20
853	$8,297,873,941	$8,089,936,770	$1,847,168,105	902,824	58,487	15.4	0.23
854	$804,756,435	$797,455,175	$170,648,509	110,226	12,280	9	0.21
855	$18,599,264	$18,254,775	$3,175,448	2,314	444	5.2	0.17
856	$1,024,808,902	$1,005,588,011	$239,806,227	130,424	8,373	15.6	0.24
857	$653,072,388	$644,665,512	$137,565,186	96,350	12,311	7.8	0.21
858	$86,110,356	$85,120,244	$17,528,436	13,087	2,711	4.8	0.21
862	$908,710,072	$896,073,297	$203,716,615	158,180	15,371	10.3	0.23
863	$724,158,419	$715,281,376	$155,828,375	149,516	27,824	5.4	0.22
864	$553,380,295	$544,890,647	$104,054,335	90,850	25,066	3.6	0.19

	1	2	3	4	5	6	7
DRG Code	Total Charges	Coveraged Charges	Medicare Reimbursement	Total Days	Number of Discharges	AVG Total Days	Cost-to-Charge Ratio
865	$123,117,545	$120,307,716	$27,719,553	18,527	2,807	6.6	0.23
866	$193,540,863	$190,087,252	$33,896,690	33,040	9,718	3.4	0.18
867	$516,223,228	$504,659,969	$117,184,801	74,831	7,043	10.6	0.23
868	$95,592,386	$94,706,071	$21,915,597	17,791	3,466	5.1	0.23
869	$17,702,590	$17,432,300	$3,856,692	3,563	1,029	3.5	0.22
870	$6,337,728,680	$6,128,915,925	$1,376,364,356	618,666	38,752	16	0.22
871	$20,483,223,245	$20,230,956,729	$4,366,876,216	2,968,878	410,011	7.2	0.22
872	$4,253,697,539	$4,220,870,972	$874,800,587	781,464	153,547	5.1	0.21
876	$95,273,176	$85,374,604	$23,863,708	23,333	1,366	17.1	0.28
880	$228,693,230	$219,712,900	$49,342,388	58,824	13,183	4.5	0.22
881	$350,389,411	$321,292,445	$101,743,119	164,251	23,547	7	0.32
882	$116,189,634	$107,337,510	$35,374,097	56,618	8,032	7	0.33
883	$84,261,585	$73,699,429	$24,092,036	41,902	3,250	12.9	0.33
884	$1,405,284,463	$1,314,788,997	$418,471,856	574,216	54,658	10.5	0.32
885	$11,604,484,478	$10,168,876,774	$3,466,233,792	6,246,875	477,555	13.1	0.34
886	$81,053,832	$70,092,004	$23,734,354	44,754	3,350	13.4	0.34
887	$28,903,746	$23,744,254	$6,486,190	16,583	1,043	15.9	0.27
894	$67,380,496	$64,895,522	$16,464,108	21,854	7,208	3	0.25
895	$246,360,435	$242,161,235	$105,311,386	166,891	14,496	11.5	0.43
896	$378,202,253	$372,985,056	$84,491,748	73,039	10,234	7.1	0.23
897	$1,075,590,211	$1,040,197,725	$269,266,221	387,338	71,194	5.4	0.26

	1	2	3	4	5	6	7
DRG Code	Total Charges	Coveraged Charges	Medicare Reimburse-ment	Total Days	Number of Dis-charges	AVG Total Days	Cost-to-Charge Ratio
901	$168,233,624	$164,722,607	$42,421,991	29,345	1,330	22.1	0.26
902	$107,665,700	$106,456,594	$27,133,984	20,031	2,265	8.8	0.25
903	$26,279,439	$25,852,870	$5,371,306	4,235	965	4.4	0.21
904	$239,500,444	$234,217,159	$55,244,364	31,627	2,757	11.5	0.24
905	$38,991,216	$38,570,834	$7,721,227	5,204	1,105	4.7	0.20
906	$33,730,752	$32,795,857	$5,540,388	3,536	974	3.6	0.17
907	$1,153,303,083	$1,124,438,310	$258,101,101	127,108	10,911	11.6	0.23
908	$651,046,101	$643,096,068	$128,683,470	77,567	12,599	6.2	0.20
909	$202,220,358	$196,250,318	$34,198,851	20,735	6,247	3.3	0.17
913	$48,464,708	$47,886,804	$11,466,324	8,894	1,369	6.5	0.24
914	$138,018,751	$135,126,522	$27,141,935	25,386	7,520	3.4	0.20
915	$96,435,977	$95,668,199	$17,736,336	11,941	2,261	5.3	0.19
916	$110,929,201	$109,437,270	$16,426,410	17,520	8,529	2.1	0.15
917	$1,225,335,518	$1,215,029,513	$247,837,660	155,253	31,242	5	0.20
918	$819,455,052	$806,844,980	$143,578,286	132,230	48,481	2.7	0.18
919	$907,161,239	$879,737,973	$200,940,489	152,457	15,936	9.6	0.23
920	$599,112,242	$589,574,955	$125,444,002	106,349	21,438	5	0.21
921	$154,142,650	$151,575,987	$27,000,392	25,558	8,864	2.9	0.18
922	$69,138,716	$68,321,673	$14,098,861	9,968	1,704	5.8	0.21
923	$84,798,796	$82,770,496	$15,998,161	13,942	4,764	2.9	0.19
927	$102,582,630	$102,555,239	$24,902,234	6,430	220	29.2	0.24

	1	2	3	4	5	6	7
DRG Code	Total Charges	Coveraged Charges	Medicare Reimburse-ment	Total Days	Number of Dis-charges	AVG Total Days	Cost-to-Charge Ratio
928	$189,603,346	$187,854,893	$48,242,314	21,131	1,345	15.7	0.26
929	$36,374,418	$36,117,921	$7,944,270	4,357	576	7.6	0.22
933	$14,980,401	$14,950,223	$3,988,789	1,238	204	6.1	0.27
934	$38,051,217	$37,520,415	$8,519,676	6,411	893	7.2	0.23
935	$105,883,444	$104,118,857	$25,907,602	16,166	2,986	5.4	0.25
939	$245,528,949	$230,369,630	$61,876,266	48,863	2,705	18.1	0.27
940	$223,344,059	$211,132,192	$53,218,072	41,627	3,776	11	0.25
941	$58,570,439	$56,283,332	$11,624,037	6,367	1,726	3.7	0.21
945	$12,480,367,065	$11,993,006,831	$5,055,039,604	4,404,528	328,351	13.4	0.42
946	$2,090,505,636	$1,998,246,142	$933,303,945	809,697	75,729	10.7	0.47
947	$513,481,587	$505,158,005	$108,955,524	88,597	18,087	4.9	0.22
948	$1,423,321,342	$1,398,986,863	$276,411,605	269,539	80,424	3.4	0.20
949	$259,605,672	$253,505,182	$75,787,869	80,934	4,385	18.5	0.30
950	$12,095,276	$11,583,429	$3,181,120	4,412	543	8.1	0.27
951	$56,880,867	$50,789,246	$18,828,973	28,125	2,007	14	0.37
955	$92,825,447	$90,812,633	$20,085,683	6,493	559	11.6	0.22
956	$540,451,430	$538,005,212	$111,374,376	49,907	5,892	8.5	0.21
957	$406,195,657	$401,132,955	$90,021,502	29,539	2,140	13.8	0.22
958	$189,633,770	$186,553,588	$36,979,275	15,152	1,643	9.2	0.20
959	$18,099,711	$17,863,975	$3,474,544	1,419	249	5.7	0.19
963	$213,270,999	$211,850,728	$47,153,265	23,722	2,611	9.1	0.22

	1	2	3	4	5	6	7
DRG Code	Total Charges	Coveraged Charges	Medicare Reimbursement	Total Days	Number of Discharges	AVG Total Days	Cost-to-Charge Ratio
964	$177,779,990	$175,571,071	$33,303,269	24,864	4,133	6	0.19
965	$32,431,300	$32,138,929	$5,969,707	4,901	1,192	4.1	0.19
969	$109,022,978	$107,612,864	$27,887,628	10,920	646	16.9	0.26
970	$7,477,321	$7,474,607	$1,709,885	737	100	7.4	0.23
974	$485,261,580	$474,351,675	$123,681,673	63,718	6,113	10.4	0.26
975	$190,633,013	$181,849,192	$44,532,326	35,861	4,602	7.8	0.24
976	$44,532,027	$40,783,720	$9,560,134	10,128	1,569	6.5	0.23
977	$122,515,616	$116,834,948	$26,078,965	24,340	3,642	6.7	0.22
981	$4,305,070,753	$4,206,074,657	$942,497,165	479,772	31,297	15.3	0.22
982	$1,715,661,066	$1,690,436,111	$350,366,964	188,310	23,195	8.1	0.21
983	$293,321,195	$274,406,734	$50,041,829	24,410	6,352	3.8	0.18
984	$58,879,239	$57,977,904	$12,240,493	8,728	634	13.8	0.21
985	$61,697,997	$60,362,655	$13,113,857	9,576	1,138	8.4	0.22
986	$15,279,195	$15,132,136	$2,817,350	1,955	540	3.6	0.19
987	$995,444,443	$948,590,051	$215,757,136	144,022	10,216	14.1	0.23
988	$615,439,686	$601,804,425	$124,656,160	93,223	12,708	7.3	0.21
989	$124,792,165	$123,359,882	$22,868,533	14,847	4,183	3.5	0.19
999	$10,484,623	$10,263,234	$6,584,294	1,054	126	8.4	0.64

Abridged life table. A means for converting mortality rates into the average life expectancy of a hypothetical cohort of 100,000 persons exposed to the mortality rates. In an abridged life table, mortality rates in n-year intervals are used to estimate the expected number of deaths in a hypothetical cohort of 100,000 persons. From these deaths, the mean number of years lived by the cohort is calculated. Although abridged life tables use larger age intervals than standard life tables, the two methods produce similar results so long as the interval is reasonably short.

Accuracy. The extent to which a measured value is representative of its real value.

Analytical horizon. The period over which all costs and outcomes are considered in an economic analysis.

Appropriate technology utilization. The prioritization of the most cost-effective technologies over less cost-effective technologies (e.g., vaccination versus heart-lung transplants).

Attribute. A given measure of health. For instance, pain on a 1-to-5 scale is a health attribute.

Baseline value. The most likely value of an uncertain parameter.

Bias. A form of nonrandom error in which some force acts to systematically influence the measurement of a given value such that it deviates from its true value. For instance, when men are asked their height, they tend to overestimate values measured by a third party.

Case-control study. An observational study that is usually retrospective that identifies patients with the disease in the present who are then matched to those without the disease and then evaluated to determine if there are specific risk factors in the past associated with the disease.

Charge. The amount billed by a given provider, including profits. A charge is almost invariably greater than the opportunity cost of the services provided.

Clinical practice guidelines. A standardized practice algorithm for diagnosing and treating disease that has been designed with the input of experts.

Community-derived preferences. Preferences for health states derived from a general population rather than from persons with the disease of interest.

Competing alternative. An alternative practice for diagnosing or treating the disease you are studying in your cost-effectiveness analysis. For instance, the competing alternative for annual screening mammography might be monthly breast self-examination.

Cost-effectiveness analysis. A type of economic analysis in which costs associated with two or more strategies are compared based on some measure of effectiveness. In the health field, cost-effectiveness and cost utility are often used interchangeably.

Cost-to-charge ratio. A ratio used to convert medical charges to something more representative of their societal opportunity cost.

Cost-utility analysis. A type of economic analysis that compares the costs associated with two or more strategies based on a measure of utility. In the reference case analysis, the measure of utility must be a quality-adjusted life-year–compatible health-related quality-of-life score.

Counterfactual. The counterfactual group is the unobservable comparison group that does not receive the intervention. In the theory of causation, the counterfactual is the "what if" scenario where the experimental group does not experience the intervention.

Cross-sectional studies. Studies that contain observational data at a single point in time. For instance, a census is a cross-sectional study of the characteristics of the general population of a country.

Crude rates. Rates unadjusted for age, gender, or other sociodemographic characteristics.

Cumulative incidence. The number of new events or outcomes that occur in a given population initially at risk for the event or outcome in a given observation period.

Data extraction tool. Software that allows users to easily obtain values from a given dataset.

Decision analysis model. A model used to calculate the expected value of a given health strategy. Decision analysis models are the most frequently used means for calculating incremental cost-effectiveness ratios.

Dimension. A given measure of health—for instance, pain on a 1-to-5 scale is a dimension of health.

Direct costs. Costs associated with goods and services consumed, such as units of influenza vaccine used in a vaccination drive.

Discounting. The process of converting future costs into present terms. The rate of discount used in cost-effectiveness analysis is 3 percent for both costs and quality-adjusted life years (QALYs).

Disutility. A preference-based measure that results in loss instead of gain in QALYs.

Domain. A given measure of health—for instance, pain on a 1-to-5 scale is a health domain.

Dominant strategy. A strategy that is more effective and less expensive than at least one competing alternative.

Dominated strategy. A strategy that is less effective and more costly than at least one competing alternative.

Double-blinded. An experimental study design in which neither the subject nor the investigator is aware of the treatment administered to a subject.

Effect size. The strength of the relationship between two variables.

Effectiveness. The performance of health interventions in the real world.

Efficacy. The performance of health interventions under controlled or exacting laboratory conditions.

Expected cost. The projected cost based on the probability of the event occurring and the total costs of the event.

Expected value. The probabilistically weighted average of a series of numbers.

Expenditure. The amount of money paid for a service.

External validity. The extent to which the results of a study are generalizable to settings other than the one in which the data were collected.

Event pathway. A pathway in the flowchart that depicts the course of different events that occur in a cost-effectiveness analysis.

False-positive test result. A false-positive test result occurs when a laboratory test indicates that disease is present when, in fact, it is absent.

Fixed costs. Costs that do not change when a health intervention is applied.

Governmental perspective. An analysis that includes costs and effectiveness benefits from the perspective of only a governmental agency. For instance, such analysis includes the cost of treatments paid for by the government but not costs incurred by patients.

Gross cost. An aggregate cost associated with a health event. For instance, the cost of hospitalization for influenza might be obtained from billing records. Such costs typically include most, but not all, products and services delivered for the particular health event.

Gross costing. The process of obtaining gross costs, usually from an electronic dataset.

Half-cycle correction. A correction factor used to address midcycle transitions that can occur in a continuous transition state model (e.g., Markov model).

Health intervention. A strategy for diagnosing or treating a disease. Examples include vaccination to prevent influenza, mammography to detect early breast cancer, and diet and exercise to prevent hypertension.

Health outcome. *See* Outcome, health.

Health state. The health status of a given person or population at a given point in time. Examples are hospitalized, ill, alive, well, and dead.

Health status. The overall state of health of an individual or group of individuals. Health status can also be defined as the sum of various health states.

Health-related quality-of-life (HRQL) score. A numerical valuation of life in a given health state anchored between 0 (death) and 1 (perfect health). These scores are used to adjust life-years to quality-adjusted life-years (QALYs). Thus, a year of life lived at an HRQL of 0.7 is equivalent to 0.7 QALYs (or 0.7 years of perfect health).

Healthy volunteer effect. Subjects who volunteer for a study are typically healthier than the average person residing in the community from which the subjects were recruited. Because healthy people are not representative of the population at large, the results of studies using such subjects may be biased.

Hypothetical cohort. A study cohort derived from statistical data rather than an actual cohort of subjects. For instance, life tables are constructed based on hypothetical numbers of deaths occurring among a group of 100,000 hypothetical subjects exposed to real-world age-specific mortality rates.

Impact statement. A statement, usually in the introduction of a manuscript, that provides information on the burden of disease (epidemiological and economic) on society (or other parties).

Incidence rate. Number of new cases divided by the amount of time the population is at risk in a given observation period.

Incremental cost-effectiveness ratio (ICER). Between two competing alternatives, it is the ratio of the change in costs and the incremental gain in benefit. For instance, a payer would need to invest $1,000 more in strategy 1 relative to strategy 2 in order to achieve a 1-unit QALY gained in benefits.

Incremental value. A cost or effectiveness value above and beyond the average value. For instance, if a woman receiving annual mammography can expect to live 11 years and a woman who does not receive mammography can expect to live 10 years, the incremental gain in life expectancy is 1 year.

Indirect costs. Costs not directly related to the consumption of goods or services. Lost productivity due to illness is an example of an indirect cost.

Intangible costs. Costs for which it is difficult to attach a monetary value. Examples of intangible costs include the cost of suffering from the loss of a loved one or the cost of missing your child's first birthday.

League table. A table of interventions listed by their incremental cost-effectiveness ratios. If the incremental cost-effectiveness ratios for most interventions are known, a league table can theoretically be used to maximize the number of lives saved within a given health budget.

Leisure time costs. The monetary valuation of time away from work. In cost-effectiveness analysis, leisure time costs are typically thought of as the time during which persons cannot enjoy the time spent away from work because they are ill.

Levels of evidence. A method used to rank the appropriateness of studies based on their research design.

Longitudinal studies. *See* Prospective studies.

Lost productivity costs. Costs associated with the time a person cannot work. In cost-effectiveness analysis, lost productivity is typically measured as time lost due to illness.

Markov model. A decision analysis model that incorporates an element of time.

Medical Expenditure Panel Survey (MEPS). An annual survey of around 40,000 households in the United States. It includes a household component with demographic and health information about the participants. It also contains a provider component that obtains the cost of medical visits from providers. This is the most important dataset for cost-effectiveness analysis available in the United States.

Meta-analysis. An analytical form of literature review in which data from two or more individual studies are combined and reanalyzed as if they were a single study.

Micro-cost. A cost obtained for a single product or service.

Micro-costing. The process of measuring, valuing, and then adding up the various cost components (goods or services) associated with a health event. For example, the cost of an influenza vaccination may include the cost of the vaccine itself, the cost of the syringe, and the time cost associated with administering the vaccine.

Misclassification bias. A form of nonrandom error associated with categorizing events. For instance, it is common for physicians to improperly categorize a patient's underlying cause of death in instances in which the patient suffered from multiple related diseases or conditions.

Monte Carlo simulation. A process that repeatedly randomly draws from a given distribution or sample. This process is then used to determine the point estimate and standard error for a model input or an individual probability of experiencing an event. Random variability in outcomes from a sample of identical patients is determined from first-order Monte Carlo simulation. Parameter uncertainty is determined from second-order Monte Carlo simulation.

Morbidity costs. The intangible costs associated with pain and suffering. In general economics, these costs are typically measured in terms of willingness-to-pay formulations. However, in cost-effectiveness analyses, they are measured in terms of changes in health-related quality of life.

Mortality costs. Costs related to human deaths. Some define these costs strictly in terms of the intangible value of human life lost, while others include tangible costs, such as burial costs, in this category.

Mortality rate. The number of deaths over a given time interval divided by the total number of people at risk of those deaths over that same time interval.

Multiattribute health status classification systems. Instruments used to generate preference scores.

Multiway sensitivity analysis. *See* Sensitivity analysis, multiway.

Net present value. The net value of future costs or returns discounted to present-day values.

Nonrandom error. *See* Bias.

Normal distribution. A probability distribution in which values are clustered toward the mean and then taper off, giving the distribution its characteristic bell-shaped curve. Also known as a bell curve or Gaussian distribution.

Odds ratios. A measure of effect size in which the odds of an event measured in one group are divided by the odds of the event occurring in another group. For instance, if the odds of death among those receiving a preventive intervention for diabetes are p and the odds of death among those who did not receive the treatment are q, then the odds ratio is $p(1 - q)/(1 - p)q$. The odds ratio is useful only when the outcome of interest is rare (occurs less than 5 percent of the time).

One-way sensitivity analysis. *See* Sensitivity analysis, one-way.

Opportunity cost. The value of the next best investment forgone.

Outcome, health. Any measure of health. Examples are diseases averted, life-years gained, and vaccine-preventable illnesses averted.

Piggyback study. A cost-effectiveness analysis conducted alongside a prospective cohort study.

Preference score. A weighted value for life lived with a given disease ranging from 0 to 1, where 0 represents death and 1 represents perfect health.

Preference-weighted generic instruments. An instrument used to generate health-related quality-of-life scores for various health states. The word *generic* indicates that the instrument is not typically applied to any disease in particular.

Prevalence. The number of people with a given disease.

Prevalence ratio. The number of people with a given disease divided by the total number of people at risk for that disease.

Prevalent cases. *See* Prevalence.

Primary cost-effectiveness analysis. A study, such as a randomized controlled trial, in which data are collected for the primary purpose of conducting a cost-effectiveness analysis.

Probabilistic sensitivity analysis. A type of sensitivity analysis in which the range of values for each variable in a decision analysis model is assigned a probability distribution (e.g., beta, gamma, triangle). Each distribution is then repeatedly sampled to obtain a mean and distribution (standard error and 95 percent confidence interval) for the overall values of interest (cost, effectiveness, or incremental cost-effectiveness) using a second-order Monte Carlo simulation.

Probability distribution. A series of values presented by the probability that they will be observed. For instance, a probability distribution of heights will have many values close to the mean and few values for people less than 3 feet (1 meter) tall or greater than 9 feet (3 meters) tall. As one approaches the mean, the probability of observing a given value increases.

Prospective studies. Studies in which subjects are followed over time. Typically, this involves following subjects with and without putative risk factors for disease to ascertain who does and does not develop the disease.

QALY. *See* Quality-adjusted life-year.

Quality-adjusted life expectancy (QALE). Life expectancy in perfect health. QALE is equal to the product of life expectancy and the age-adjusted health-related quality-of-life score.

Quality-adjusted life-year (QALY). A year of life lived in perfect health.

Random error. Variance in a parameter estimate due to sampling error.

Randomized controlled trial. A form of experimental study in which subjects are randomly assigned to treatment conditions.

Recursive event. An event that repeats itself over time.

Reference case analysis. A standardized set of methods and theoretical frameworks for capturing costs, quality of life, and life expectancy in cost-effectiveness analysis. The reference case guidelines were forwarded by the Panel on Cost-Effectiveness in Health and Medicine.

Relative risk. *See* Risk ratio.

Reliable. An estimate that can be reproduced with relatively similar results from one study to the next.

Reproducible. *See* Reliable.

Retrospective cohort study. A retrospective study design that identifies risk factors in the past first in order to find associations with the outcome of interest in the present (or sometime after the exposure to the risk factor).

Retrospective studies. An observational study design in which the outcome of interest has already occurred with the goal of determining the risk factors associated with the outcome.

Risk ratio. The ratio of the probability of an event occurring in an exposed group relative to the probability of the event's occurring in the unexposed group.

Robust analysis. An analysis in which one alternative remains dominant even after testing it over the high and low range of values in a sensitivity analysis.

Rollback. The term sometimes used when a decision analysis model is instructed to calculate the expected value of each strategy.

Sensitivity analysis. An analysis that varies model inputs over their plausible range of real-world value in order to examine how they might influence model outputs.

Sensitivity analysis, multiway. A test of the effect of error on model outputs in which three or more variables of interest are simultaneously varied over a range of plausible values while holding all other variables constant.

Sensitivity analysis, one-way. A test of the effect of error on model outputs in which the variable of interest is varied over a range of plausible values while holding all other variables constant.

Sensitivity analysis, tornado. A test of the effect of error on model outputs in which each variable of interest within the model is sequentially varied over a range of plausible values while holding all other variables constant. Graphs of the variables are stacked according to their overall influence on the model, so the output assumes the appearance of a tornado.

Sensitivity analysis, two-way. A test of the effect of error on model outputs in which two variables of interest are simultaneously varied over a range of plausible values while holding all other variables constant.

Simple decision analysis tree. A decision analysis tree that calculates the expected value of a series of probabilistically weighted events based on outcomes presented in present terms. This contrasts with a Markov model, which calculates changes in health states or costs from one year to the next.

Societal perspective. An analysis that includes all costs and benefits of a health intervention regardless of who is paying for it.

Standard deviation. A measure of the spread of a given set of numbers, calculated as the root mean squared deviation of these values from their mean.

Standard gamble. A method for calculating preference scores in which subjects are asked to trade life with a particular disease for a gamble between perfect health and death.

Standard life table. A means for converting mortality rates into the average life expectancy of a hypothetical cohort of 100,000 persons exposed to the mortality rates. In a standard life table, age-specific mortality rates in one-year intervals are used to estimate the expected number of deaths in a hypothetical cohort of 100,000 persons. From these deaths, the mean number of years lived by the cohort is calculated.

Standard of care. The best practice based on current scientific evidence.

State transition model. A decision analysis model that incorporates an element of time. Also known as a Markov model.

Statement of need. A statement, usually in the introduction of the manuscript, that provides justification and rationality for conducting a research study.

Statistical power. The likelihood that a statistical test will correctly identify a statistically significant difference between two means. In more technical terms, it is the probability that a test will reject a false null hypothesis.

Status quo. What is typically done in current medical practice. This can be a mix of treatments or diagnostic modalities.

Stochastic uncertainty. A type of uncertainty that focuses on random variability in outcomes across individuals who are identical. A first-order Monte Carlo simulation is usually performed to evaluate stochastic uncertainty.

Structural uncertainty. Also known as model uncertainty. A type of sensitivity analysis where the structure of the decision model is modified (adding or removing branches and changing pathways) in order to test its assumptions.

Systematic bias. *See* Bias.

Threshold analysis. A one-way sensitivity analysis conducted with the purpose of determining the point at which the incremental cost, effectiveness, or cost-effectiveness of two competing alternatives is neutral.

Time costs. Costs associated with the time a patient spends receiving a medical intervention or receiving medical care.

Time horizon. *See Analytical horizon.*

Time preference. The rate of discounting applied to future events by any given person.

Time trade-off. A method for calculating preference scores in which subjects are asked to condense the quantity of life with a particular disease to achieve perfect health.

Tornado diagram. *See* Sensitivity analysis, tornado.

Triangular distribution. An artificial probability distribution in which the most likely value of a variable is assigned the highest probability of occurring, and the lowest and highest plausible value are assigned a probability of 0. All values in between are linearly interpolated.

Two-way sensitivity analysis. *See* Sensitivity analysis, two-way.

Variable costs. Costs that change when a health intervention is applied.

Willingness to pay. The incremental cost-effectiveness threshold that a patient, payer, or society is willing to pay for an intervention versus a competing alternative.